Progress in Drug Research
Fortschritte der Arzneimittelforschung
Progrès des recherches pharmaceutiques
Vol. 47

Progress in Drug Research
Fortschritte der Arzneimittelforschung
Progrès des recherches pharmaceutiques
Vol. 47

Edited by / Herausgegeben von / Rédigé par
Ernst Jucker, Basel

Authors / Autoren / Auteurs
Kurt R. H. Repke, Kathleen J. Sweadner, Jürgen Weiland, Rudolf Megges and Rudolf Schön · Silvano Sozzani, Paola Allavena, Paul Proost, Jo Van Damme and Alberto Mantovani · J. Paul Hieble and Robert R. Ruffolo, Jr · E. Leong Way, Yong Qing Liu and Chieh-Fu Chen · Jeanne Fürst Jucker and Gary P. Anderson · Gaetano Cardi, Thomas L. Ciardelli and Marc S. Ernstoff · Pushkar N. Kaul · Leo E. Hollister and Enrique S. Garza-Trevino

1996   Birkhäuser Verlag
Basel · Boston · Berlin

Editor:

Dr. E. Jucker
Steinweg 28
CH-4107 Ettingen
Switzerland

© 1996 Birkhäuser Verlag, P.O. Box 133, CH-4010 Basel, Switzerland
Softcover reprint of the hardcover 1st edition 1996

Printed on acid-free paper produced from chlorine-free pulp. TCF ∞

ISBN-13:978-3-0348-9862-1   e-ISBN-13: 978-3-0348-8998-8
DOI: 10.1007/978-3-0348-8998-8

9 8 7 6 5 4 3 2 1

Contents · Inhalt · Sommaire

Foreword

Volume 47 of „Progress in Drug Research" contains eight reviews and the various indexes which facilitate its use and establish the connection with the previous volumes. The articles in this volume deal with inotropic steroids, with chemokines and their involvement in a wide range of inflammatory diseases, with the subclassification and nomenclature of α_1- and α_2-adrenoceptors, with Chinese traditional medicine, with drug targets in the molecular pathogenesis of asthma, with cytokines and their therapeutic application in immunosuppression and immunostimulation, with alternative medicine and with the potential use of calcium blockers in psychiatry.

These reviews and the quotations of original articles provide the reader with valuable information on several new developments in the world-wide search for new and better medicines. In 1959, when the Editor started this series of monographs, it was his intention to help disseminate information on the vast and fast growing domain of drug research. Already at that time, it was not possible to follow the major individual publications in this field, and the reader was thereby provided with a tool to keep abreast of the latest developments and trends. This goal remained unchanged over the last 37 years, and I believe that the reviews in PDR are useful to the non-specialist who can obtain an overview of a particular field of drug research in a relatively short time. The specialist readers of PDR will appreciate the reviews' comprehensive bibliographies and, in addition, they might even get fresh impulses for their own research. Finally, the readers can use the 47 volumes with 450 reviews as an encyclopedic source of information.

In the 37 years of PDR's existence, the Editor has enjoyed much appreciated help from the authors, the readers, many colleagues and, last but not least, from the reviewers. To all of them I would like to express my gratitude.

In addition to the thanks expressed above, I would like to extend my thanks to Birkhäuser Verlag and, in particular, to Mrs. Elizabeth Beckett, Dr. Petra Gerlach, Mrs. L. Koechlin and Mssrs. H.-P. Thür, E. Mazenauer and G. Messmer. Their personal involvement, assistance and advice was of great importance for the successful production of PDR Volume 47.

Basel, October 1996   DR. E. JUCKER

Vorwort

Der vorliegende 47. Band der Reihe «Fortschritte der Arzneimittelforschung» enthält acht Beiträge sowie die verschiedenen Register, welche das Arbeiten mit diesem Band erleichtern und den Zugriff auf die vorhergehenden Bände ermöglichen. Die Artikel des 47. Bandes behandeln wiederum verschiedene aktuelle Themen des komplexen Gebietes der Arzneimittelforschung. Der erste Beitrag befasst sich mit Steroiden, die analog z.B. den Digitalis-Glykosiden bei Herz-Kreislauf-Störungen eingesetzt werden könnten. Der nächste Artikel behandelt C–C Chemokine aus der immunobiologischen Sicht und im Hinblick auf eine mögliche pharmakologische Intervention. Die dritte Übersicht behandelt die Subklassifikation und die Nomenklatur der α_1- und α_2-Adrenorezeptoren aus der Sicht potentieller Möglichkeiten ihres Einsatzes als Arzneimittel. Dem grossen Interesse, das zunehmend der alternativen Medizin entgegengebracht wird, Rechnung tragend, finden sich im vorliegenden Band je ein Beitrag über die traditionelle chinesische Medizin und über die alternative Medizin im allgemeinen. Die zunehmende Verbreitung der asthmatischen Beschwerden macht eine Intensivierung der Erforschung dieser Krankheit notwendig. Aus dieser Sicht ist der Beitrag über die molekulare Pathogenese, mit Schwerpunkt auf Immunologie und Zellbiologie, von ganz besonderer Aktualität. Der Übersichtsartikel über die therapeutische Anwendung der Cytokine ist die Fortsetzung des ersten Beitrages in PDR 39 (1992), wobei dem heutigen Stand des Wissens entsprechend das Schwergewicht auf die immunomodulatorische Therapie am Menschen gelegt wird. Der letzte Beitrag fasst die heutigen Kenntnisse der Anwendung von Calcium-Blockern in der Psychiatrie zusammen.

Seit der Gründung der Reihe sind mehr als 37 Jahre vergangen. Damals, 1959, war es die Absicht des Herausgebers, den Fachkollegen ein Hilfsmittel zur Verfügung zu stellen, welches es erlaubt, sich verhältnismässig rasch über ein Gebiet der Arzneimittelforschung zu informieren. Schon damals war es dem Einzelnen nicht mehr möglich, die Flut der Originalliteratur auch nur annähernd zu studieren und das Wichtigste aufzunehmen. Diesem Zustand sollten die «Fortschritte» abhelfen. Das Echo aus dem Leserkreis und die Rezensionen waren durchaus positiv, und die Reihe blieb der damals definierten Zielsetzung treu. So kann sich der Leser, der an der Arzneimittelforschung allgemein interessiert ist, über einzelne Gebiete mühelos informieren, der Spezialist hingegen findet in den einzelnen Übersichten nicht nur die Summe des Wissens und der Erfahrung des betreffenden Autors, sondern darüber hinaus auch eine äusserst umfassende Bibliographie, die ihm das Eindringen in die Original-arbeiten erleichtert.

In all den Jahren der Herausgabe der «Fortschritte» habe ich auf die Hilfe und den Rat vieler Fachkollegen zählen dürfen. Besonders wertvoll waren auch die Rezensionen, zeigten sie doch oft weitere, neue Richtungen für die Berichterstattung auf. So möchte ich hiermit den Autoren, den Lesern, den Fachkollegen und den Rezensenten meinen Dank aussprechen. Dieser Dank geht aber auch an den Birkhäuser Verlag und im besonderen an die Damen Elizabeth Beckett, Dr. Petra Gerlach und Leslie Koechlin; sie und die Herren H.-P. Thür, E. Mazenauer und G. Messmer sind massgeblich am Zustandekommen des 47. Bandes beteiligt.

Basel, Oktober 1996   DR. E. JUCKER

Progress in Drug Research, Vol. 47 (E. Jucker, Ed.)
© 1996 Birkhäuser Verlag, Basel (Switzerland)

In search of ideal inotropic steroids: Recent progress*

By Kurt R.H. Repke[1], Kathleen J. Sweadner[2], Jürgen Weiland[1], Rudolf Megges[1] and Rudolf Schön[3]

[1]Max Delbrück Center of Molecular Medicine, Robert-Rössle-Straße 10, D-13122 Berlin-Buch, Germany; [2]Massachusetts General Hospital, Laboratory of Membrane Biology, Charlestown, MA 02129-2060, USA; [3]Humboldt-Universität Berlin, Universitätsklinikum Charité, Klinik für Innere Medizin, Schumannstraße 20/21, D-10117 Berlin, Germany

---

*   Abbreviations and definitions:
Na⁺/K⁺-ATPase, Na⁺/K⁺-transporting adenosine triphosphate phosphohydrolase
(EC 3.6.1.37); digitalis, generic name of steroids inhibiting Na⁺/K⁺-ATPase by
intercalation in the digitalis binding matrix of the receptor enzyme.

1   Way of looking at the problem

1.1   Aim of review

The need for new inotropic drugs follows from the prevalence of congestive heart failure in the developed countries, and from the fact that the cardiac drugs currently available are clearly inadequate to restore health or even to minimize discomfort and disability (review in [1]). In 1990, Kellermann [2] expected for the coming years that every effort must and will be made to further develop and create new compounds. These should not only beneficially affect the hemodynamic and functional impairment of patients with congestive heart failure, but also hopefully contribute to reaching an achievable goal, namely, the prevention of the clinical manifestations of heart failure. The arduous research, on the part of the pharmaceutical industry, to find a nonsteroidal "digitalis replacement" cannot be regarded as having been accomplished [3]. The present review deliberately excludes the great number of cardioactive compounds of nonsteroidal types and divergent points of attack because they do not appear to promise progress in the treatment of cardiac failure (review in [4, 5]). Taking the above demand as our challenge, we review in this chapter where we presently are in the search for ideal inotropic steroids. Earlier stages of this endeavor, documented elsewhere [6–8], will but cursorily be cited here. Our more recent approach has been derived from the hypothesis that the earlier failures in the synthetic further development of inotropic steroids with improved therapeutic range were based on the use of C/D-cis connected steroids as lead compounds which form the core in the medicinally used cardiac glycosides. Hence, we felt it promising to explore the suitability of C/D-trans steroids, constituting the core in steroid hormones, to serve as lead structures. The results of this novel approach will form the major part of present review.

1.2   Scope of review

1.2.1   Qualification of Na^+/K^+-ATPase as the digitalis receptor
The marking of the enzyme Na^+/K^+-ATPase as digitalis receptor, proved by the senior author [9, 10] has sometimes been found inappropriate [11]. Specifically, in the need to differentiate entities thought to be pharmacological receptors from enzymes, it has been stipulated that the recognition unit (the enzyme) should not chemically alter the endogenous ligand (the enzyme's substrate) [12]. This stipulation is clearly not met by Na^+/K^+-ATPase. However, the two main criteria for the operational term receptor, i.e., the functions of recognition and transduction [12], do fully apply.

As required, recognition of Na^+/K^+-ATPase by digitalis-like acting steroids shows selectivity and saturable binding [13–15]. The transduction of the message includes the increase of the intracellular Na^+ activity, resulting from the digitalis-produced reduction of the Na^+/K^+ pumping capacity of the cell by inhibition of a portion of total Na^+/K^+-ATPase. This primary event [16] produces via Na^+/Ca^{2+} exchange an increase of intracellular Ca^{2+} activity which is the final regulator of cardiac contractility (reviewed in [6, 17]). The knowledge of Na^+/K^+-ATPase as the only "cardiovascular" digitalis receptor has made it possible to use Na^+/K^+-ATPase from human tissues for primary screening in the search for novel digitalis-like acting steroids (reviewed in [6–8, 18–20]. The evaluation of the digitalis-like potency of diverse C/D-trans steroids of the hormone type reported here was hence primarily performed in tests with Na^+/K^+-ATPase (see sections 4.1 and 5). Methodological details in carrying out the 'macroscopic' and 'microscopic' variants of testing (defined in [7]) have been reported elsewhere [7, 14, 15, 18–21] and will thus not be treated here.

1.2.2   The quest for the three-dimensional structure of the digitalis intercalating matrix in the receptor

As shown recently by us [22], the interface between two catalytic α-subunits in the Na^+/K^+-ATPase protodimer $(\alpha\beta)_2$ is likely to provide the cleft for inhibitory digitalis intercalation. Thus, the inability of the digitalis-intercalated enzyme to perform the reaction-transport cycle may result from disruption of the interprotodimeric interaction between the various effectors (ATP, Mg^{2+}, Na^+, K^+) bound to the catalytic subunits that is otherwise the prerequisite of Na^+/K^+-ATPase function [23–25]. Generally, an understanding of protein-protein interaction in dimeric receptors has been held to be a condition for targeted design of drugs which act through interdimeric intercalation and thus interfere with transmembrane signaling [26–28]. Hence, we model here (section 2) the three-dimensional structure of the digitalis intercalating matrix of Na^+/K^+-ATPase and reveal the interacting structural features of both protein matrix and digitalis compound.

1.2.3   Different digitalis actions due to the diversity of roles of Na^+/K^+-ATPase in various tissues

Although the Na^+/K^+ pump is in all cells involved in a multitude of physiological processes, the digitalis-evoked inhibition of Na^+/K^+-ATPase will differently affect the function of specialized cells (reviewed in [29]). Even a modest decrease of the pump capacity of the cell is likely to have a significant effect on the Na^+ electrochemical gradient over the plasma membrane, which may have a rather complex impact on neurotransmitter release and uptake, and on many other Na^+ gradient-dependent transport processes. Via the Na^+/Ca^{2+} exchanger the pump participates in the control of intracellular Ca^{2+} concentration and thus generally of cell activity as in cardiac muscle, neurons, glia and vascular smooth muscle. In addition, the cardiotonic steroids have direct effects on the Na^+/K^+ pump in the kidney such that they can promote natriuresis.

1.2.4 Isoforms of the receptor enzyme in human tissues
The species-variant digitalis affinity of Na^+/K^+-ATPase was discovered by Repke et al. [30] already in 1965 and shown to account for the huge *in vivo* species differences in digitalis sensitivity. Since the finding of Sweadner in 1979 [31] that a Na^+/K^+-ATPase preparation from rat brain contains two isoenzymes of very different ouabain susceptibility, many authors have reported that three isoenzymes, now mostly called α1, α2 or α3 according to the structural differences of the catalytic subunits (which enclose the digitalis binding matrix [22]) exist in most mammals and in various tissues of a species (review in [32]). In humans, the major form in kidney is α1 and in skeletal muscle α2, while all three forms appear to be expressed in the brain and heart muscle [33–37]. As stated by Lingrel and coworkers [35], the finding that all three α isoforms are expressed in adult human heart poses the interesting question whether all three isoenzymes serve as receptors for the therapeutic effects of digitalis compounds or whether their therapeutic (or toxic) action is due to the selective inhibition of one or two of the isoenzymes based either on their cellular location in the heart or on intrinsically different affinities to digitalis compounds. This question will be treated in broader context in section 3.

1.2.5 The issue of endogenous digitalis
The widespread belief in the existence of endogenous digitalis has been fueled by the discovery of endorphins, the endogenous ligands for the opiate receptors. The belief is also supported by the evolutionary conservation of the digitalis binding matrix in the receptor enzyme. Hence, a number of laboratories have struggled to isolate and to functionally as well as structurally identify the supposed endogenous equivalent of digitalis. Despite the considerable efforts of a number of laboratories (reviews on historical background [11, 29, 38–41]), a consensus on the existence, origin and chemical nature of the putative endogenous digitalis has not yet been reached. The present state of contradictions and uncertainties as well as the conclusions for the search of ideal inotropic steroids will be evaluated in section 4.

2   Design of the three-dimensional structure of the digitalis intercalating matrix in Na+/K+-ATPase protodimer

2.1   Starting points for the design

In 1973, we deduced the hypothesis that Na+/K+-ATPase works in the plasma membrane in form of a dimer of two functionally identical sub-units [42]. In 1983, Askari and coworkers [23] confirmed by chemical cross-linking studies that Na+/K+-ATPase exists in the plasma membrane as non-covalent dimer of the α,β-protomer, i.e., as the protodimer $(\alpha\beta)_2$. Their findings that enzyme phosphorylation from ATP favored the formation of crosslinked α,α-dimer, and enzyme ligation with K+ and ATP reduced cross-linking, indicated function-linked changes in the juxtapositions of the appropriate reactive groups at the α,α-domain of two associated α,β-protomers.

In 1985, our group [13] derived from various findings that the digitalis binding matrix in Na+/K+-ATPase protein is the cleft between two neigh-boring lobes of the catalytic α-chain, that communicates with the extra-cellular space and is approximately 20 Å deep. We further concluded that the interactive energy surfaces become locked on intercalation of a car-diac glycoside so as to envelope: its lactone side chain, lying at the bot-tom of the cleft, its steroid nucleus, and its sugar residue bound next to the steroid carrier, lying near the mouth of the cleft [13]. Newer sets of information uncovered that the interface between two interacting α-sub-units in the Na+/K+-ATPase protodimer $(\alpha\beta)_2$ provides the deduced cleft for inhibitory digitalis intercalation (recently reviewed in [22]). Specifi-cally, it has been shown that ATP, through enzyme phosphorylation, favors protomer-protomer association and that ouabain, through interprotodi-meric intercalation, makes the protomer association much stronger and enormously stabilizes the $(\alpha\beta)_2$ protodimer structure [43, 44]. Our present endeavor to model the three-dimensional structure of the digitalis bind-ing cleft (short report in [45]) has been rendered possible through the sig-nificant progress reached in the elucidation of the topological determi-nants of the tertiary and quaternary structure of membrane-spanning pro-teins [26, 46–49].

2.2   Modeling of the three-dimensional structure of the digitalis binding cleft

Since 1979, various types of analysis have supported oligomeric models for Na+/K+-ATPase-driven Na+/K+ transport with an $(\alpha\beta)_2$ diprotomeric structure being favored [50–56]. Most recently, studies with a series of Na+/K+-ATPase – H+/K+-ATPase chimeras [57] have shown that a cytoplasmic mid region in the α-subunit of Na+/K+-ATPase (arginine 350 – proline 785) is necessary for specific, stable α,α-association, whereas the N-terminal and C-terminal transmembrane regions *alone* are incapable of supporting stable α,α-association. Chemical cross-linking studies with proteolytic fragments of Na+/K+-ATPase have allowed to localize the dimerizing domains to the C-terminal sides of alanines 439 [58]. The process of oligomerization appears to be completed by the specific association of complementary surfaces of contacting intramembrane helices from the N-terminal portions of two dimerized α-subunits. In line with this interpretation, the intramembrane helices from the amino terminal portions of two α-subunits, visualized in two-dimensional crystals, are found to be in contact [59]. Since the bordering helices, called H1 and H2 (H stands for hydrophobic), are pairwise linked by a short extramembraneous amino acid sequence ("loop") [60], the interface cleft in the dimer may be lined by the surfaces of four helix segments from the two H1·H2 pairs.

Based on the hydropathy profile of the amino acids involved, it has been concluded that H1 could stretch from Q88 to T114 and H2 from N122 to Q143 in the α1 subunit from human Na+/K+-ATPase [61], in which these intramembrane segments are connected by an extracellularly disposed loop as specified in Fig. 1. Raman spectroscopic data demonstrated that the intramembrane peptide sequences are in the α-helical configuration [62]. Remarkably enough, the transition of enzyme conformation from E1 to E2, characterizing major changes in the functional behavior of the enzyme [24, 63], does not alter the α-helical configuration of the intramembrane sequences [64]. Apparently, the E1 and E2 enzyme conformations differ only in the orientation relationships of the α-helices such that this transition could produce opening and closing of the extracellularly disposed digitalis binding cleft as well as alter (see [64]) the conformation of the intracellular domains of the catalytic protein.

In an approach to define the surroundings of the intramembrane helices of the H1·H2 pairs, we have chosen a model, which divides the surface of each helix into four differently disposed regions (cf. [65]). This model, visualized in Fig. 1, is admittedly simplistic, but in the absence of definite structural information, a more detailed model would not be justified. Four regions with different surroundings are to be specified.

First, the regions, suggested to be in contact with the hydrophobic core of the lipid bilayer, appear to include all amino acids usually regarded as hydrophobic (A, V, L, I, F, W) plus serine and tyrosine. Serine can satisfy its hydrogen bonding potential by bonding within the helix chain and thus

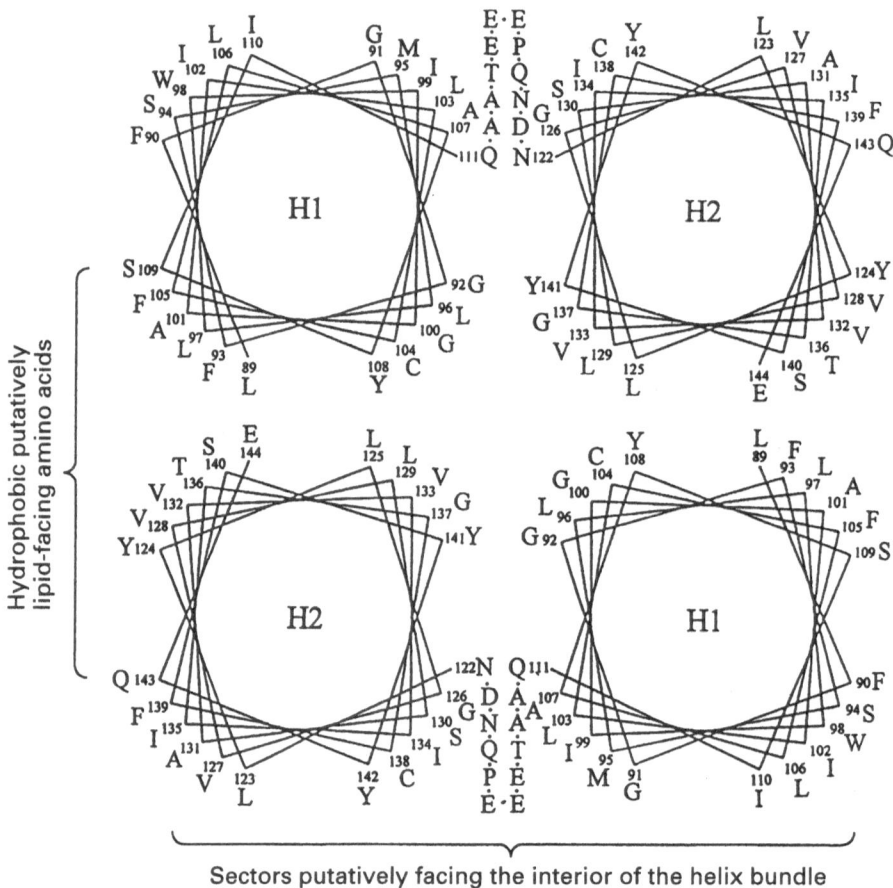

Sectors putatively facing the interior of the helix bundle

Fig. 1
Presumed topological arrangement of first and second transmembrane helix (H1 and H2) in
two dimerized α1 subunits of human Na^+/K^+-ATPase visualized by helical wheel projection of
C_α positions, assuming a periodicity of 3.9 residues per turn. L89 at the beginning of H1 and
E144 at the end of H2 thus are at the inner surface of the plasma membrane, whereas the loop
between the helices protrudes from the outer membrane surface. This method of projection
can be misleading since the position of the side-chains may deviate from the periodicity. In
numbering the amino acids, the highly conserved cysteine 104 [66] has been chosen for stan-
dardization throughout this paper. The pictorial design of the helical wheel follows the plot
given for the transmembrane helix of glycophorin [65].

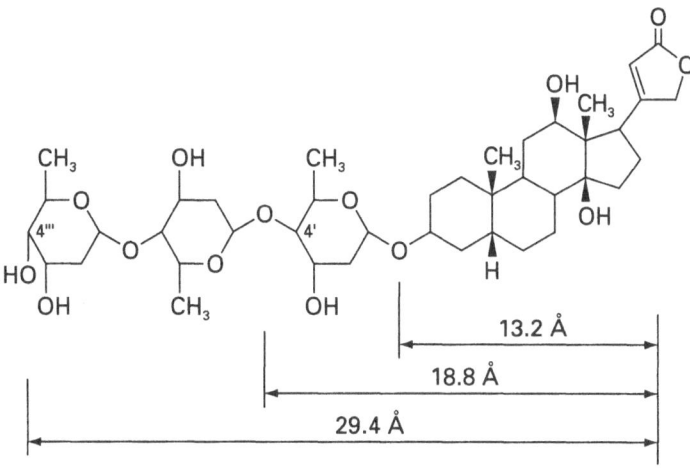

Fig. 2
Structural formula and dimension of digoxigenin tridigitoxoside (digoxin) used to measure the
length of the digitalis intercalating cleft between two dimerized α-subunits. The distances are
derived from X-ray crystallographic analysis [69].

can be on its lipid-facing surface. Tyrosine residues are known to occur
on lipid-facing surfaces mainly between the non-polar and the polar parts
of the membrane.

Second, the regions of H1 and H2, involved in the interaction with neigh-
boring helix bundles (probably H10 and H8, respectively [67]), would be
thought to be located in the outer boundaries of the H1·H2 pairs as marked
in Fig. 1. In line with this suggestion appears to be the absence of highly
polar groups and the preponderance of amino acids with hydrophobic side
chains such that their precise packing interactions between the helices
can provide the energy for the stable interaction of the helix bundles in
the α-subunit (cf. [68]).

Third, a quarter of each helix wheel appears to contribute to form the
interprotodimeric cleft in which cardiac glycosides intercalate to inter-
rupt the catalytic cycle of Na+/K+-ATPase. This hypothesis is supported
by the direct involvement of cysteine 104 and tyrosine 108 as well as glu-
tamic acid 117 in the digitalis binding process (see next section). The depth
of the cleft would span then about 19 Å (cf. Fig. 2) and stretch between

E117 and C104. The part of the cleft residing in the membrane would then be formed by G92, L96, G100, C104 and Y108 from the H1 helix, and by L125, L129, Y133, G137 and Y141 from the H2 helix. These amino acids show either a positive or a low negative hydropathy index [70] and hence appear fit for hydrophobic bonding of the apolar cyclopentano-perhy-drophenanthrene core of digitalis compounds. As derived below, the C12β-OH of digoxin appears to form a H-bond with the phenolic OH of tyro-sine in the C104Y mutated enzyme. This would mean that the β-surface of the steroid core interacts with the H1 helix, while the α-surface inter-acts with the H2 helix. Due to the burial of molecular surface area of the steroid core, the "hydrophobic energy" is the driving force for the bimo-lecular association, whereas the electrostatic interactions simply confer specificity (cf. [71]).

Fourth, if all this applies, the interprotodimeric interaction forces would extend beyond C104, i.e., between the side chains of G100, L96, G92, V133, G137, Y141 in the corresponding two H1 and two H2 helix sections. The amino acids with relatively hydrophobic side chains (glycine, leucine and valine) could contribute to interprotodimeric hydrophobic bonding. Due to the phenolic OH's, the two tyrosines would be able to form interpro-todimeric hydrogen bonds.

2.3   Interpretation of the inhibitory digitalis interaction with Na+/K+-ATPase in terms of the three-dimensional structure model of the digitalis binding cleft

As reasoned by us for many years, based on various arguments, one of the first steps in the formation of the inhibitory digitalis-enzyme complex should be hydrogen bonding between the partners (for recent reviews see [6, 7]). The capacity of the carbonyl and bridge oxygens in the butenolide and pentadienolide side chains of digitalis compounds to accept two hydro-gen bonds is well supported by the presence of deep negative potential wells around these oxygens and their marked electronegativity (reviewed in [6, 7]). The above deduction has generally been ignored as yet, since the hydrogen donors were not identified. Fortunately, the outcome of mutational amino acid substitutions published recently has opened the way to their identification.

In 1992, Rossier and colleagues [72] discovered that the replacement of cysteine 104 in H1 of the wild type enzyme by tyrosine (C104Y) or by phenylalanine (C104F) much increased the inhibition constant K_i of oua-bain. The dissociation rate constants with the glycoside ouabain and the aglycone strophanthidin were much alike so that the authors hypothesized that the mutations alter the binding of the genin moiety. In 1993, Schultheis and Lingrel [73] reported that the mutations C104A and C104F confer graded losses of ouabain sensitivity to the enzyme. The I_{50} value for the wild-type enzyme increased from 0.032 µM to 0.2 µM in case of C104A substitution and to 4.8 µM in case of C104F substitution. The surprisingly large increase by phenylalanine substitution could be due to steric hindering of mutual interaction between its bulky side chain and the lactone residue (cf. below). The smaller increase by alanine substitution, corresponding to a decrease of $\Delta G^{0'}$ from –44.5 kJ/mol to –38.8 kJ/mol, appears to us to indicate the loss of two hydrogen bonds (the value for one bond lies between –1.2 and –4.3 kJ/mol [74]).

In 1994, Askew and Lingrel [75] discovered that the amino acid substitution C104Y conferred different sensitivity for digitoxin and digoxin. They proposed that the differential resistance of the C104Y receptor enzyme for these ligands is a consequence of altering two features of the ligand-receptor interaction; one, a disruption of a common hydrogen bond with C14 hydroxyl resulting in general loss of affinity for cardiac glycosides and the other, after reorientation of the ligand-receptor interface, formation of a new H-bond between the C12 hydroxyl of digoxin and the receptor, thus specifically augmenting the stability of this ligand receptor complex. In the light of the above-mentioned H-bond acceptor capacities of the oxygens in the lactone side chain of both glycosides we suggest here that the common hydrogen bond, lost in C104Y substitution, is formed between the lactone oxygens of either cardiac glycoside and the SH of cysteine 104, and the new H-bond forms between the C12 hydroxyl of digoxin and the phenolic OH of tyrosine 104. The exceptional role of cysteine 104 emerges also from the findings that the exchanges of cysteine 138, C138F [73] and C138S [72], do not alter ouabain affinity.

The strongly bent shape of the lead structure in digitalis compounds, i.e., 5β,14β-androstane-14,17β-diol, which is due to the cis-junction of the rings A and B as well as C and D, implies that the digitalis recognition matrix is primarily a widely open cleft, the closure of which is elicited only after slippage of the lead into the cleft [7]. This possibly explains the report that N-hydroxysuccinimidyl-digoxigenin-3-methylcarbonyl-ε-amino-caproate forms a thioester with cysteine 104 [76, 77]. Regularly, however, cysteine 104 does not play a role in binding of the usual side chain at C3 of cardiac glycosides, i.e., their sugar moiety. This emerges from the observation that the I_{50} ratio for ouabagenin to ouabain remains unchanged after replacement of the cysteine 104 by phenylalanine [78]. Normally, instead, the digitalis compounds enter into the binding cleft not with the side chain at C3, but with the lactone ring at C17 ahead. This derives from the findings that linkage of the sugar chain of ouabain or digoxin with a large protein or sepharose via a long polyamide or hydrocarbon bridge allows the development of the inhibitory action of the digitalis derivatives [79, 80], associated, as we propose, with H bridge bonding between the lactone ring and cysteine 104 as derived above.

The steroid binding subsite of the cleft binds $5\beta, 14\beta$-androstane-14, 17β-diol, 5α, 14α-androstane, estradiol-17β and progesterone with similar Gibbs energies of interaction [7]. The steroid subsite thus displays a surprisingly great adaptability to the molding interaction with the strongly different molecular surfaces of the various steroids. It appears to involve a change of the rotational relationship of the intramembrane helices between the local minima in the unliganded and liganded state as referred to below. This renders it at first difficult to locate and identify the amino acid residues finally interacting with the steroid nucleus. Interestingly, the exchange Y108A in H1 increases the I_{50} value of ouabain from 0.032 μM to 0.29 μM [73] corresponding to a loss of Gibbs interaction energy by -5.7 kJ/mol. For comparison, the $\Delta G^{0'}$ value of the lead structure in digitalis compounds (5β, 14β-androstane-3β,14-diol) amounts to -22.6 kJ/mol [13]. Clearly, further amino acid residues are involved in binding of the steroid nucleus (cf. below). Anyhow, tyrosine 108 appears to participate therein since its substitution by phenylalanine does not drop the I_{50} value. Phenylalanine is, like tyrosine, known to form hydrophobic bonds especially to other extended molecules. Additional hydrophobic bonds to interact with the apolar steroid skeleton appear to be provided by the ten, mostly apolar amino acids from the H1 and H2 helix which seem to line that part of the cleft which resides in the membrane (see above). Indeed, the involvement of H2 in ouabain binding is suggested by the findings that mutations Y124C, I135V or S140C cause ouabain resistance [81].

The location of the sugar binding subsite of cardiac glycosides was clearly marked through two independent analytical approaches. First, the Gibbs energies of interaction with Na^+/K^+-ATPase were found to decrease in the order genin-monosaccharide > genin-disaccharide > genin-trisaccharide [7]. This gradation indicates that only the proximate sugar provides atom groupings for an attractive interaction with the binding subsite. The decrease of the $\Delta G^{0'}$ values by the second and third sugar would result from the increase of rotational and translational entropies of the glycosides by the unbound extreme ends of the sugar chain. Second, photoaffinity labeling of Na^+/K^+-ATPase with 4'-ethyldiazomalonyl-digitoxigenin monodigitoxoside or with 4'''-ethyldiazomalonyl-digitoxigenin tridigitoxoside revealed that either the α-subunit or the β-subunit becomes labeled [82]. Taken together with the above findings, the labeling data indicate that the proximate sugar is immobilized in the mouth of the cleft, whereas the remote sugar is free to rotate and thus able to allow the photolabel to react with the β-subunit.

Concerning the chemical identity of the sugar binding subsite, the following conclusions could be reached. As shown by Lingrel and coworkers [78], the mutational substitution of C104, Q111, A112, D121 or N122 does not change the I_{50} ratio for ouabagenin to ouabain. Apparently, these amino acids do not participate in the binding of the rhamnose moiety of ouabain so that it should bind to residues in the H1·H2 region which have not been tested. The most likely candidates appear to be the three glutamates (E115, E116, E117) in the H1 helix cap of the α1 isoenzyme (cf. Fig. 1) about 19 Å away from C104 (cf. Fig. 2). This derives from our following findings [7]. All highly potent cardenolide monosaccharides have α-L-rhamnose or its 4'-amino-4'-deoxy derivative as the sugar component. Since $-NH_2$ serves better than $-OH$ at C4' in generating high interaction energy, a hydrogen bond-accepting reaction with an acidic proton likely underlies the maximum efficacy of the carrier cardenolides. Because this involves an acid partner, that linkage would be a particularly strong hydrogen bond [83]. The involvement of carboxyl side-chains in the sugar binding subsite is also suggested by the findings that, through electrostatic repulsion, acid substituents at C3β-OH of cardenolides as glucuronide or dicarbonic acid as well as sulphate esters decrease or eliminate the activity of the parent genin [7].

Between the above three potential partners of sugar residue binding, glutamates 115 and 116 are replaceable by serine [84] or glutamine [85], respectively, with only modest or no loss of ouabain affinity. However, replacement of glutamate 117 by asparagine is accompanied by a strong drop of ouabain sensitivity [86, 87]. The Gibbs energy of inhibitory interaction decreases from –42.1 kJ/mol to –30.5 kJ/mol such that the $\delta\Delta G^{0'}$ value even surpasses the usual decrement effected by removal of the α-L-rhamnosyl side chain from ouabain amounting to –10 kJ/mol [7]. Apparently then, in the human α1 isoenzyme glutamate 117 is a good candidate to be the binding partner of the rhamnose side chain of ouabain. Rhamnose, like other sugars, is by itself without inhibitory effect, that is, the sugar binding subsite does not pre-exist, but is created in the process of cleft closure induced by cardiac glycoside binding [7].

There are a number of observations on the outcome of amino acid replacements which cannot be interpreted in terms of an involvement in direct, attracting or rejecting interaction with digitalis structure components. So, in the C-terminal end of the helix H1, the substitution of glutamine 111 by arginine conferred ouabain resistance to the enzyme [88]. The initial interpretation that glutamine is somehow involved in ouabain binding [89] could not be maintained because its replacement by alanine [90] or leucine [91] did not produce a ouabain-resistant enzyme. Further in the C-terminal end of the H1-H2 loop, the exchanges of aspartate 121 for conservative (glutamate), isosteric (asparagine) and nonconservative (alanine or serine) amino acids all decreased the ouabain affinity to the enzyme nearly 100fold [92]. The authors suggested an involvement of the carboxyl residue of D121 in ouabain binding and the necessity for its precise positioning. However, it does not relate to rhamnose binding since the D121E substitution decreases the inhibitory potency of ouabagenin and ouabain by the same ratio [78]. The substitution of asparagine 122 by alanine [90] does not reduce ouabain affinity at all.

Double substitutions as N120D and N122H [93], Q111D and N122R [88, 90, 94], Q111R and N122D [88, 91], or Q111K and N122K [88, 90] produce the highest decreases of ouabain potency [88, 90, 91, 93, 94]. Remarkably, the combined exchange Q111A and N122A [90], involving uncharged amino acids, does not confer ouabain resistance. From these findings, Lingrel and associates have drawn the following conclusions (reviewed in [66]). Substitution of glutamine 111 and asparagine 122, which have uncharged side chains, by amino acids with charged side chains, positive or negative, invariably produces an enzyme of reduced ouabain affinity. The nature and combination of charges does not appear to be particularly important. These findings have led to the postulate that the introduced charges would alter the ouabain-induced conformational change which otherwise effectively prevents rapid ouabain dissociation from a sensitive enzyme [78, 88] and hence increases ouabain potency.

As shown before, the substituted amino acids, listed above, do not directly participate in ouabain binding. Interestingly enough, they are all located in the border positions of the H1-H2 loop. The puzzling mechanism of the impact of changes in its amino acid composition on the 'conformational change' [78, 88], which appears to us to design the shape of the protodimer interface cleft, may be deduced from the knowledge that extramembraneous loops can constrain the spatial relationship between the caps of transmembrane helices and thus determine their orientational relationship [46, 48]. The closure of the digitalis binding cleft upon ouabain binding could parallel the response of the aspartate receptor in which the binding pocket residues are brought closer together upon ligand complexation by a rigid body rotation of the helix bundles about an axis perpendicular to the dimer interface (cf. reviews [46, 48]). In this way, the transmembrane helices may undergo a transition from one local energy minimum (in the unliganded state) to another (in the liganded state), resulting in both an altered relationship between the *intracellular* domains of the receptor and an effective transmembrane signaling by such receptors [46, 48]. These interconnections help to realize the inhibitory action of a digitalis compound on Na^+/K^+-ATPase via its attack from the extracellular space and its interprotodimeric intercalation followed by loss of the affinity of the intracellularly disposed catalytic center to ATP [95]. Reciprocally, phosphate binding to the catalytic phosphorylation site, aspartate 369, induces a conformational change in the enzyme, which increases its affinity to ouabain. Thus, catalytic ATPase activity and ouabain binding are linked through this phosphorylation site [96].

2.4   Modeling of the mechanism for transmembrane signaling

A detailed understanding of the interaction between effector molecules and receptor proteins is believed to be a suitable basis for a rational drug design strategy. However, due to various methodological limitations (reviewed in [28]), the application of the diverse methods to ligand-protein docking has revealed that the "successes" have been limited to lead compound design [28]. On the other hand, interactive molecular graphics methods with incorporated energy minimization procedures appear to be well suited to explore the mechanism of transmembrane signaling via membrane receptor proteins [46, 97, 98]. Thanks to the knowledge on the position of the three structural components of digitalis glycosides in the receptor matrix derived in section 2.3, the procedure appears to be largely devoid of personal biases [28].

2.5   Conclusions concerning the rational design of novel
         inotropic steroids

Due to the high conformational adaptability of the digitalis intercalating matrix in Na^+/K^+-ATPase, documented above, its three-dimensional structure could be roughly deduced here. The task of rational design of novel drugs when based on this knowledge offers a daunting prospect (cf. [28]). The existence of the three isoenzymes in human heart muscle and human brain [33–37, 99, 100] appears to open a new avenue for the discovery of novel drugs which would inhibit only the one or the other isoenzyme and thus could limit toxic side reactions [100, 101]. What is clearly needed now is the in-depth analysis of the fundamental connection between configuration of steroidal compounds and predicted specificity of their inhibitory interaction with the α1-, α2-, and α3-isoforms of human Na$^+$/K$^+$-ATPase as comprehensively derived elsewhere [7, 8].

3   The significance of differential digitalis affinity of the Na$^+$/K$^+$-ATPase isoforms for the targeted design of ideal inotropic steroids

3.1   Expression of the isoenzymes in human digitalis target tissues

Since 1988, the mRNA expression of all three isoenzymes have been described for brain [33–35] and cardiac muscle [34–37]. The most striking observation was that the α3-isoform is a major form in adult heart [35]. On the other hand, the major isoenzymes were α1 in kidney [33–35] and α2 in skeletal muscle [34, 35]. The information on the relative abundance of the isoforms in cardiac muscle given in [35–37] are not cited here due to their large variability. Moreover, the mRNA levels do not immediately allow prediction of the protein levels because of the isoform-specific translational rates and the complexities of hetero-protodimer formation [101]. Only Sweadner has unequivocally demonstrated, by analysis with isoenzyme-specific antibodies in human myocardium and brain [102] as well as in rat brain [103], the co-existence of all three isoform proteins. In the central nervous system, a wide spectrum of region- and cell-type-specific isoform distribution has been found so that a formidably complex picture emerged [104].
As concluded by Farley et al. [101] in 1995, knowing which isoform is the 'therapeutic receptor' in the heart will put investigators in a position to design isoform-specific inhibitors interacting with the isoenzymes linked to positive inotropy but not those linked to toxicity.

3.2   Approaches to derive the digitalis affinity of the α-subunits of the three isoenzymes from their primary structure as deduced from the cDNA sequences

We have tried two approaches to the identification of the amino acids that may cause differences in ouabain affinity between human isoenzymes (cf. section 3.3).
First, we compared the amino acid sequences of α1 [61], α2 [105] and α3 [106]. In the region between amino acids 95 and 996, we found 100 differences in the amino acid composition between both α1 versus α2 (46

conservative and 54 non-conservative replacements) and between α1 versus α3 (53 conservative and 47 non-conservative replacements). As defined by Fambrough et al. [107], the conservative replacements, not expected to alter protein conformation markedly, include the conservation of: a) charged residues of same sign, b) polar uncharged residues, and c) hydrophobic residues.

The non-conservative amino acid differences between α1:α2:α3, expected to alter protein conformation markedly, include:

1) the exchange of uncharged by charged residues (present in positions 167 Asn:Glu:Glu; 202 and 226 Asn:His:His; 398 and 490 Asn:Asp:Asp; 439 Ala:Asp:Asp;);
2) replacement of charged versus uncharged residues (present in positions 286 His:Gln:Gln; 307 Glu:Gly:Gly; 496 His:His:Tyr; 517 His:Gln:Gln; 528 Lys:Gln:Lys; 550 His:Gln:His; 555 Asp:Ser:Glu; 556 Glu:Gly:Glu; 676 Lys:Lys:Gln; 832 Lys:Gln:Arg; 874 His:Arg:Asn);
3) change of sign of charge (present in positions 462 Glu:Lys:Leu; 487 Lys:Glu:Glu; 525 Glu:Lys:Glu; 560 Glu:Arg:Gln);
4) deletion of amino acids (in positions 324 Gap:Asn:Asn; 491 Thr:Gap:Pro);
5) inclusion of proline (in positions 409 Ala:Pro:His; 434 Pro:Ser:Pro; 467 Ala:Pro:Lys; 493 Glu:Pro:Asp; 494 Pro:Gln:Asn; 572 Pro:Pro:Thr; 831 Pro:Ser:Pro; 977 Pro:Val:Pro).

The sequence comparisons among the three human [61, 105, 106] and avian isoenzymes [107] reveal the following similarities. The isoform-characteristic divergencies occur mainly in the NH_2-terminal half of the α chain. The putative membrane spanning regions H1–H10 (cf. Fig. 2 in [66]) are all regions of comparatively little sequence variation. Taken together, no unique difference in the amino acid composition of human α1-, α2- and α3-isoforms could be singled out, that could *singularly* be related to the postulated differences in ouabain affinity.

In the second approach, we searched in the human α-subunits for amino acids and amino acid combinations which were identified by mutagenesis in Na^+/K^+-ATPases from other species to confer ouabain resistance [72, 73, 75, 78, 81, 84–86, 88–94, 108–110]. These included Y124C, I135V and S140C [81] in the H2 transmembrane helix; Y308C [108] in the H3–H4 extracellular loop; E327L or E327Q [109] in the H4 transmembrane helix; T797L or T797V [110] in the H5 helix; N880P [85] in the H7–H8 loop, and D925Q or D925L [109] in the H8 helix, respectively. The mentioned resistance-favoring amino acids do not occur in the indicated positions of human α-subunits. The most informative exception concerns position 135 in which isoleucine is present in human α1 and α3, but valine in α2. Since the α2 isoenzyme appears to be ouabain-sensitive (cf. above), the realization of resistance does not necessarily result from the exchange of a single amino acid, but appears to require its allosteric cooperation with the digitalis binding matrix through the communication with a special amino acid sequence not present in α2.

Taken together the results of the two lines of approach, we conclude that ouabain affinity is difficult to predict simply from the primary structure, because *apart from the digitalis binding matrix*, distant amino acids can indirectly control the geometry and flexibility of the digitalis intercalating matrix via the bordering transmembrane helices and the interconnecting extra- and intracellular loops. The latter connection, not to be treated here, emerges from the well-documented impact of the ligand occupancy of the intracellularly disposed catalytic center on digitalis affinity (cf. review in [95]). The above conclusions are in accord with the general knowledge that localized sequence changes can exert long-range effects on the global behavior of enzymes including delocalized structural reorganizations, which render topological interpretations dubious [111–113]. Remarkably enough, our failure to identify the amino acid(s) responsible for the probable differences of digitalis sensitivity between the three Na+/K+-ATPase isoforms parallels the failure to define the domain for binding of progesterone, glucocorticoid, estrogen, and vitamin D to their receptors through deletion of amino acids, insertional mutations or point mutations (reviewed in [114]). All this has been shown to result in loss of hormone binding capacity, hence indicating the sensitivity of the domain to single amino acid mutations anywhere in the region. Because of this sensitivity it has not been possible to more closely define the domain by site-directed mutagenesis.

3.3   Attempts to correlate ouabain IC_{50} values of Na+/K+-ATPase
        isoforms with isoenzymes' identity

The value for half-maximum inhibition of Na+/K+-ATPase activity in enzyme preparations from human cardiac muscle or brain cortex amounts to 0.027 μM and 0.033 μM, respectively [115]. The concentration-inhibition curves show no multiphasic shape as found with enzyme preparations from rat heart [116]. However, monophasic curves as observed with the above human enzyme preparations do not exclude the co-existence of isoenzymes when they have ouabain affinity differences of less than one order of magnitude and occur in a near 1:1 ratio (cf. reference [117]). Mathematical simulation (Fig. 3) reveals that a clear diagnosis of the occurrence of two isoenzymes in a preparation requires, even when they

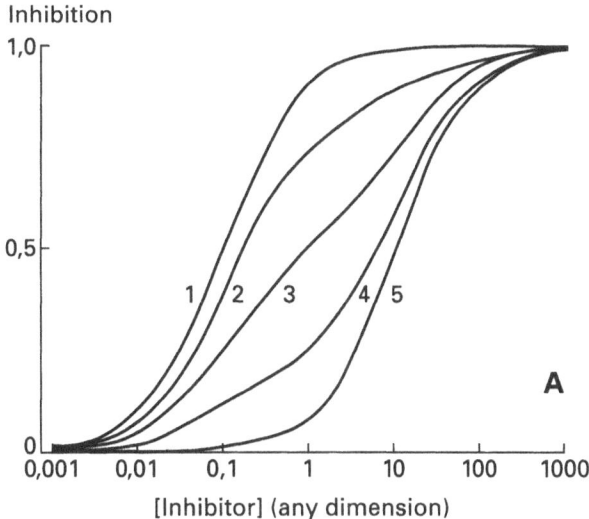

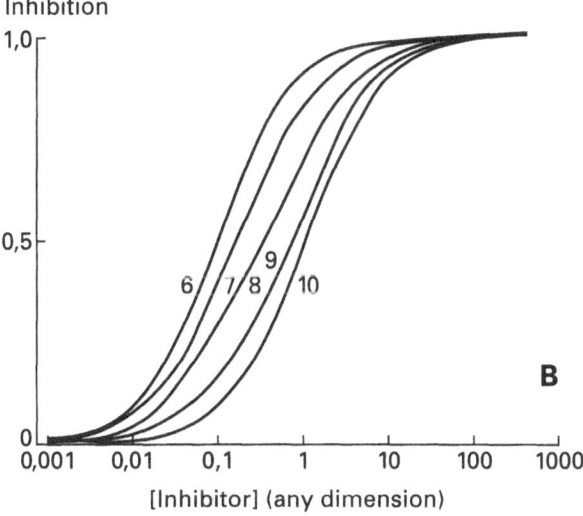

Fig. 3
Simulation of the curves describing the relation between varying digitalis concentration and degree of Na^+/K^+ATPase inhibition.
Case A: Response of a mixture of two isoenzymes differing in digitalis affinity by a factor of hundred. Curve 3 applies for a 1:1 mixture.
Case B: Response of a mixture of two isoenzymes differing in digitalis affinity by a factor of ten. Curves 8 and 10 apply for 50% or 1% apportionment of the higher affinity isoenzyme, respectively.

differ in digitalis affinity by a factor of 100, that the high affinity form comprises say between 80% and 20%. On the other hand, when the affinity difference between two isoenzymes is only ten and the low affinity form makes up say 20% to 80%, the presence of the high affinity isoenzyme does not deform the monotonic curve shape, but produces only a shift of the concentration-inhibition curve to a lower concentration region.

The latter case appears to apply to the isoenzyme population in some human Na^+/K^+-ATPase preparations. This emerges from the fact that the IC_{50} ouabain value of the $\alpha 1$-isoform is 0.1 μM [89], i.e., 3- to 4-fold higher than the above IC_{50} values found with Na^+/K^+-ATPase preparations from cardiac muscle and brain cortex. According to the simulated curves, this means that co-existing $\alpha 2$- or/and $\alpha 3$-isoenzymes have a higher ouabain affinity than $\alpha 1$, but occur in a lower percentage, say 20% of total.

In line with this interpretation, the elusive determination of the inhibitory action of ouabain on a Na^+/K^+-ATPase preparation from human cardiac muscle revealed IC_{50} values of 0.125 μM and 0.01 μM comprising 66% or 33% of total population [118]. In view of the measured affinity for human $\alpha 1$, we deduce that the higher value belongs to the $\alpha 1$-isoenzyme so that the lower value indicates the admixture of the $\alpha 2$- or/and $\alpha 3$-isoenzyme distinguished from $\alpha 1$ by an at least ten-fold higher ouabain affinity.

3.4   Significance of the inferred higher digitalis affinity of the $\alpha 2$- or/and $\alpha 3$-Na^+/K^+-ATPase isoform for understanding and avoidance of the toxic digitalis effects

3.4.1   Pathogenesis of digitalis toxicity

The major determinant of the total digitalis dose that can be administered is the development of cardiac arrhythmias. The sympathetic neuroexcitatory effect of digitalis drugs is a major contributing factor to their arrhythmogenic action [119]. Neural digitalis effects in humans arise from various sites in the central nervous system which increase central sympathetic outflow leading, with high digitalis doses, to ventricular tachyarrhythmias and arterial as well as coronary vasoconstriction [120]. Moreover, myocardial tissue contains substantial norepinephrine stores in β-adrenergic nerve terminals which also contain Na^+/K^+-ATPase [121]. Ouabain enhances norepinephrine release via inhibition of Na^+/K^+-ATPase [122] and blocks norepinephrine re-uptake at ouabain concentrations in the nanomolar range [29]. Actually, the Na^+/K^+-ATPase isoform of β-adrenergic nerves appears to show an about 100-fold higher ouabain sensitivity than the isoenzyme involved in the inotropic reaction of cardiac muscle; this indirectly emerges from the ouabain concentrations required for the inotropic responses of myocardium before and after catecholamine depletion [123,124]. Finally, the above neurohormonal actions of digitalis are particularly important as the progression of heart failure appears to be related to excessive activation of the sympathetic nervous system [125, 126] which thus carries prognostic importance [127].

Hence, a desirable agent to treat heart failure is likely one that improves hemodynamics without further activation of the neurohormonal system [125, 128]. Eisner and Smith [129] asked in 1992, if naturally occurring or synthetic digitalis compounds can be found with better separation between therapeutic and toxic effects, benefit could be drawn from the fact that sympathetic neuroexcitatory mechanisms are important in the mediation of most unwanted cardiac and extracardiac effects of cardiac glycosides. In other words, the way to increase the therapeutic/toxic dose ratio is to search for digitalis replacements with greater discrimination between the Na^+/K^+-ATPase isoform involved in the inotropic action and that responsible for the neuroexcitatory toxicity. As stated by Farley et al. [101] in 1995, knowing which isoforms are "the therapeutic and toxic receptors" will put investigators in a position to design isoform-specific agents. Already, ten years earlier, Erdmann et al. [130] had stated that, if two types of digitalis receptors can be distinguished in human heart, then there is hope for the development of new, more specific and possibly safer drugs to be used in myocardial failure.

3.4.2   *Tentative assignment of the cardiac and neural actions of cardiac glycosides to their interaction with particular isoforms of Na^+/K^+-ATPase*

As referred to above, the three isoforms are expressed in human cardiac muscle and nerve cells. All three could hence in principle be able to participate in eliciting the inotropic and neural effects of cardiac glycosides if they had similar digitalis affinities. However, this does not appear to apply as already addressed above.

The human $\alpha 1$-isoform from wild-type HeLa cells or from human kidney shows ouabain IC_{50} values near 100 nM [89]. The EC_{50} value for eliciting the positive-inotropic effect on human papillary muscle strips from non-failing hearts amounts to 80 nM ouabain [131]. As in the strips norepinephrine stores may have become exhausted during the long procedure of their preparation, this clearly favors the $\alpha 1$-isoenzyme as a major target for eliciting the inotropic ouabain action under conditions of exclusion of neurohormonal interference. In the same vein, Somberg and Smith

[132] showed in experiments with cats that the transection of the spinal cord at the atlanto-occipital junction significantly protects against neurally mediated digitalis toxicity.

The digitalis affinities of human α2- and α3-isoforms have not yet separately been determined, but certainly lie below 10 nM (cf. above). If the gradation of ouabain affinities in terms of K_i, found with rat α1 (4300 nM), rat α2 (170 nM) and rat α3 (31 nM) [133], can be extended to the human isoenzymes, the human α2- and α3-isoforms could be inferred to exhibit digitalis affinities two orders of magnitude lower than that of α1 (100 nM). This tentative inference appears to be supported by the knowledge that the therapeutic range for digoxin treatment of cardiac failure lies between 1.3 nM and 2.6 nM [134]. The digoxin concentrations found in the blood serum of patients with cardiac failure varied between 0.77 and 4.86 nM [135]. Rising from 2.56 nM, the probability of intoxication increased so that at 4.86 nM all patients showed signs of toxic neural actions. Remarkably enough, the disparity between the digitalis concentrations producing inotropic effects in isolated human papillary muscle strips (near 80 nM ouabain [131]) and those eliciting therapeutically beneficial actions in patients with cardiac failure (near 2 nM digoxin [134]) suggests the conclusion that the therapeutic cardiovascular effects of cardiac glycosides result, in part, from their neurohormonal actions [122, 136, 137].

A comparison of the mentioned latitudes of doses applicable to cardiac muscle strips and to patients with cardiac failure indicates that in the former case high affinity isoforms of Na+/K+-ATPase do not narrow the dose regimen (as accounted for above), whereas in the latter case the α3-isoenzyme, probably having the highest digitalis affinity, appears to be causally affected in eliciting increased sympathetic outflow. At high doses it can mediate ventricular tachyarrhythmias and arterial vasoconstriction [136].

3.5   Conclusions

Since the α1-isoenzyme is the major form expressed in kidney, Na+/K+-ATPase preparations from this tissue have been used here by us in a first approach to explore the structure-activity relationships in various C/D-trans steroids (see section 5). This will be followed by comparative determinations on the α3-isoenzyme with the aim to discover C/D-*trans* steroid derivatives which favorably differ from C/D-*cis* steroid derivatives in their affinity to the α1-isoenzyme. Since the α3-isoform cannot easily be prepared from cardiac muscle and brain due to its coexistence with the α1- and α2-forms, the indicated follow-up study has to wait for the availability of α2- and α3-Na$^+$/K$^+$-ATPase forms from a correspondingly transfected cell line.

4   Present knowledge on origin, property and structure of the putative endogenous digitalis

4.1   Criteria for classification of steroidal Na$^+$/K$^+$-ATPase inhibitors

In a comprehensive review in 1992, Goto et al. [39] set up nine requirements ("criteria") for classifying a substance as an endogenous digitalis-like factor. The list included: inhibition of Na$^+$/K$^+$-ATPase; inhibition of [^{3}H]-ouabain binding; inhibition of Na$^+$/K$^+$ pump activity; reversibility; high affinity; selectivity; competition with KCl; species sensitivity difference; positive inotropic effect. A smaller or greater part of these criteria were shown to be met by: eight lipids, ten steroidal compounds, eight peptides, seven substances of unknown identity, as well as by ascorbic acid, lignans, urodienolone and hemin. This huge diversity of chemical entities suggests the conclusion that most, if not all of these "criteria" reflect properties which are not unique to digitalis compounds. As stated already in 1988 by Haupert [38], the term digitalis-like is best considered a convenient metaphor, whilst remaining something of a misnomer. Apparently, the straightforward search for endogenous digitalis and novel digitalis-like acting steroids requires the application of strictly specific criteria. As experimentally substantiated by us [6–8, 13, 15, 19–21], the search for endogenous digitalis-like acting steroids should be confined to the isolation of compounds which competently intercalate in the digitalis binding matrix of Na$^+$/K$^+$-ATPase. The competent intercalation is proven first by the demonstration of characteristic species, tissue and/or isoenzyme differences in digitalis sensitivity, or/and second by the positive outcome of the phosphorylation promotion test with orthophosphate and Mg^{2+}, i.e., the negentropy-driven synthesis of the high-energy phosphoenzyme with an aspartyl phosphate residue in the catalytic center (methodic details in [15, 21, 138, 139]). In the end, applying these criteria, the pertinent literature data only on biologically and/or physicochemically characterized steroids will be evaluated below. This review will not address the wide range of questions concerning the potential role of putative endogenous digitalis as a mediator of responses to altered fluid balance and as a regulator of cardiovascular function in health and disease (reviewed in [29, 140]).

4.2   Origin and properties of putatively endogenous steroidal inhibitors of Na+/K+-ATPase

4.2.1   Cardiac glycosides from regular rat diet

Tamura and colleagues [141] found large amounts of several specific inhibitors of Na+/K+-ATPase and Na+/K+ pump in the urine of rats raised on a regular chow diet. The inhibitors disappeared from the urine within a week after switching the diet to a pure synthetic one, thus demonstrating their non-endogenous origin. Two of the inhibitors were isolated and identified as periplogenin rhamnoside and a stereoisomer of convalloside.

4.2.2   "Ouabain" (the endogenous digitalis-like factor EDLF) from human blood plasma

Between 1989 and 1991, Hamlyn and colleagues presented a large array of properties of an isolated compound that strongly suggested to them its identity with authentic ouabain. The pieces of biological evidence included promotion of enzyme phosphorylation by orthophosphate in the presence of Mg^{2+}, inhibition of Na+/K+-ATPase and Na+/K+ pump activity, inhibition of [^{3}H]-ouabain binding, high affinity to the enzyme, reversibility, and positive-inotropic action [142–145].

Total parenteral nutrition of blood donors for at least a week did not decrease the circulating level of "ouabain", proving its endogenous origin [146]. The physicochemical evidence comprised identification by mass spectrometry, high-performance liquid chromatography, and immunoreactivity [147–149].

However, Hamlyn's group reported in 1988/89 also on a variety of pieces of evidence that appear to be incompatible with the identity of the compound with authentic ouabain. The species differences in the sensitivity were found to be much smaller than the differences seen with ouabain [150]. The compound interacted with the Na+/K+-ATPase as a function of its ligation with an affinity 10–200 times higher than ouabain [142,143]. Its association rate constant was ~13-fold greater than that of ouabain [142]. Its molar absorption coefficient at 220 nm was at least 10 times greater than that of ouabain [142]. Without referring to the incompatibilities, Hamlyn more recently stated [151]: "A significant difference in any response would indicate that the human ouabain has a unique stereochemical configuration."

Accepting this interpretation of features distinguishing the compound from authentic ouabain, the ouabain-like compound isolated from human plasma has been put here in quotation marks. Actually, most recently, Haupert and coworkers have been able to prove by an ingenious physicochemical comparison that EDLF and authentic ouabain are not identical, whereas bovine HIF (see below) and human EDLF are indistinguishable [152].

4.2.3   Ouabain isomer (hypothalamic inhibitory factor HIF) from bovine hypothalamus

A series of experimental observations (reviewed in [153]) strongly suggested that lesions in the region of the anteroventral third ventricle of the brain prevent the secretion of a Na^+/K^+ transport inhibitor. Because the midbrain has been implicated in the control of circulating Na^+/K^+-ATPase inhibitors, the brain has been a favored source of tissue for studying this issue. Since 1984, in the course of efforts to identify the hypothalamic inhibitory factor, Haupert and associates have succeeded in isolating and characterizing the factor [154–160]. HIF was shown to inhibit Na^+/K^+ transport like ouabain from the extracellular surface and to reversibly suppress Na^+/K^+-ATPase activity with a K_i of 1.4 nM. Unlike ouabain, the factor does not promote enzyme phosphorylation with orthophosphate in the presence of Mg^{2+}, but instead it blocks the ouabain-supported phosphorylation. The latter action appears to indicate that the factor does intercalate in the digitalis binding matrix of the interprotodimeric cleft between the catalytic subunits and inhibits in this way enzyme and transport activities. Further unlike ouabain, HIF crosses the cell membrane [158], shows a single binding site for Na^+/K^+ pump inhibition in rat cardiac myocytes and rapid reversibility of an inotropic effect [157], makes no distinction in inhibitory potency with Na^+/K^+-ATPases from different species, and modulates the Na^+/K^+-ATPase: norepinephrine interplay leading to vasoconstriction [160].

During the course of isolation, no physical or chemical evidence was found to differentiate HIF from ouabain [159]. Both were indistinguishable by HPLC retention time, by susceptibility to naringinase hydrolysis and by molecular weight of both the aglycones and rhamnosides as derived from gas chromatographic and mass spectrometric analyses [159] To clarify the question of identity, naphthoylation of the hydroxyl groups was used as a means of amplifying any structural differences. An authentic sample of ouabain 1,19,2',3',4'-pentanaphthoate gave a clearly split CD curve with a positive Cotton effect, whereas HIF pentanaphthoate exhibited no distinct CD Cotton effect. Since HIF yielded additionally two hexanaphthoates, it appeared likely that the position of two hydroxyl groups in HIF is altered relative to ouabain [159]. This subtle structural difference has significant effects on biological activity as partially already mentioned above. Additionally, HIF was shown to have positive inotropic effects equipotent with ouabain in cultured rat myocytes, but at doses nearly three orders of magnitude lower than those required for ouabain [157]. These studies also showed that, at the same intracellular Ca^{2+}-concentration, ouabain was toxic whereas HIF was not. More recently, Haupert, Haber and their associates, partly members of the Brystol-Myers Squibb Pharmaceutical Research Institute [159], stated that the determination of the exact structure of the ouabain isomer HIF is desirable since it would probably reveal a general strategy for improving the therapeutic index of cardiac glycosides.

Concerning the origin of HIF (the ouabain isomer), the bulk of available evidence suggested to Haupert [153] that the brain, specifically the hypothalamus, represents an enriched source, if not the site of biosynthesis. The latter possibility no longer seems unlikely in the light of the recent demonstration that the hypothalamus is able to synthesize steroids (as pregnenolone, progesterone, pregnanedione and pregnanolone) independent of endocrine function [161].

4.2.4   *Ouabain-like factor (OLF) from rat hypothalamus*
Ferrandi and associates [162] reported recently that OLF from the hypothalamus of ox and rat have similar characteristics concerning both those that are close to ouabain and those that do not resemble ouabain. The latter include the ~100–1000 times greater potency of OLF to inhibit the low-affinity Na^+/K^+-ATPase isoform from rat kidney. The yield of OLF was greater from hypertensive than from normotensive rats. These findings represented the first direct evidence that a higher amount of OLF is present in tissues from genetically hypertensive rats than in those from their inbred normotensive controls, maintained under the same dietary and environmental conditions. This appears to support the role of OLF in the pathogenesis of genetically determined hypertension [162].

4.2.5   *"Ouabain" (EDLF) from the adrenal gland*
As reviewed in 1992 by Hamlyn and Manunta [140], in all mammalian species studied including man the adrenal gland is highly enriched in "ouabain". When the adrenal glands are removed from rats, the plasma levels of "ouabain" are lower than in matched pair-fed controls. After selective removal of the adrenal medulla, the plasma levels of "ouabain" are normal, suggesting that the adrenal cortex is a source of circulating "ouabain". Cultured human and bovine adrenocortical cells were shown to secrete "ouabain" in the culture fluid [163]. Collectively, these data suggested to the authors that the adrenal cortex is a major source of plasma "ouabain" and that "ouabain" is a probable "endogenous digitalis" in mammals.

Unexpectedly, "ouabain" secretion was unaltered by hemorrhage and re-infusion of shed blood in marked contrast to the large changes elicited in both cortisol and aldosterone secretion.

4.2.6   Ouabain isomer (OLF) from the adrenal gland
Ferrandi et al. [162] reported in 1992 that, besides hypothalamus, the adrenals could be a site of OLF production. The yield of OLF from the adrenals of the hypertensive rat strain was found to be significantly higher than that from the adrenals of the normotensive strain, again suggesting a role of OLF in the pathogenesis of hypertension in the studied rat strain.

4.2.7   Digoxin-like immunoreactive factor (DLIF) from adrenal cortex
Valdes et al. [164] measured DLIF concentrations in tissue extracts from rats as follows: adrenal glands, 44.3; serum, 6.3; liver, 5.2; kidney, 1.2; heart, brain or lungs, <1.4 ng of digoxin equivalent per g of protein. Human tissues showed similar results. Bovine adrenal cortex contained 7 times more DLIF per g of tissue than the adrenal medulla. In high performance liquid chromatography, none of 14 hormone steroids nor 7 cardiac glycoside congeners co-eluted with the major DLIF activity. Purified DLIF showed a molecular mass of 780 daltons (digoxin m.w. 781) comprised of one 390-dalton aglycone component (digoxigenin m.w. 391) plus several sugar moieties. The UV spectrophotometric absorbance properties were almost identical with that of digoxin. Taken together, the findings suggested some structural similarity with digoxin.

4.2.8   Ouabain-like activity (OLA) from the pituitary
In the brain of hamsters and rats, very high concentrations of OLA were noted in the pituitary, whereas the hypothalamus, pons, and cortex were 10- to 20-fold less compared with the pituitary [165]. Heart failure was described to be associated with significant increases in plasma OLA. Several new findings pointed to the concept that brain OLA mediates the sympathetic hyperactivity in congestive heart failure [165].

4.2.9   Independent attempts to confirm the existence of endogenous
ouabain
Recently, Doris et al. [166] attempted to confirm some of the observations reviewed above. The blood plasma from healthy volunteers and intensive care patients showed no ouabain immunoreactivity in most subjects. The low-level immunoreactivity with some probes was largely attributable to cross-reactivity with diverse substances different from ouabain. Bovine adrenocortical cells showed some ouabain-like immunoreactiv-

ity, but chemical blockade of steroidogenesis had no consistent effect on ouabain immunoreactivity. Stimulation of steroidogenesis did not produce any increase in the ouabain immunoreactivity. Examination of ouabain immunoreactivity in serum-supplemented medium conditioned by a murine adrenocortical tumor cell line indicated higher levels of immuno-reactivity, but the major portion eluted during high-performance liquid chromatography with much lower polarity than authentic ouabain. The authors stated that the discrepancies between their findings and others cannot be attributed to significant differences in methodologies, because they carefully emulated the solid-phase extraction procedures of Ham-lyn et al. [145]. These attempts to verify major findings of Hamlyn's group led Doris et al. [166] to the conclusion that ouabain is unlikely to be an endogenous mammalian cardiotonic steroid.

4.3   Critical evaluation of the present state of insight

In a recent review, Doris [167] listed 14 issues which he felt comprised the problems to be solved for the validation of ouabain as a relevant endoge-nous inhibitor of the Na^+/K^+ pump. What is more important, recent results [159, 160] and the present analysis lead to the conclusion that the inhibi-tor in question is certainly not identical with authentic ouabain, but appears to be, both functionally and chemically, a near relative of ouabain, pos-sibly a ouabain isomer as reviewed in subsections 4.2.2–4.2.6 and 4.2.8. The structure of the hypothalamic inhibitor HIF allowed the naphthoylation of one hydroxyl group more than with ouabain, in which C11α-OH is not accessible. Its epimerization would further decrease the accessibility for esterification, so that the sixth OH in HIF must be located elsewhere.
The explored metabolic pathways for the biosynthesis of steroids in mam-mals lead to steroids with trans-, but not with cis-junction of the rings C and D as present in ouabain. The obvious possibility of isomerism in HIF could be at the C/D cis- to trans-junction. However, this would mean loss of inhibitory potency, if (as likely, but not proven) HIF carries a buteno-lide side chain in C17β-position (cf. review [8]). Taken together, the present pieces of information offer no clue as to HIF structure.

4.4   Conclusion as to the search for ideal inotropic steroids

The impact of the reported biological properties of the hypothalamic inhib-itory factor (HIF) on the search for ideal inotropic steroids appears to be quite inconsistent. The most inviting observation on cultured rat myocy-tes has been that the ouabain isomer, at a dose producing similar inhibition of the Na^+/K^+ pump and greater elevations in $[Ca^{2+}]_{in}$ than the toxic dose of 1 μM ouabain, does not produce this toxicity [157]. This divergence cannot easily be explained.

Three other properties of HIF appear to be quite unfavorable. In contrast to ouabain, HIF modulates the interplay between Na^+/K^+ pump and adrenergic neuroeffectors leading to potentiation of norepinephrine action on smooth muscle, resulting in vasoconstriction [160]. The curve describing the relationship between concentration and inhibition of Na^+/K^+-ATPase is much steeper with HIF than with ouabain [160]. An even more important disadvantage of HIF compared to ouabain appears to be that HIF equally strongly inhibits ouabain-insensitive and -sensitive Na^+/K^+-ATPase forms from ouabain-resistant or ouabain-sensitive tissues and species, respectively [160]. This feature appears to be incompatible with the desired improvement of the therapeutic index through increased selectivity of interaction with human isoforms of Na^+/K^+-ATPase.

The ouabain-like activity (OLA) from the pituitary appears to cause (like ouabain) progressive sympathetic hyperactivity in congestive heart failure [165]. Hence it does not seem to offer a promising model for the design of ideal inotrop steroids.

5 Steroidal compounds designed to differentially interact with isoforms of Na^+/K^+-ATPase

5.1 Current state of knowledge

As the result of our targeted search, the lead structure in cardiac glycosides was recognized in 1985 to be the common steroid nucleus 5β,14β-androstane [13–15]. Hence, the often raised demand for the synthetic further development of digitalis compounds appeared to be resolved into the task of lead optimization. This has since been attempted by us through systematic derivatization of the lead structure, including change of the *cis*-junction of the rings A and B as well as C and D into *trans*-junction, introduction of double bonds or substituents in various positions of steroid skeleton as well as variation, derivatization or replacement of the C17β-lactone side chain and the C3β-O sugar residue (reviewed in [6–8]). This work revealed that the lactone side chain can provide a major increment of potency and the sugar residue can strongly modulate not only potency, but also receptor kinetics and pharmacokinetics, whereas the geometry of the steroid nucleus serves as the sensor for isoforms of Na^+/K^+-ATPase in man and experimental animals, and thus determines the selectivity of interaction [115, 168]. This suggested to us the conclusion that the cause of failure in all previous attempts to discover inotropes with improved therapeutic range by modifying cardiac glycosides was the preservation of the C/D-*cis* junction of steroid backbone unique to digitalis steroids.

Hence, we decided to test the suitability of C/D-*trans* steroids of hormone type to function as digitalis-like acting inhibitors of Na^+/K^+-ATPase. This possibility is supported by the early findings that progesterone, cortisone, deoxycorticosterone, spirolactone as well as aldosterone can produce significant increases in contractile force of cat papillary muscle preparation [169, 170]. Hence, one may conclude that their inotropic potency is not related to their intrinsic hormonal action. Actually, toxic doses of both deoxycorticosterone and digitoxin were found to produce similar shifts in intracellular cations [170]. Our above decision has crucially been supported by our data which demonstrated that $5\beta,14\alpha$-androstane can serve as a lead structure [7,21,138,139]. Here, we report on a series of chemical derivatizations of this lead with the *primary* aim to increase its low basal potency.

5.2   Parameters for data analysis

As a rational way of quantitatively correlating potency and structure, we have performed the extrathermodynamic analysis of the inhibitor constant which is numerically equivalent to the dissociation constant K'_D of the inhibitor-enzyme complex. Essentially, the extrathermodynamic derivation of structure-activity relationships is based on a division of the inhibitor molecule into substructural elements, the contribution of which to the integral Gibbs energy of interaction $\Delta G^{0'}$ with Na^+/K^+-ATPase is to be evaluated ($\Delta G^{0'} = RT \cdot \ln K'_D$). The $\Delta G^{0'}$ quantity is assumed to be the result of favorable and unfavorable energetic contributions of the individual structure components. Hence, the procedure involves calculation of the $\delta \Delta G^{0'}$ value for a pair of compounds differing in only one structural feature to give the increment or decrement of $\Delta G^{0'}$ caused by the substructural variable concerned.

Interpretation of the $\delta \Delta G^{0'}$ value in terms of the inhibitor substructure and the binding subsite chemotopography is, in principle, admissible since the extrathermodynamic relationships implicitly contain the connection between the "macroscopic" quantity ($\Delta G^{0'}$) and the "microscopic" properties as the atomic structure, geometry, hydropathy, charge distribution and electric field (cf. [171]). However, any such interpretation has to consider that the observed $\Delta G^{0'}$ value is a composite quantity:

$$\Delta G_{obs} = \Delta G_{int} + \Delta G_D - T\Delta S_{int}$$

where ΔG_{int} = intrinsic Gibbs energy of binding, ΔG_D = unfavorable Gibbs energy due to steric and electronic hindrances, and $T\Delta S_{int}$ = intrinsic entropy changes (cf. [172]). This makes difficult a clear-cut interpretation of the $\delta\Delta G^{0'}$-values so that the approach, while potentially very informative, also invites validation or rejection. The $\delta\Delta G^{0'}$-values are used here as the basis for the primary evaluation. As a complementary tactic for possibly more rigorous interpretation of structure-activity relationships, we have also utilized the rates of formation (k_{on}) and dissociation (k_{off}) of the inhibitor-enzyme complexes as a function of the inhibitor structure [7, 168].

5.3   Limited significance of present test data

As repeatedly stated by us [7, 168], one of the major obstacles in making full use of Na^+/K^+-ATPase in primary screening is the fact that the enzyme preparations from human cardiac muscle and brain cortex used till now consist of mixtures of three isoenzymes, the proportions and the properties of which are still largely unknown (cf. section 3). Since the isolation of pure isoenzymes from those tissues appears at present to be problematic, we have to wait for the availability of the individual isoenzymes from cell lines transfected with the cDNAs coding for the isoenzymes. In the meantime, we have applied Na^+/K^+-ATPase preparations from human kidney cortex which contain essentially the $\alpha1$-isoenzyme only [34–36]. The primary aim of testing the properties of partialsynthetic derivatives of $5\beta,14\alpha$-androstane derivatives with that $\alpha1$-isoenzyme has been to find out those derivatizations which grossly change the values of $\Delta G^{0'}$, k_{on} and k_{off} in the one or the other direction. This insight into the characteristic determinants of interaction can advantageously be applied when it is clear whether the inhibition of the $\alpha1$-isoenzyme or $\alpha3$-isoenzyme is involved in eliciting the medicinally desired or unwanted actions, respectively. As comparative measures, the constants for the $5\beta,14\beta$-androstane derivatives digitoxin, digoxin and 16-epi-gitoxin will be considered.

5.4   Derivatization of C/D-trans steroids: impact on the $\Delta G^{0'}$ values of interaction with kidney Na^+/K^+-ATPase (Table 1 and Fig. 4)

Most precursor steroids as 5β-androstan-3β-ol-17-one (4), canrenone (17), 5β-pregnan-21-ol-3,20-dione (60), progesterone (61) and 4-pregnene-17α,21-diol-3,20-dione (80) show interaction energies around –20 kJ/mol. This is much below the $\Delta G^{0'}$ values evolved by the medicinally used gly-

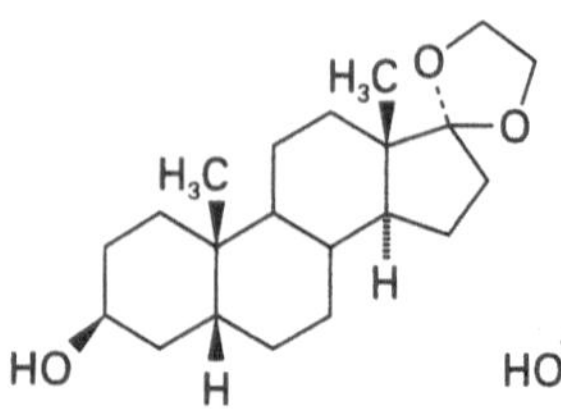

6

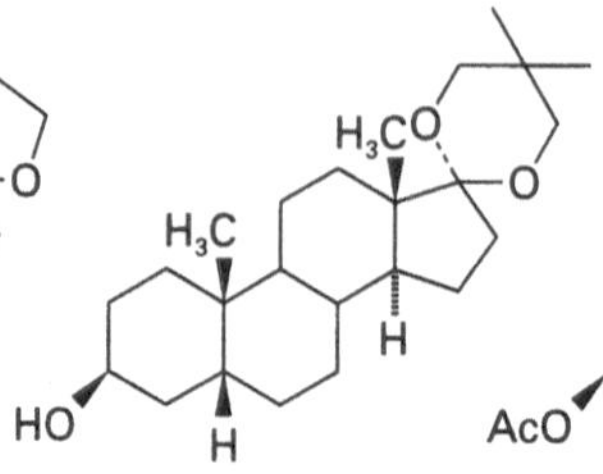

7

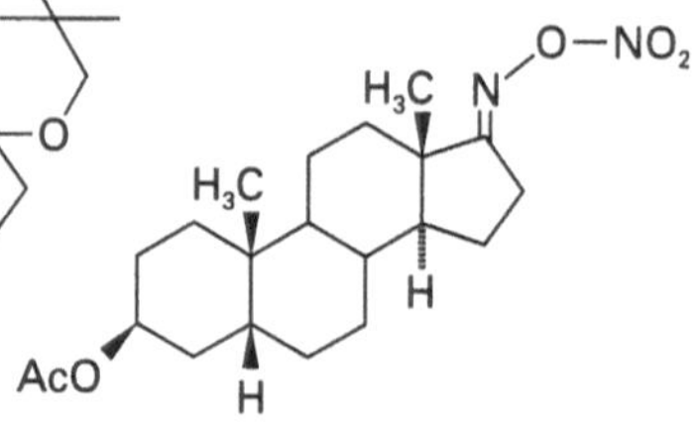

11

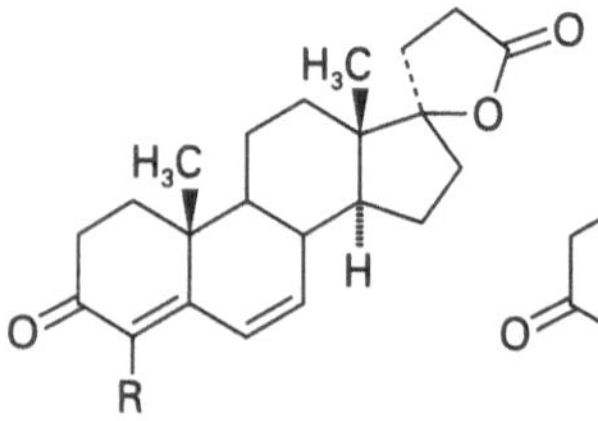

17: R=H
19: R=NO$_2$

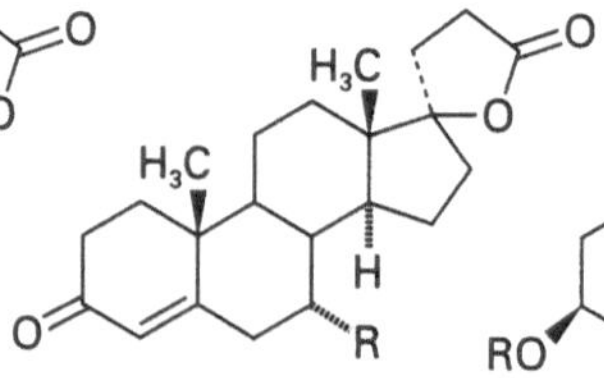

20: R=SH
21: R=CN

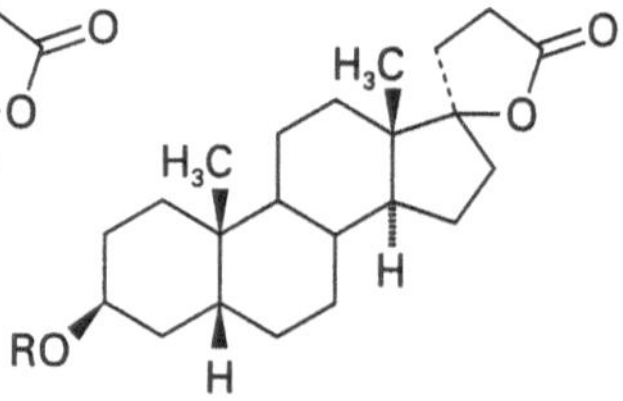

24: R=CF$_3$CO
25: R=NO
26: R=NO$_2$

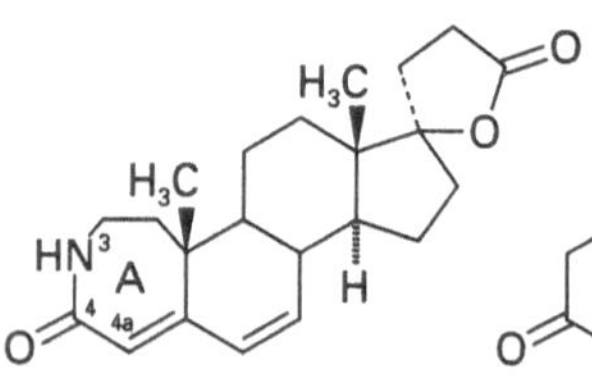

27

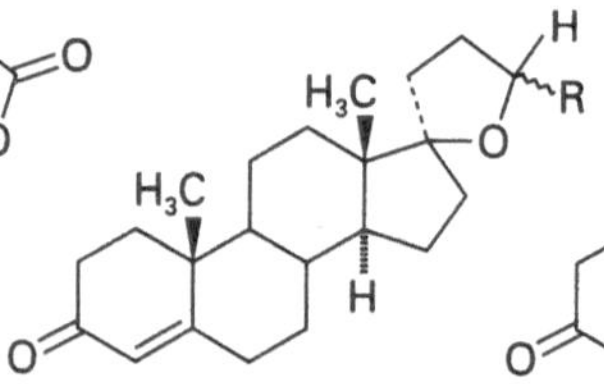

28: R=OH
29: R=F (apolar isomer)
30: R=F (polar isomer)

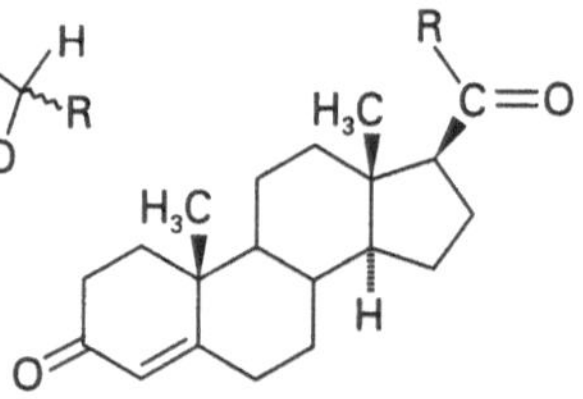

68: R=CHO
74: R=COOH

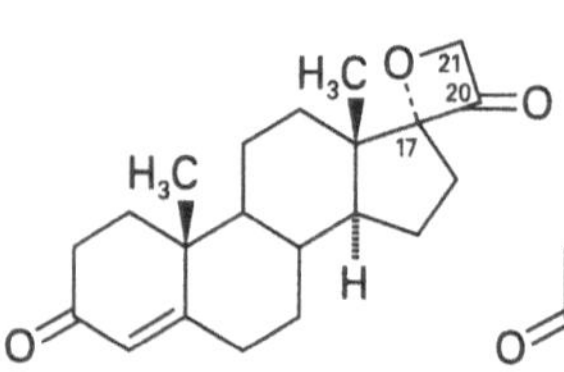

82

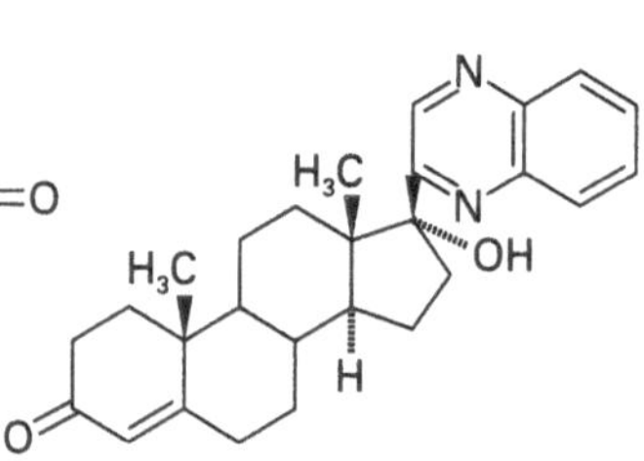

86

Fig. 4
Structural formulas of some of the investigated steroids. The numbering refers to Table 1.

cosides of the C/D-cis steroids digoxin (–43.1 kJ/mol) and digitoxin (–46.3 kJ/mol). A prospective pharmacological evaluation would require $\Delta G^{0'}$ values of at least –27 kJ/mol. In case of 3β-O-rhamnosyl-chlormadinol acetate, such value was namely found to be sufficient for *in vivo* evaluation [138]. Although many of the new derivatives evolve $\Delta G^{0'}$ values above that limit, for pharmacokinetic reasons (i.e. sufficient life time in the body) only the rhamnosyl pregnanes (40–43) appear to be suitable for *in vivo* testing.

The outcome of any derivatization can vary with the configuration and substitution of the precursor steroid and is hence not easily predictable. Surprisingly, already simple oxidation of a hydroxy group at C17 (1→4) or C21 (65→68) increases the potency. Quite unexpected are also the findings that the introduction of a nitro group at C4 (17→19) or a fluorine (17→29, 17→30) as well as the enlargement of the steroid ring A through insertion of a hetero atom (17→27) raise the interaction energy. Also surprising is the dramatic potency loss resulting from the replacement of 3β-acetoxy by 3β-trifluoracetoxy (53→54). The most favorable substitution sites for increasing $\Delta G^{0'}$ are C3β (e.g. 37→40), C17β (e.g. 8→51), C21 (e.g. 61→72) and C23 (e.g. 17→30). Somewhat smaller effects result from substitution at C4 (17→19), C6α (61→62) and C7α (17→20).

The present observations document but a small part of the large potential of possibilities for increasing the interaction energy of C/D-trans steroids by derivatization. They invite for more targeted modifications, which then will allow the generalizing evaluation of structure-activity relationships in physicochemical terms.

5.5   Derivatization of C/D-trans steroids: impact on the kinetics
         of interaction with kidney Na^+/K^+-ATPase (Table 1)

As derived earlier [168], the quantities of the association and dissociation rate constants, k_{on} and k_{off}, found for digitalis compounds grossly reflect the range of protein conformational changes associated with their inhibitory interaction with and their re-activating release from the enzyme. These interrelationships appear to be likewise valid for the C/D-trans steroids. The k_{on} values range from 0.46 $\mu M^{-1} \cdot min^{-1}$ (43) to 0.0002 $\mu M^{-1} \cdot min^{-1}$ (13), while the k_{Off} values range from 2.2 min^{-1} (4) to 0.1 min^{-1} (85). The half-life time ($\tau = \ln 2/k_{off}$) of the inhibitory complex with the most active derivative (43) amounts to 0.9 min and is thus much shorter than that of digitoxin (46.2 min) and digoxin (34.6 min), and even shorter than that of 16-epi-gitoxin (2.8 min). This accounts for the fact, that therapeutic advantages of the latter can be utilized to a limited extent only [5].

6   Conclusions for future work

– Derivatization of further precursor steroids as nor-, homo- and heteroro-steroids which, due to their peculiar surfaces, promise to evolve differential affinities to the isoforms of Na^+/K^+-ATPase.
– Comparative biochemical and pharmacological analysis of the most promising steroid glycosides concerning discrimination between Na^+/K^+-ATPase isoforms associated with the generation of the beneficial or toxic actions.
– Synthesis of glycosides from the aglycones with the highest isoenzymes' discrimination that should show half-life times long enough for comprehensive pharmacological/clinical evaluation.

7   Acknowledgment

This work was supported by the Deutsche Forschungsgemeinschaft until May 1995. Surprisingly, the support was then stopped for financial reasons.

Table 1.
Kinetic and equilibrium parameters of interaction of 94 C/D-trans steroid derivatives calculated from the time course of inhibition of human kidney Na$^+$/K$^+$-ATPase at 37° C and pH 7.4. Steroids listed were either obtained from commercial sources or synthesized in the author's laboratory. For methodical details see [168].

No	Systematic / trivial name	k_{on} [μM^{-1} min^{-1}]	k_{off} [min^{-1}]	K'_D [μM]	$\Delta G^{0'}$ [kJ M^{-1}]
1	5β-androstane-3β,17α-diol	0.0013	0.55	~450	~19.9
2	5β-androstane-3α-ol-17-one	0.0033	0.77	232	21.6
3	5β-androstane-3β,17β-diol	0.0062	1.15	185	22.2
4	5β-androstane-3β-ol-17-one	0.0076	2.2	289	21.0
5	5β-androstane-3β-ol-17-oxime	0.0051	1.04	202	21.9
6	5β-androstane-3β-ol-17-(1,2-ethyleneketal)			~140	~22.9
7	5β-androstane-3β-ol-17-(2,2-dimethyl)-1,3-propyleneketal			92	24.0
8	5β-androstane-3β-acetoxy-17-one	0.0095	1.28	137	23.0
9	5β-androstane-3β-acetoxy-17-oxime	0.021	0.53	25	27.3
10	5β-androstane-3β-acetoxy-17-methoxime			~200	~22.0
11	5β-androstane-3β-acetoxy-17-oxime nitric acid ester			~200	~22.0
12	5β-androstane-3β-acetoxy-17-hydrazone			>1000	<17.8
13	5β-androstane-3β-acetoxy-17-N,N-dimethyl-hydrazone	0.0002	0.32	1600	16.6
14	5β-androstane-3β-acetoxy-17(β?)-amine			~140	~22.2
15	5β-androstane-3β-acetoxy-17(β?)-nitro			>500	<19.6
16	5β-androstane-3β-O-rhamnosyl-17-oxime	0.0106	0.46	44	25.9
17	21,24-bis-nor-17α-chola-4,6-diene-17β,23-oxido-3,23-dione / canrenone	0.0012	0.58	472	19.8
18	canrenone-3-oxime			~280	~21.1
19	canrenone-4-nitro	0.0021	0.105	50	25.5
20	6,7-dihydro-canrenone-7α-thiol	0.0048	0.81	170	22.4
21	6,7-dihydro-canrenone-7α-nitril			>1000	<17.8
22	5β-H-4,5,6,7-tetrahydro-canrenone-2α-ol	~0.0009	~0.45	~500	~19.6

No	Systematic / trivial name	k_{on} [μM^{-1} min^{-1}]	k_{off} [min^{-1}]	K'_D [μM]	$\Delta G^{0'}$ [kJ M^{-1}]
23	5β-H-4,5,6,7-tetrahydro-canrenone-2α-O-acetate	~0.0014	~0.97	~700	~18.7
24	5β-H-3,3,4,5,6,7-hexahydro-canrenone 3β-O-trifluoroacetate			>1000	<17.8
25	5β-H-3,3,4,5,6,7-hexahydro-canrenone-3β-O-nitrite			>1000	<17.8
26	5β-H-3,3,4,5,6,7-hexahydro-canrenone-3β-O-nitrate			>>500	<19.6
27	A-homo-21,24-bis-nor-17α-chola-4a,6-diene-3-aza-17β,23-oxido-4,23-dione			99	23.8
28	21,24-bis-nor-17α-chol-4-ene-3-one-17β,23-oxido-23-ξ-ol	0.0027	0.62	230	21.6
29	21,24-bis-nor-17α-chol-4-ene-3-one-17β,23-oxido-23ξ-fluoride (apolar isomer)	0.0028	0.13	47.7	25.7
30	21,24-bis-nor-17α-chol-4-ene-3-one-17β,23-oxido-23ξ-fluoride(polar isomer)	0.0054	0.14	25.8	27.2
31	21-nor-5β-pregnane-3ξ-ol-20-oxime	0.0033	0.18	53.4	25.4
32	21-nor-5β-pregnane-3ξ-ol-20-amine (apolar isomer)	0.0011	0.67	>800	<18.4
33	21-nor-5β-pregnane-3ξ-ol-20-amine (polar isomer)	0.0027	0.95	>350	<20.5
34	21-nor-5β-pregnane-3ξ-ol-20-nitro (apolar isomer)			>800	<18.4
35	21-nor-5β-pregnane-3ξ-ol-20-nitro (polar isomer)			>900	<18.1
36	5β-pregnane-3β,20β-diol	0.021	1.33	62	25.0
37	5β-pregnane-3β-ol-20-one	0.0152	0.61	40	26.1
38	5β-pregnane-3β-ol-20-oxime	0.026	0.68	26	27.2
39	5β-pregnane-3β,21-diol-20-one	0.0038	0.86	225	21.7
40	5β-pregnane-3β-rhamnosyloxy-20-one	0.27	1.1	4.1	32.0
41	5β-pregnane-3β-rhamnosyloxy-20-oxime	0.076	0.6	7.9	30.3
42	5β-pregnane-3β-rhamnosyloxy-6α-methyl-17α-acetoxy-20-oxime	0.35	1.14	3.3	32.5
43	5β-pregnane-3β-rhamnosyloxy-6α-methyl-17α-acetoxy-20-one	0.46	0.8	1.7	34.3
44	5β-pregnane-3β-acetoxy-20α-ol	0.09	1.4	15.6	28.5
45	5β-pregnane-3β-acetoxy-20β-ol	0.011	0.26	23.3	27.5
46	5β-pregnane-3β,20β-di-O-acetate			>500	<19.6

#	Compound				
47	5β-pregnane-3β-O-acetate-20β-O-nitrate			>>500	<19.6
48	5β-pregnane-3β-O-acetate-20α-O-nitrate			>>500	<19.6
49	5β-pregnane-3β,20β-di-O-nitrite			>>500	<19.6
50	5β-pregnane-3β,20β-di-O-nitrate	0.0033	0.177	53	25.3
51	5β-pregnane-3β-acetoxy-20-oxime	0.065	0.53	8.1	30.2
52	5β-pregnane-3β-acetoxy-20-oxime acetate			18.5	28.1
53	5β-pregnane-3β-acetoxy-20-one	0.113	1.03	9.1	29.9
54	5β-pregnane-3β-trifluoroacetoxy-20-one			>500	<19.6
55	5β-pregnane-3β-formoxy-20-one	0.06	1.08	17.9	28.2
56	5β-pregnane-3β-propionoxy-20-one			53	25.4
57	5β-pregnane-3β-nitryloxy-20-one	0.0077	0.47	61	25.0
58	5β-pregnane-3,20-dione	0.0088	0.71	80	24.3
59	5β-pregnane-3,20-dione-17α-O-acetate			>200	<22.0
60	5β-pregnane-3,20-dione-21-ol	0.0029	0.84	290	21.0
61	4-pregnene-3,20-dione / progesterone	0.003	0.6	202	21.9
62	4-pregnene-3,20-dione-6α-methyl			60	25.1
63	4-pregnene-3,20-dione-16α-ol			~450	~19.9
64	4-pregnene-3,20-dione-16α-O-acetate			~350	~20.5
65	4-pregnene-3,20-dione-21-ol / deoxycorticosterone	0.0067	1.97	290	21.0
66	4-pregnene-3,20-dione-21-O-acetate	0.0084	1	118	23.3
67	4-pregnene-3,20-dione-21-fluoride			~200	22.0
68	4-pregnene-3,20-dione-21-al	0.0032	0.107	33.7	26.6
69	4-pregnene-3,20-dione-21-oxime	0.0116	0.63	54	25.3
70	4-pregnene-3,20-dione-21-oxime formiate	0.043	0.29	69	24.7
71	4-pregnene-3,20-dione-21-oxime acetate	0.0036	0.26	73.5	24.5
72	4-pregnene-3,20-dione-21-oxime trifluoroacetate			~22	~27.9
73	4-pregnene-3,20-dione-21-methoxime	0.063	1.44	23	27.5
74	4-pregnene-3,20-dione-21-carbonic acid	0.0003	0.22	650	18.9
75	4-pregnene-3,20-dione-17α-ol			>1000	<17.8
76	4-pregnene-3,20-dione-17α-O-acetate	0.0058	0.48	82	24.3

No	Systematic / trivial name	k_{on} [M^{-1} min^{-1}]	k_{off} [min^{-1}]	K'_D [μM]	$\Delta G^{0'}$ [kJ M^{-1}]
77	4-pregnene-3,20-dione-17α-O-nitrate			25.6*	27.3
78	4-pregnene-3,20-dione-6α-methyl-17α-ol	0.0025	0.46	184	22.2
79	4-pregnene-3,20-dione-6α-methyl-17α-O-acetate	0.029	1.09	37	26.3
80	4-pregnene-3,20-dione-17α,21-diol / Reichstein S	0.001	0.49	470	19.8
81	4-pregnene-3,20-dioxime-17α-ol	0.0011	0.47	450	19.9
82	4-pregnene-3,20-dione-17α,21-oxetane	0.0014	0.47	340	20.6
83	4-pregnene-3,20-dione-17α-ol-21-oxime	0.112	0.47	42	26.0
84	4-pregnene-3,20-dione-17α-ol-21-O-trifluoroacetate	0.0003	0.25	740	18.6
85	4-pregnene-3,20-dione-17α-ol-21-O-nitrate	0.0004	0.099	250	21.4
86	4-pregnene-3-one-17α-ol-20,21-chinoxaline			>500	<19.6
87	4-pregnene-3,20,21-trioxime	0.0075	0.37	50	25.5
88	5-pregnene-3β-acetoxy-20-one	0.01	1.02	102	23.7
89	5-pregnene-3β-acetoxy-20-oxime			60	25.1
90	5,16-pregnadiene-3β-acetoxy-20-one			190	22.0
91	5-pregnene-3β-acetoxy-16α-cyano-20-one			~120	~23.3
92	5-pregnene-3β-acetoxy-16α-nitromethyl-20-one			~150	~22.7
93	5-pregnene-3β,16α-diacetoxy-20-one			187	22.1
94	5-pregnene-3β,16α-diol-20-one	0.005	0.38	75.2	24.5

*Probably unstable under measuring conditions.

References

1 M. Packer: Circulation *79*, 198–204 (1989).
2 J.J. Kellermann: Am. Heart J. *120*, 1529–1531 (1990).
3 P.W. Erhardt: J. Med. Chem. 30, 231–237 (1987).
4 J.N. Cohn: N. Engl. J. Med. *320*, 729–731 (1989).
5 K.-O. Haustein and R. Bauer: Int. J. Clin. Pharmacol. Ther. *32*, 299–304 (1994).
6 K.R.H. Repke, W. Schönfeld, J. Weiland, R. Megges and A. Hache, in: Design of Enzyme Inhibitors as Drugs (M. Sandler and H.J. Smith, Eds.), pp. 435–502. Oxford University Press, Oxford, 1989.
7 K.R.H. Repke, J. Weiland, R. Megges and R. Schön: Prog. Med. Chem. *30*, 135–202 (1993).
8 K.R.H. Repke, R. Megges, J. Weiland and R. Schön: Angew. Chem. Int. Ed. Engl. *34*, 282–294 (1995).
9 K.R.H. Repke and H.J. Portius: Experientia (Basel) *19*, 452–458 (1963).
10 K.R.H. Repke and W. Schönfeld: Trends Pharmacol. Sci. *5*, 393–397 (1984).
11 R.A. Kelley and T.W. Smith: Adv. Pharmacol. *25*, 263–288 (1994).
12 T.P. Kenakin, R.A. Bond and T.I. Bonner: Pharmacol. Rev. *44*, 351–362 (1992).
13 W. Schönfeld, J. Weiland, C. Lindig, M. Masnyk, M.M. Kabat, A. Kurek, J. Wicha and K.R.H. Repke: Naunyn-Schmiedeberg's Arch. Pharmacol. *329*, 414–426 (1985).
14 K.R.H. Repke: Trends Pharmacol. Sci. *6*, 275–278 (1985).
15 W. Schönfeld, K.-H. Menke, R. Schönfeld and K.R.H. Repke: J. Enzyme Inhib. *2*, 37–45 (1987).
16 K.R.H. Repke: Klin. Wochenschr. *42*, 157–165 (1964).
17 A.J. Levi, M.R. Boyett and C.O. Lee: Prog. Biophys. Molec. Biol. *62*, 1–54 (1994).
18 K.R.H. Repke and H.J. Portius: Planta Med., *Suppl. 4*, 66–78 (1971).
19 K.R.H. Repke and J. Weiland: Pharmacol. Res. Commun. *20*, 425–450 (1988).
20 K.R.H. Repke, W. Schönfeld, R. Schönfeld and K.-H. Menke: Pharmazie *45*, 237–239 (1990).
21 J. Weiland, W. Schönfeld, K.-H. Menke and K.R.H. Repke: Pharmacol. Res. *23*, 27–32 (1991).
22 K.R.H. Repke, R. Megges, J. Weiland and R. Schön: FEBS Lett. *359*, 107–109 (1995).
23 S.M. Periyasamy, W.-H. Huang and A. Askari: J. Biol. Chem. *258*, 9878–9885 (1983).
24 K.R.H. Repke: Biochim. Biophys. Acta *864*, 195–212 (1986).
25 A. Askari: J. Bioenerg. Biomembr. *19*, 359–374 (1987).
26 C.-H. Heldin: Cell *80*, 213–223 (1995).
27 S. Jones and J.M. Thornton: Prog. Biophys. Molec. Biol. *63*, 31–65 (1995).
28 T.P. Lybrand: Curr. Opinion Struct. Biol. *5*, 224–228 (1995).
29 M.P. Blaustein: Am. J. Physiol. *264*, C1367–C1387 (1993).
30 K.R.H. Repke, M. Est and H.J. Portius: Biochem. Pharmacol. *14*, 1785–1802 (1965).
31 K.J. Sweadner: J. Biol. Chem. *254*, 6060–6067 (1979).
32 K.J. Sweadner: Biochim. Biophys. Acta *988*, 185–220 (1989).
33 E.D. Sverdlov, N.S. Akopyanz, K.E. Petrukhin, N.E. Broude, G.S. Monastyrskaya and N.N. Modyanov: FEBS Lett. *239*, 6568 (1988).
34 N.S. Akopyanz, N.E. Broude, N.G. Vinogradova, Yu.A. Balabanov, G.S. Monastyrskaya and E.D. Sverdlov, in: Soc. Gen. Physiol. Ser., Vol. 46, Part 2: The Sodium Pump: Recent Developments (J.H. Kaplan and P. De Weer, Eds.), pp. 189–193. The Rockefeller University Press, New York, 1991.
35 O.I. Shamraj, D. Melvin and J.B. Lingrel: Biochem. Biophys. Res. Commun. *179*, 1434–1440 (1991).

36   P.D. Allen, T.A. Schmidt, J.D. Marsh and K. Kjeldsen, in: Cellular and Molecular Alterations in the Failing Human Heart (G. Hasenfuss, Ch. Holubarsh, H. Just and N.R. Alpert, Eds.), pp. 87–94. Steinkopff, Darmstadt, 1992.

37   R. Zahler, M. Gilmore-Hebert, J.C. Baldwin, K. Franco and E.J. Benz, Jr.: Biochim. Biophys. Acta 1149, 189–194 (1993).

38   G.T. Haupert, Jr., in: The Na$^+$/K$^+$-Pump, Part B: Cellular Aspects (J.C. Skou, J.G. Nørby, A.B. Maunsbach and M. Esmann, Eds.), pp. 297–320. Alan R. Liss, Inc., New York, 1988.

39   A. Goto, K. Yamada, N. Yagi, M. Yoshioka and T. Sugimoto: Pharmacol. Rev. 44, 377–399 (1992).

40   J.M. Hamlyn, J. Laredo, Z.-R. Lu, B. Hamilton, G. Lighthall and P. Manunta: Hypertension 24, 641–644 (1994).

41   N.K. Hollenberg and S.W. Graves: Hypertens. Res. 18, 1–6 (1995).

42   K.R.H. Repke and R. Schön: Acta biol. med. germ. 31, K19–K30 (1973).

43   M. Inaba and Y. Maede: Biochim. Biophys. Acta 818, 267–270 (1985).

44   K. Mimura, H. Matsui, T. Takagi and Y. Hayashi: Biochim. Biophys. Acta 1145, 63–74 (1993).

45   K.R.H. Repke, J. Weiland, R. Megges and R. Schön: J. Enzyme Inhib. 10, 147–157 (1996).

46   W.A. Hendrickson: Curr. Biol. 2, 57–59 (1992).

47   D.L. Stokes, W.R. Taylor and N.M. Green: FEBS Lett. 346, 32–38 (1994).

48   M.A. Lemmon and D.M. Engelman: FEBS Lett. 346, 17–20 (1994).

49   T. Haltia and E. Freire: Biochim. Biophys. Acta 1228, 1–27 (1995).

50   J.C. Ellory, J.R. Green, S.M. Jarvis and J.D. Young: J. Physiol. (Lond.) 295, 10–11 (1979).

51   M. Esmann, C. Christiansen, K.A. Karlsson, G.C. Hansson and J.C. Skou: Biochim. Biophys. Acta 603, 1–12 (1980).

52   A. Askari, W.-H. Huang and J.M. Antieau: Biochemistry 19, 1132–1140 (1980).

53   W.-H. Huang and A. Askari: Biochim. Biophys. Acta 645, 54–58 (1981).

54   B. Vilsen, J.P. Andersen, J. Petersen and P.L. Jørgensen: J. Biol. Chem. 262, 10511–10517 (1987).

55   J.G. Nørby and J. Jensen in: The Sodium Pump: Recent Developments (P. De Weer and J.H. Kaplan, Eds.), pp. 173–188. Rockefeller University Press, New York, 1991.

56   W. Schoner, D. Thönges, E. Hamer, R. Antolovic, E. Buxbaum M. Willeke, E.H. Serpersu and G. Scheiner-Bobis in: The Sodium Pump: Structure Mechanism, Hormonal Control and its Role in Disease (E. Bamberg and W. Schoner, Eds.), pp. 332–341. Steinkopff, Darmstadt, 1994.

57   J.C. Koster, G. Blanco and R.W. Mercer: J. Biol. Chem. 270, 14332–14339 (1995).

58   M. Ganjeizadeh, N. Zolotarjova, W.-H. Huang and A. Askari: J. Biol. Chem. 270, 15707–15710 (1995).

59   M. Mohraz, M.V. Simpson and P.R. Smith: J. Cell Biol. 105, 1–8 (1987).

60   N. Modyanov, S. Lutsenko, E. Chertova and R. Efremov, in: Soc. Gen. Physiol. Ser., Vol. 46: The Sodium Pump: Structure, Mechanism, and Regulation (J.H. Kaplan and P. De Weer, Eds.), pp. 99–115. The Rockefeller University Press, New York, 1991.

61   K. Kawakami, T. Ohta, H. Nojima and K. Nagano: J. Biochem. 100, 389–397 (1986).

62   Yu.A. Ovchinnikov, E.A. Arystarkhova, N.M. Arzamazova, K.N. Dzhandzhugazyan, R.G. Efremov, I.R. Nabiev and N.N. Modyanov: FEBS Lett. 227, 235–239 (1988).

63   K.R.H. Repke and R. Schön: Biol. Rev. 67, 31–78 (1992).

64   I.R. Nabiev, K.N. Dzhandzhugazyan, R.G. Efremov and N.N. Modyanov: FEBS Lett. 236, 235–239 (1988).

65   M.A. Lemmon, J.M. Flanagan, H.R. Treutlein, J. Zhang and D.M. Engelman: Bio-
     chemistry 31, 12719–12725 (1992).
66   J.B. Lingrel and T. Kuntzweiler: J. Biol. Chem. 269, 19659–19662 (1994).
67   N.A. Sarvazyan, N.M. Modyanov and A. Askari: J. Biol. Chem. 270, 26528–26532
     (1995).
68   M.A. Lemmon and D.M. Engelman: Curr. Opinion Struct. Biol. 2, 511–518 (1992).
69   K. Go and G. Kartha: Acta Cryst. C39, 376–383 (1983).
70   J. Kyte and R.F. Doolittle: J. Mol. Biol. 157, 105–132 (1982).
71   R.M. Jackson and M.J.E. Sternberg: J. Mol. Biol. 250, 258–275 (1995).
72   C.M. Canessa, J.-D. Horisberger, D. Louvard and B.C. Rossier: EMBO J. 11, 1681–1687
     (1992).
73   P.J. Schultheis and J.B. Lingrel: Biochemistry 32, 544–550 (1993).
74   A.R. Fersht: Trends Biochem. Sci. 12, 301–304 (1987).
75   G.R. Askew and J.B. Lingrel: J. Biol. Chem. 269, 24120–24126 (1994).
76   R. Antolovic, D. Linder, J. Hahnen and W. Schoner: Eur. J. Biochem. 227, 61–67 (1995).
77   R. Antolovic, W. Schoner, K. Geering, C. Canessa, B.C. Rossier and J.D. Horisber-
     ger: FEBS Lett. 368, 169–172 (1995).
78   W.J. O'Brien, E.T. Wallick and J.B. Lingrel: J. Biol. Chem. 268, 7707–7712 (1993).
79   T.W. Smith, V.P. Butler and E. Haber: Biochemistry 9, 331–337 (1970).
80   T.B. Okarma, P. Tramell and S.M. Kalman: Mol. Pharmacol. 8, 476–480 (1972).
81   L.G. Cantley, X.-M. Zhou, M.J. Cunha, J. Epstein and L.C. Cantley: J. Biol. Chem.
     267, 17271–17278 (1992).
82   C.C. Hall and A.E. Ruoho, in: Current Topics in Membranes and Transport, Vol. 19:
     Structure, Mechanism, and Function of the Na/K Pump (J.F. Hoffman and B. For-
     bush III, Eds.), pp. 265–270. Academic Press, New York, 1983.
83   E. Srocco, and J. Tomasi: Adv. Quantum Chem. 11, 115–194 (1978).
84   R.M. Lebovitz, K. Takeyasu and D.M. Fambrough: EMBO J. 8, 193–202 (1989).
85   P.J. Schultheis, E.T. Wallick and J.B. Lingrel: J. Biol. Chem. 268, 22686–22694 (1993).
86   Y. Hara, O. Urayama, K. Kawakami, H. Nojima, H. Nagamune, T. Kojima, T. Ohta,
     K. Nagano and M. Nakao: J. Biochem. 102, 43–58 (1987).
87   S. Fahn, G.J. Koval and R.W. Albers: J. Biol. Chem. 241, 1882–1889 (1966).
88   E.M. Price, D.A. Rice and J.B. Lingrel: J. Biol. Chem. 265, 6638–6641 (1990).
89   E.M. Price and J.B. Lingrel: Biochemistry 27, 8400–8408 (1988).
90   J.B. Lingrel, J. Orlowski, E.M. Price and B.G. Pathak, in: Soc. Gen. Physiol. Ser., Vol.
     46: The Sodium Pump: Structure, Mechanism, and Regulation (J.H. Kaplan and P.
     De Weer, Eds.), pp. 1–16. The Rockefeller University Press, New York, 1991.
91   E.A. Jewell and J.B. Lingrel: Ann. N.Y. Acad. Sci. 671, 120–133 (1992).
92   E.M. Price, D.A. Rice and J.B. Lingrel: J. Biol. Chem. 264, 21902–21906 (1989).
93   F. Holzinger, C. Frick and M. Wink: FEBS Lett. 314, 477–480 (1992).
94   F. Jaisser, C.M. Canessa, J.-D. Horisberger and B.C. Rossier: J. Biol. Chem. 267,
     16895–16903 (1992).
95   O. Hansen: Pharmacol. Rev. 36, 143–163 (1984).
96   T. Kuntzweiler, E.T. Wallick, C.L. Johnson and J.B. Lingrel: J. Biol. Chem. 270, 16206–
     16212 (1995).
97   M.V. Milburn, G.G. Privé, D.L. Milligan, W.G. Scott, J. Yeh, J. Jancarik, D.E. Kosh-
     land, Jr. and S.-H. Kim: Science 254, 1342–1347 (1991).
98   D.L. Milligan and D.E. Koshland, Jr.: Science 254, 1651–1654 (1991).
99   O.I. Shamraj, I.L. Grupp, G. Grupp, D. Melvin, N. Gradoux, W. Kremers, J.B. Lingrel
     and A. De Pover: Cardiovasc. Res. 27, 2229–2237 (1993).

100   K.J. Sweadner: Trends Cardiovasc. Med. *3*, 2–6 (1993).
101   A.A. McDonough, J. Wang and R.A. Farley: Mol. Cell. Cardiol. *27*, 1001–1009 (1995).
102   K.J. Sweadner, V.L.M. Herrera, S. Amato, A. Moellmann, D.K. Gibbons and K.R.H. Repke: Circ. Res. *74*, 669–678 (1994).
103   K.M. McGrail, J.M. Phillips and K.J. Sweadner: J. Neurosci. *11*, 381–391 (1991).
104   K.J. Sweadner: Can. J. Physiol. *70*, S255–S259 (1992).
105   M.A. Shull, D.G. Pugh and J.B. Lingrel: J. Biol. Chem. *264*, 17532–17543 (1989).
106   Yu.A. Ovchinnikov, G.S. Monastyrskaya, N.E. Broude, Yu.A. Ushkaryov, A.M. Melkov, Yu.V. Smirnov, I.V. Malyshev, R.L. Allikmets, M.B. Kostina, I.E. Dulubova, N.I. Kiyatkin, A.V. Grishin, N.N. Modyanov and E.D. Sverdlov: FEBS Lett. *233*, 87–94 (1988).
107   K. Takeyasu, V. Lemas and D.M. Fambrough: Am. J. Physiol. *259*, C619–C630 (1990).
108   C.M. Canessa, J.-D. Horisberger and B.C. Rossier: J. Biol. Chem. *268*, 17722–17726 (1993).
109   E.A. Jewell-Motz and J.B. Lingrel: Biochemistry *32*, 13523–13530 (1993).
110   J. Feng and J.B. Lingrel: Biochemistry *33*, 4218–4224 (1994).
111   T.G. Consler, S.H. Woodard and J.C. Lee: Biochemistry *28*, 8756–8764 (1989).
112   P. Schimmel: Biochemistry *29*, 9495–9502 (1990).
113   M.-D. Tsai and H. Yan: Biochemistry *30*, 6806–6818 (1991).
114   M.A. Carson-Jurica, W.T. Schrader and B.W. O'Malley: Endocr. Rev. *11*, 201–220 (1990).
115   W. Schönfeld, R. Schönfeld, K.-H. Menke, J. Weiland and K.R.H. Repke: Biochem. Pharmacol. *35*, 3221–3231 (1986).
116   A. De Pover, G. Grupp, A. Schwartz and I.L. Grupp: Heart Failure (December 1990/ January 1991), 201–211 and 258 (1991).
117   L.B. Hough, H. Weinstein and J.P. Green, in: Receptors for Neurotransmitters and Peptide Hormones (G. Pepeu, M.J. Kuhar and S.J. Enna, Eds.), pp. 183–192. Raven Press, New York, 1980.
118   S. Decollogne, J.J. Mercadier, Ph. Lechat, P. Allen and L.G. Lelièvre, in: The Sodium Pump: Structure Mechanism, Hormonal Control and its Role in Disease (E. Bamberg and W. Schoner, Eds.), pp. 812–815. Steinkopff, Darmstadt, 1994.
119   D.G. Pace and R.A. Gillis: Arch. int. Pharmacodyn. Ther. *255*, 103–116 (1982).
120   T.W. Smith, E.M. Antman, P.L. Friedman, C.M. Blatt and J.D. Marsh: Prog. Cardiovasc. Diseases *26*, 495–523 (1984).
121   V.K. Sharma and S.P. Banerjee: Molec. Pharmacol. *13*, 796–804 (1977).
122   R. Kranzhöfer, M. Haass, T. Kurz, G. Richardt and A. Schömig: Circ. Res. *68*, 1628–1637 (1991).
123   T.J. Hougen, N. Spicer and T.W. Smith: J. Clin. Invest. *68*, 1207–1214 (1981).
124   P. Lechat, C.R. Malloy and T.W. Smith: Circ. Res. *52*, 411–422 (1983).
125   M. Gheorghiade and D. Ferguson: Circulation *84*, 2181–2186 (1991).
126   G. Grassi, G. Seravalle, B.M. Cattaneo, A. Lanfranchi, S. Vailati, C. Giannattasio, A. Del Bo, C. Sala, G.B. Bolla, M. Pozzi and G. Mancia: Circulation *92*, 3206–3211 (1995).
127   T.S. Rector, M.T. Olivari, T.B. Levine, G.S. Francis and J.N. Cohn: Am. Heart J. *114*, 148–152 (1987).
128   R.A. Gillis and J.A. Quest: Pharmacol. Rev. *31*, 19–97 (1980).
129   D.A. Eisner and T.W. Smith, in: The Heart and Cardiovascular System. Second Edition (H.A. Fozzard et al., Eds.), pp. 863–902. Raven Press, New York, 1992.
130   E. Erdmann, K. Werdan and L. Brown: Trends Pharmacol. Sci. *6*, 293–295 (1985).
131   R.H.G. Schwinger, M. Böhm and E. Erdmann: J. Cardiovasc. Pharmacol. *15*, 692–697 (1990).

132 J.C. Somberg and T.W. Smith: Science *204*, 321–323 (1979).

133 G. Blanco, G. Sánchez and R.W. Mercer: Biochemistry *34*, 9897–9903 (1995).

134 F.I. Marcus, L.H. Opie and E.H. Sonnenblick, in: Drugs for the Heart. Third Edition (L.H. Opie, Ed.). W. Saunders, Philadelphia, 1991.

135 K. Kochsiek: Münch. med. Wschr. *127*, 950–955 (1985).

136 R.A. Gillis and J.A. Quest, in: Cardiac Glycosides 1785–1985 – Biochemistry, Pharmacology, Clinical Relevance (E. Erdmann, K. Greeff and J.C. Skou, Eds.), pp. 347–356. Steinkopff Verlag, Darmstadt and Springer-Verlag, New York, 1986.

137 D.W. Ferguson: Am. J. Cardiol. *69*, 24G–33G (1992).

138 J. Weiland, K. Schwabe, D. Hübler, W. Schönfeld and K.R.H. Repke: J. Enzyme Inhib. *2*, 31–36 (1987).

139 K.R.H. Repke, J. Weiland and K.-H. Menke: J. Enzyme Inhib. *5*, 25–32 (1991).

140 J.M. Hamlyn and P. Manunta: J. Hypertension *10* (Suppl. 7), S99–S111 (1992).

141 M. Tamura, T.M. Harris, D. Phillips, I.A. Blair, Y.F. Wang, C.G. Hellerqvist, S.K. Lam and T. Inagami: J. Biol. Chem. *269*, 11972–11979 (1994).

142 J.M. Hamlyn, D.W. Harris and J.H. Ludens: J. Biol. Chem. *264*, 7395–7404 (1989).

143 J.M. Hamlyn, D.W. Harris, M.A. Clark, A.C. Rogowski, R.J. White and J.H. Ludens: Hypertension *13*, 681–689 (1989).

144 S. Bova, M.P. Blaustein, J.H. Ludens, D.W. Harris, D.W. DuCharme and J.M. Hamlyn: Hypertension *17*, 944–950 (1991).

145 J.M. Hamlyn, M.P. Blaustein, S. Bova, D.W. DuCharme, D.W. Harris, F. Mandel, W.R. Mathews and J.H. Ludens: Proc. Natl. Acad. Sci. USA *88*, 6259–6263 (1991).

146 D.W. Harris, M.A. Clark, J.H. Ludens, D.W. DuCharme and J.M. Hamlyn: Hypertension *16*, 337 (1990).

147 J.H. Ludens, M.A. Clark, D.W. DuCharme, D.W. Harris, B.S. Lutzke, F. Mandel, W.R. Mathews, D.M. Sutter and J.M. Hamlyn: Hypertension *17*, 923–929 (1991).

148 W.R. Mathews, D.W. DuCharme, J.M. Hamlyn, D.W. Harris, F. Mandel, M.A. Clark and J.H. Ludens: Hypertension *17*, 930–935 (1991).

149 D.W. Harris, M.A. Clark, J.F. Fisher, J.M. Hamlyn, K.P. Kolbasa, J.H. Ludens and D.W. DuCharme: Hypertension *17*, 936–943 (1991).

150 J.M. Hamlyn, D. Ashen, B. Forrest, A.C. Rogowski and R.J. White: Prog. Biochem. Pharmacol. *23*, 22–34 (1988).

151 J.M. Hamlyn, in: The Sodium Pump Structure Mechanism, Hormonal Control and its Role in Disease (E. Bamberg and W. Schoner, Eds.), pp. 722–731. Steinkopff, Darmstadt, 1994.

152 N. Zhao, L.-C. Lo, N. Berova, K. Nakanishi, A.A. Tymiak, J.H. Ludens and G.T. Haupert, Jr.: Biochemistry *34*, 9893–9896 (1995).

153 E. Haber and G.T. Haupert, Jr.: Hypertension *9*, 315–324 (1987).

154 G.T. Haupert, Jr., C.T. Carilli and L.C. Cantley: Am. J. Physiol. *247*, F919–F924 (1984).

155 C.T. Carilli, M. Berne, L.C. Cantley and G.T. Haupert, Jr.: J. Biol. Chem. *260*, 1027–1031 (1985).

156 G.T. Haupert, Jr., in: Atrial Hormones and other Natriuretic Factors, pp. 143–156. American Physiological Society, 1987.

157 H.A. Hallaq and G.T. Haupert, Jr.: Proc. Natl. Acad. Sci. USA *86*, 10080–10084 (1989).

158 B.M. Anner, H.G. Rey, M. Moosmayer, L. Meszoely and G.T. Haupert, Jr.: Am. J. Physiol. *258*, F144–F153 (1990).

159 A.A. Tymiak, J.A. Norman, M. Bolgar, G.C. DiDonato, H. Lee, W.L. Parker, L.-C. Lo, N. Berova, K. Nakanishi, E. Haber and G.T. Haupert, Jr.: Proc. Natl. Acad. Sci. USA *90*, 8189–8193 (1993).

160 G.T. Haupert, Jr., in: The Sodium Pump: Structure Mechanism, Hormonal Control and its Role in Disease (E. Bamberg and W. Schoner, Eds.), pp. 732–742. Steinkopff, Darmstadt, 1994.

161 E.-E. Baulieu and P. Robel: J. Steroid Biochem. Molec. Biol. *37*, 395–403 (1990).

162 M. Ferrandi, E. Minotti, S. Salardi, M. Florio, G. Bianchi and P. Ferrari: Am. J. Physiol. *263*, F739–F748 (1992).

163 B.R. Boulanger, M.P. Lilly, J.M. Hamlyn, J. Laredo, D. Shurtleff and D.S. Gann: Am. J. Physiol. *264*, E413–E419 (1993).

164 I.M. Shaikh, B.W.C. Lau, B.A. Siegfried and R. Valdes, Jr.: J. Biol. Chem. *266*, 13672–13678 (1991).

165 F.H.H. Leenen, B.S. Huang, H. Yu and B. Yuan: Circ. Res. *77*, 993–1000 (1995).

166 P.A. Doris, L.A. Jenkins and D.M. Stocco: Hypertension *23*, 632–638 (1994).

167 P.A. Doris: Proc. Soc. Exp. Biol. Med. *205*, 202–212 (1994).

168 R. Schön, J. Weiland, R. Megges and K.R.H. Repke: Naunyn-Schmiedeberg's Arch. Pharmacol. *351*, 282–292 (1995).

169 R.D. Tanz: J. Pharmacol. Exp. Ther. *135*, 71–78 (1962).

170 R.D. Tanz: Rev. Can. Biol. *22*, 147–163 (1963).

171 R. Osman, H. Weinstein and J.P. Green, in: Computer-Assisted Drug Design (E.C. Olson and R.E. Christoffersen, Eds.), ACS Symposium, vol. 12, pp. 21–77. American Chemical Society, Washington, 1979.

172 T.J. Franklin, in: Towards Understanding Receptors (J.W. Lamble, Ed.), pp. 8–15. Elsevier, Amsterdam, 1981.

Progress in Drug Research, Vol. 47 (E. Jucker, Ed.)
© 1996 Birkhäuser Verlag, Basel (Switzerland)

Chemokines as targets for pharmacological intervention

By Silvano Sozzani[1], Paola Allavena[1], Paul Proost[3], Jo Van Damme[3] and Alberto Mantovani[1,2]

[1]Istituto di Ricerche Farmacologiche "Mario Negri", Milan; [2]Section of Pathology and Immunology, Dept. Biotechnology, University of Brescia, Italy; [3]Rega Institute, Leuven, Belgium

1   Introduction

Chemokines are a complex superfamily of mediators mainly involved in immune and inflammatory processes [1, 2]. Structurally, they are characterized by 4 conserved Cys residues, the first 2 of which are in tandem. Based on the relative position of the Cys tandem a Cys-X-Cys and Cys-Cys family are distinguished, with IL-8 and monocyte chemotactic protein-1 as prototypic molecules. Recently a new molecule called lymphotactin with only one C residue was identified [3]. Chemokines act via 7 transmembrane domain, serpentine-type, receptors.
Chemokines play a central role in the multistep process of leukocyte recruitment and are involved in a variety of disease processes ranging from inflammation to neoplasia. As such, they have become an important target for therapeutic intervention and drug design. Given the explosive growth of information and complexity of this family which may include as many as 30 molecules and genes, we will focus this review on the immunobiology of C–C chemokines and then discuss current strategies of therapeutic intervention.

2   C–C chemokines

Several independent lines of work lead to the identification of monocyte chemotactic protein-1 (MCP-1) and related molecules. Already in the early '70s it had been noted that supernatants of activated blood mononuclear cells contained attractants active on monocytes and neutrophils [4]. Subsequently a chemotactic factor active on monocytes was identified in culture supernatants of mouse [5] and human [6, 7] tumor lines and called tumor-derived chemotactic factor (TDCF) [6–8]. TDCF was at the time rather unique in that it was active on monocytes but not on neutrophils [7] and had a low (12 kDa) molecular weight [6, 7]. Moreover, correlative evidence suggested its involvement in the regulation of macrophage infiltration in murine and human tumors [6, 7, 9]. A molecule with similar cellular specificity and physicochemical properties was independently identified in the culture supernatant of smooth muscle cells (SMDCF) [10]. The JE gene had been identified as an immediate-early PDGF-inducible gene in fibroblasts [11, 12]. Thus, in the mid '80s a gene (JE) was in search of function and a monocyte-specific attractant was waiting for molecular definition. In 1989, MCP-1 was successfully purified from supernatants of a human glioma [13], a human monocytic leukemia [14] and a human sarcoma [15–17]: sequencing and molecular cloning revealed its relationship with the long known JE gene [18–20].

The number of related monocyte chemotactrants as well as their spectrum of action, cellular source and role *in vivo* now extend well beyond those of the initial studies. It is now apparent that MCP-1, -2 and -3 are produced by different cell types and play a role in a variety of pathophysiological conditions, which include neoplasia and vascular diseases as originally viewed. Most notably, the spectrum of action of these molecules has enlarged considerably, to include T cells, NK cells, basophils and, for MCP-3, eosinophils and dendritic cells.

3   Cellular sources and induction of MCPs

Originally it was thought that several C–C chemokines were selectively expressed by specific cell types, e.g. T cells for RANTES (Regulated on Activation, Normal T cell Expressed and Secreted), hu MIP-1α/LD78, hu MIP-1β/Act-2 and T-cell activation gene 3 (TCA3)/I-309. Although human LD78 and Act-2 were identified from lymphocytes, the mouse counterparts (macrophage inflammatory proteins-1α and 1β) were isolated from macrophages stimulated with LPS. However, mouse JE was first isolated from fibroblasts [11], whereas human MCP-1 was initially derived from tumor cell lines [13, 14, 16, 17]. In fact, there exists a variety of cell types in which this C–C chemokine can be expressed. Alternatively, certain cell types (e.g. osteosarcoma cells) are reported to secrete several C–C chemokines including MCP-1, -2, -3, RANTES as well as a number of CXC chemokines (IL-8, GRO, IP-10, GCP-2) [for review 1, 2, 21, 22].

Expression studies on MCP-1/JE have demonstrated that monocytes, fibroblasts and endothelial cells are the predominant normal cellular sources for this chemokine [16, 23–27]. More recent reports indicate that MCP-1 is produced by still other cell types and by various tumor cell lines (Table 1). Although mouse JE has been identified as a PDGF-induced gene [11], human MCP-1 was found to be predominantly induced in cells by the cytokines IL-1, TNF-α or IFN-γ [28–33]. Expression of mouse JE and human MCP-1 have been independently studied in virus or double-stranded RNA-treated cells [11, 34]. MCP-2 was found to be coexpressed with MCP-1 in fibroblasts and mononuclear leukocytes, but lower production levels were observed for MCP-2 [24, 35]. Similarly, MCP-3 is co-inducible with MCP-1 in mononuclear leukocytes by PHA and IFN-γ [36]. In mouse mast cells immunoglobulin E plus antigen challenge induces

MARC [37], a chemokine that represents the mouse equivalent of human MCP-3 [38]. It becomes clear that for MCP-1, -2 and -3 there exists no specific cellular origin and that several normal cell types each coproduce these chemokines if appropriately stimulated. The fact of such significant inducibility of chemokines has led to the earlier designations SIS (Small Inducible Secreted) and SIG (Small Inducible Genes) for these molecules. The physiological or pathological inducers for MCPs production can be classified in several groups. First, cytokines such as IL-1, TNF-α and IFN-γ are reported as potent stimulators of several C–C chemokines including MCP-1, MCP-2 and MCP-3. Furthermore, an additional number of cytokines such as IL-4, IL-10, GM-CSF, PDGF and TGF-β induce expression of MCP-1 in certain cell types [39–42]. Synergy between cytokines (e.g. IL-1β and IFN-γ) for MCP induction has been observed. Second, several types of infections (viral, bacterial) and products derived from bacteria (e.g. LPS) viruses (e.g. dsRNA) and plants (e.g. mitogen), as well as various other immunomodulators have been found to directly or indirectly induce MCP-1 and MCP-2 (Table 1). In addition, production of MCP-1 and MCP-3 can also be downregulated by inhibitory cytokines (e.g. IL-13) or by glucocorticoids such as dexamethasone [36, 42]. Although often coproduced, the expression of MCP-1, -2 and -3 can be differently regulated, both qualitatively and quantitatively, depending on the inducer and the cellular source. For example, in connective tissue cells IL-1β was found to be the best inducer of MCP-1, but IFN-γ was relatively superior as an inducer of MCP-2. MCP-2 is produced at a lower absolute concentration than MCP-1 by these cells [24].

4   Protein and gene structure

Human MCP-1 is a glycoprotein of 76 residues with four cysteines forming two intramolecular disulfide bridges [18, 19]. Using a combination of sequencing of proteolytic fragments and mass spectrometry, the complete amino acid sequence of human MCP-1 could be determined [43]. Except for some minor amino-terminal processed forms [44, 45], the amino-terminus of mature MCP-1 protein is blocked for Edman degradation by a pyroglutamic acid residue. One N-glycosylation site is located close to the amino-terminus (Fig. 1), and several glycosylated forms of MCP-1 have been reported ranging from 9 kDa to 17 kDa on SDS-PAGE. The addition of O-linked sugar and sialic acid residue contributes to the different molecular weight forms of MCP-1 [13, 43, 44, 46]. MCP-1 is a basic protein (pI = 10.6) that shows affinity for heparin.

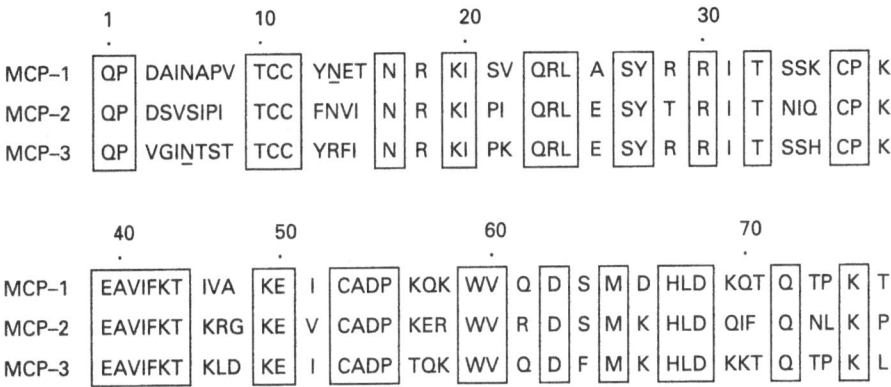

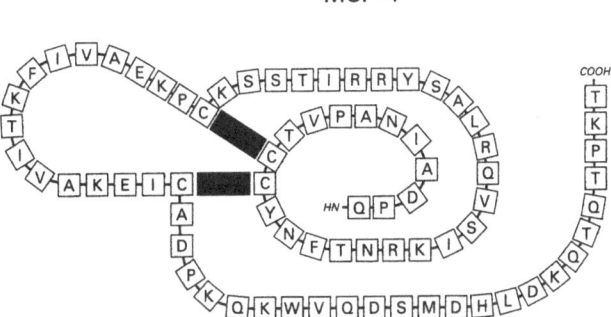

MCP–1

Fig. 1

NMR studies on the solution structure of IL-8 and MIP-1β revealed a number of structural differences between C–C and C–X–C chemokines [47, 48]. IL-8 was found to be globular in shape, whereas for MIP-1β a more cylindrical structure is proposed. In contrast to the IL-8 α-helices, both MIP-1β α-helices were found to be located at opposite sites of the molecule. Thus, the MIP-1β monomer structure is similar to the IL-8 structure but the interface and quaternary-structure are completely different. Recent studies using size exclusion HPLC, sedimentation equilibrium and chemical cross-linking have shown that, at physiological (low nanomolar) concentrations, MCP-1 as well as IL-8 and I-309 occur as monomers instead of dimers [49]. MCP-1 as well as IL-8 form an equilibrium between the monomeric and dimeric form. At concentrations above 100 μM almost all MCP-1 is in the dimeric condition, but at physiologically active concentrations (<100 nM) MCP-1 nearly exclusively occurs as monomer.

Natural MCP-2 and -3 proteins were first copurified from conditioned medium of osteosarcoma cells and identified by amino acid sequence analysis [50]. MCP-2 and MCP-3 contain 76 amino acids, including four cysteines which are characteristic for the chemokine family (Fig. 1). Both peptides display high sequence similarity to MCP-1 (62% and 71% identity, respectively). MCP-2 and MCP-3 are slightly more basic than MCP-1 (pI = 10.6) with theoretical pI's of 10.8 and 10.9, respectively. Similar to all other animal MCPs isolated so far, human MCP-2 and MCP-3 also appeared to be blocked at the amino-terminus but protein sequence data were obtained by Edman degradation of proteolytic fragments [50]. The MCP-2 sequence does not contain N-glycosylation sites. Based upon the theoretical relative molecular mass (8893 Da) and on the apparent molecular weight of 7.5 kDa on SDS-PAGE [50, 51], no O-glycosylation is to be expected for MCP-2. Natural human MCP-3 occurred as an 11 kDa protein on SDS-PAGE [50]. Although the cDNA-derived protein sequence contains one amino-terminally located N-glycosylation site (Fig. 1) [36, 38], natural 11 kDa MCP-3 did not appear to be N-glycosylated [52]. Moreover, folded synthetic MCP-3 also appeared as an 11 kDa protein on SDS-PAGE, although the theoretical relative molecular mass is only 8935 Da [51]. In addition to the unglycosylated MCP-3 form, Minty et al. [36] detected multiple forms (11, 13, 17 and 18 kDa) after expression in COS cells. Here, both N- and O-glycosylation were involved. Electrospray mass spectrometry (MS) of the unglycosylated protein confirmed the amino-terminal pyroglutamate and the existence of two disulfide bridges.

The MCP-1 and MCP-3 genes with the locus symbols SCYA2 and SCYA7 (small inducible cytokine genes number 2 and 7), respectively, were assigned to the C–C chemokine gene cluster on human chromosome 17q11.2-12 [53–55]. For the MCP-2 protein, so far, neither the cDNA nor the genomic DNA sequence are publicly available.

The MCP-1 gene consists of three exons and two introns [35, 56]. The translated MCP-1 mRNA codes for a 99 amino acid precursor protein including a 23 amino acid long, mainly hydrophobic leader sequence. The promoter region contains the TATA box, 96 bp upstream of the translation initiation site. The polyadenylation site (AATAA) is located 353 bp downstream of the stop codon. The GGAAGATCCCT consensus sequence for the kB enhancer element (position −148), which is possibly involved in lipopolysaccharide (LPS) and tumor necrosis factor (TNF) responses, and the ATTTGCGT consensus sequence for the octamer transcription factor (OTF at position –282) were found further in the promoter region [56]. In addition to a GC-box (at –126 bp), two TPA-responsive elements (TRE) for the binding of transacting factor AP-1 (-TGACTCC and TCACTCA) are found at positions –128 and –156, respectively. Several other kB binding sites and TREs were discovered in the enhancer region, between 2 and 3 kbp upstream from the translation initiation site [57]. Promoter and enhancer regions thus contain ciselements which are possibly important for the regulation of MCP-1 gene transcription. The two cis-elements, essential for the MCP-1 induction and for the maintenance of basal MCP-1 transcriptional activity, were found to be the Sp-1 binding GC-box at position –126 in the promoter region and the kB binding site at position –2672 in the enhancer region, respectively. All other kB binding sites and TREs are to be nonfunctional. The essential nuclear factor-kb (NF-kB) and Sp-1 binding sites can, however, not completely explain the MCP-1 gene transcription since, e.g. in lymphocytes virtually no MCP-1 mRNA is found [25], although the Sp-1 expression is rather high [57].

Much like for the MCP-1 gene, three exons and two introns are included in the MCP-3 gene. Similar to the MCP-1 exons, the MCP-3 exons encode a protein of 99 residues, which includes a 23 amino acid signal sequence. The promoter region of the MCP-3 gene contains two tandem dinucleotide repeats (TDR), $(CA)_{17}$ and $(GA)_7$, a property which is shared with the MIP-1α and I-309 gene sequences. Direct and indirect repeats (DR and IR) as well as palindromic sequences (Pal), which might enhance DNA recombinatorial events, are also clustered in this region. Other interesting features like the CAAT-box, the TATA-box, a Cap-signal, the transcription initiation site and at the 3' end a mRNA hairpin loop, an AT-rich mRNA destabilizing region and the polyadenylation site are described by Opdenakker et al. [55].

The murine equivalent of human MCP-1 has been identified as the competence gene JE, regulated by PDGF [11, 58]. Surprisingly the JE gene codes for an NH_2-terminally blocked protein with an additional COOH-terminal tail (49 amino acids) compared to human MCP-1. The corresponding biologically active protein has been isolated from virally infected fibroblasts [34]. The murine homologue of MCP-3 has been isolated from macrophages using a cDNA probe for human MCP-3 [59]. The sequence was found to be identical to that of MARC, derived from mast cells challenged with immunoglobulin E and antigen [37] and FIC isolated from fibroblasts stimulated with serum [60]. Mouse JE and MARC show 55% and 59% amino acid sequence similarity with human MCP-1 and MCP-3, respectively [38].

5   Signal transduction

The molecular mechanisms responsible for cell activation by chemokines have been recently discussed elsewhere [21, 61]. Here, only a brief overview of the most recent findings will be discussed. Elevation of intracellular calcium concentration has been reported to be one of the earliest events after receptor engagement by most of the C–C chemokines [60, 62–76]. This response is rapid, transient and sensitive to *Bordetella pertussis* toxin (PTox) [60, 65, 67, 72, 77] suggesting that chemokine receptors are associated with PTox-sensitive GTP-binding proteins. In support of this observation it was reported that monocyte chemotaxis in response to MCP-1, MCP-3, RANTES, and MIP-1α is inhibited in a concentration-dependent manner by PTox [62, 69, 72], while in the same experimental conditions Cholera toxin (CTox) was ineffective [62, 72]. However, the chemotactic response of monocytes to MCP-2 [62] and of IL-2-activated NK cells to MCP-1, RANTES and MIP-1α [78] were recently reported to be sensitive to the action of CTox, suggesting that chemokine receptors can be associated with both PTox and CTox sensitive GTP-binding proteins. Inhibition of forskolin-induced cyclic AMP generation by MCP-1 was recently reported also to be a precocious effect of MCP-1β receptor activation [77]. This finding is consistent with the activation of a $G_{\alpha i}$ GTP-binding protein. The role of cyclic AMP metabolism in chemokine-induced biological responses awaits further investigation.

In initial studies it was found that in human monocytes activated with MCP-1 the influx of Ca^{2+} across plasma membrane rather than the release of Ca^{2+} from intracellular stores appeared to be the main mechanism responsible for intracellular Ca^{2+} elevation [62, 69]. In parallel, MCP-1-stimulation of human monocytes did not result in a detectable metabolism of phosphatidyl inositol biphosphate [69]. More recently, single cell analysis of human monocytes selected by avid adherence has shown that MCP-1 also mobilizes Ca^{2+} from intracellular stores [79]. In addition, MCP-1β receptor expressed in 293 cells induces the discharge of intracellular calcium stores, though this effect was not associated with inositol trisphosphate production [77].

Calcium influx was required for arachidonate accumulation by MCP-1 in human monocytes [80]. Arachidonic acid release by C–C chemokines (MCP-1, MCP-3, RANTES and MIP-1α was rapid (< 15 sec), reached the plateau at 2–3 minutes and was inhibited by PTox [62, 80, 81]. Platelet activating factor (PAF), a product of membrane phospholipid metabolism, increased in a synergistic fashion both arachidonic acid release and chemotactic response by MCP-1, MCP-3, RANTES and MIP-1α [80, 81].

Recently, it was observed that also 5-oxo-ETE, a product of 5-hydroxyei-cosanoid dehydrogenase, could strongly increase both monocyte migration and arachidonic acid release by MCP-1 and MCP-3, but not by FMLP [S. Sozzani, unpublished]. These results, together with the finding that PLA_2 inhibitors block both monocyte polarization and chemotaxis [80] support the role of arachidonic acid as a second messenger for monocyte migration to chemokines.

Elevation of intracellular calcium concentration might be required also to sustain receptor-induced protein kinase activation. Staurosporine, C–I and H-7, inhibitors of serine/threonine kinases and genistein and erbstatin, inhibitors of tyrosine kinases, were found to inhibit monocyte migration in response to MCP-1, RANTES, MIP-1α, MCP-2 and MCP-3 [62, 72]. These results indicate a possible role for protein kinases in the induction of monocyte migration. The exact role and nature of the protein kinases involved await further investigation.

Three C–C chemokine receptors have been molecularly identified. The first, C–C CKR-1, binds to MIP-1α, RANTES as well as to MCP-1 and MIP-1β [70, 71]. The other two, MCP-1Rα and MCP-1Rβ differ for their alternatively spliced carboxyl tails and bind MCP-1 [76]. However, also MCP-1β is a promiscuous receptor, shown to bind with high affinity MCP-3 [81A]. Earlier studies based on cross-desensitization of calcium transients and chemotactic response were used to investigate receptor usage by MCPs in monocytes [61, 62, 69]. Based on these studies, a model of at least two receptors was proposed: the first shared by MCP-1 and MCP-3 and the second specific for MCP-2. MCP-2, at higher concentrations, could displace labeled-MCP-1 from human monocytes suggesting either that MCP-2 could interact with MCP-1 binding site(s) with an affinity about 30-fold lower than MCP-1 and MCP-3 or that MCP-2 shared with MCP-1 a subset of binding sites [62]. More recently, Uguccioni and colleagues have proposed that MCPs activate monocytes through the same receptor [82]. The reason for this discrepancy is at present unknown and could be related to the different preparations of synthetic MCP-2 used in the two studies. It is also possible that MCP-2 interacts with high affinity with its own receptor and at higher concentrations (over one log higher than MCP-1 [82]) will bind with low affinity to MCP-1 and/or MCP-3 receptor(s).

6   *In vitro* effects

Chemotaxis, the eponimous function of chemokines, is the activity of these molecules which has been studied most extensively. Functions such as expression of cytokines, enzymes and adhesion molecules have been studied in a less extensive and systematic fashion. Table 2 is an attempt to summarize in a concise way the spectrum of action of C–C chemokines, as emerging from studies with human molecules. The activity of human IL-8, the prototypic C–X–C chemokine, is also shown by way of comparison with the C–C molecules. Chemokines of animal origin have been studied less extensively [83–85]; the discordancy of the results on the effect of MIP-1 on neutrophils in mouse versus man raises the possibility that significant differences in the spectrum of action of chemokines may exist among species. In a number of *in vitro* or *in vivo* experiments human C–C chemokines have been studied in rodents [6, 15, 59, 86, 87]. Studies conducted mainly with MCP-1, but to some extent also with MCP-3 and RANTES, suggest that, while the mouse molecules are fully active in humans, human C–C chemokines are considerably less active in the mouse [83, 84]. These results caution against underestimating the potential of these molecules in heterologous systems.

6.1   Monocytes

All members of the C–C chemokine family which have been adequately tested in this respect share the capacity to induce leukocyte migration with distinct, but overlapping, spectrum of action (Table 2). Human and, to the extent tested, murine MCP-1, MCP-2, MP-3, RANTES, I309 elicit directional migration of mononuclear phagocytes and are inactive on neutrophylic granulocytes [1, 2, 88]. Interestingly substitution of 2 amino acids (Tyr^{28} and Arg^{30}) decreases the activity of MCP-1 on monocytes and induces the appearance of activity on PMN [89]. On the contrary, substitution of the two equivalent residues which point upward the central β-sheet of IL-8 (Leu^{25} and Val^{27}) introduces a novel monocyte chemoattractant activity in IL-8 [90]. MCP-1 affects several functions of mononuclear phagocytes related to recruitment or to effector activity (Table 3). Natural and recombinant MCP-1 was reported to augment expression of the integrins CD11b and c in human monocytes [91, 92]. Interaction and localized digestion of extracellular matrix components is essential for phagocyte extravasation and progression in tissues. MCP-1 induces production of gelatinase and of urokinase-type plasminogen activator (uPA). Concomitantly, MCP-1 augments expression of the cell surface receptor for uPA [93]. Induction of gelatinase was also observed with MCP-2 and -3 [38, 50]. Thus, C–C chemokines arm monocytes with the molecular tools which allow localized and polarized digestion of extracellular matrix components during recruitment. In tumor tissues, the release of lytic enzymes by MCP-1-stimulated tumor-associated macrophages (TAM) may provide a ready-made pathway for invasion of tumor cells [94] and thus contribute to augmented metastasis associated with inflammation [95]. MCP-1 induces a respiratory burst in human monocytes, though it is a weak stimulus compared to other agonists [15, 74]. MCP-1 was reported to induce low levels of IL-1 but not TNF production [91, 96]. Natural MCP-1 was also reported to induce IL-6 [91]. However, in another study recombinant MCP-1 had little effect on IL-6 release [Sironi M. et al., unpublished data]. Human MCP-1 induced monocyte cytostasis for a tumor line [15] or synergized with bacterial products, (but not with IFNγ) in stimulation of mouse macrophage cytotoxicity [97] or human monocytes [96]. In an interesting and intriguing recent study, human MCP-1 inhibited induction of the NO synthase in the macrophage cell line J774 [98]. If confirmed, this finding would suggest that MCP-1 could account for both recruitment and concomitant partial functional deactivation of TAM (see below).

Early descriptions of the chemokine subsequently identified as MCP-1 showed its selective activity on mononuclear phagocytes versus PMN as a distinctive and, at the time, unique property [5, 6]. However, more recent studies have shown that MCPs are active on multiple leukocyte populations.

6.2   Basophils and eosinophils

Unlike RANTES and MIP-1α, MCP-1 is not active on human eosinophils [66]. However, MCP-1 appeared to have chemotactic properties for basophils [99]. It was active from 3 nM onwards with an optimal concentration of 10–30 nM (Table 4). RANTES was active at the same concentration but resulted in a higher number of migrating cells, whereas MIP-1α caused comparable basophil migration to MCP-1 at 3 times lower concentrations [100]. MCP-1 (10 nM to 1 µM) was also able to induce histamine release from human basophils. This effect could be partially inhibited by preincubation with IL-8 or RANTES [101, 102]. When basophils were pretreated with IL-3, IL-5 or GM-CSF, the histamine-releasing effect of MCP-1 was doubled, and basophils were also activated to release leukotriene C4 (LTC$_4$) [67, 103]. MCP-1 was found to be a stronger basophil agonist than IL-8, RANTES, MIP-1α, MIP-1β, complement fragment 3a (C3a) and anti-IgE receptor antibodies, but was somewhat weaker than C5a. Trigging of basophils with 30 nM MCP-1 induced a significant increase in [Ca^{2+}]i.

MCP-2 induced *in vitro* chemotaxis of eosinophils from 30 nM onwards, out was less potent than RANTES [104]. Like MCP-1, MCP-2 was found to be chemotactic for basophils (from 10 nM onwards). MCP-2 (100 nM) was also able to induce enhanced (Ca^{2+} dependent) histamine secretion from human basophils. No effect could be detected on mouse peritoneal mast cells [105]. Synthetic [51] as well as recombinant [36] MCP-3 were found to be potent (minimal effective concentration of 3 nM) chemotactic proteins for eosinophil and basophil granulocytes. MCP-3 also induced an increase in $[Ca^{2+}]_i$ in these cells [68, 105]. MCP-3 caused an enhanced histamine release from both unprimed and IL-3-treated basophils. Moreover, MCP-3 induced the release of LTC_4 from IL-3-treated basophil granulocytes [68, 105].

6.3   T lymphocytes

MCP-1, -2 and -3 were reported to induce directional migration of CD4+ and CD8+ freshly isolated T lymphocytes and T cell clones, *in vitro* [106, 107]. In T clones, MCPs induced calcium fluxes that were sensitive to the action of pertussis toxin [106]. MCP-1 also was purified as the main attractant for T lymphocytes from cultures of mitogen-activated peripheral mononuclear cells [108]. Natural purified MCP-1 induced transendothelial migration of T lymphocytes with a memory phenotype (CD45RO+) in a four-hour assay [108] and induced T lymphocytes accumulation *in vivo* when inoculated in SCID mice [107]. These findings propose MCPs as important determinants in T lymphocyte distribution in physiopathological conditions.

6.4   NK cells

NK cells were tested by our group, for their ability to migrate in response to MCP-1, MCP-2 and MCP-3 [109]. In this study purified NK cells (>80% CD16+ and CD56+ and <2% CD3+ and CD14+) were tested in a new double filter assay. Freshly isolated NK cells showed only a minor response to MCP-1, however, if NK cells were cultured *in vitro* in the presence of IL-2 (7–10 days) they acquired a strong response to MCP-1. Migration to MCP-1 showed a typical bell-shaped concentration curve with maximal migration observed at 50 ng/ml MCP-1. At peak concentration, a consistent fraction (~30%) of the input cell population responded to the agonist. These results were confirmed and extended by Maghazachi and coworkers [78] who showed that IL-2-activated NK cells and NK 3.3 cells migrate in response to MCP-1, MIP-1α and RANTES. MCP-1 and RANTES also induced chemokinesis of NK cells [78]. IL-2-cultured NK cells showed specific binding sites for labeled MCP-1 and cell migration was inhibited in a concentration-dependent manner by both CTox and

PTox. Collectively, these results show that NK cells express specific receptors for MCP-1. By reverse transcriptase polymerase chain reaction, we recently found that IL-2-cultured NK cells express MCP-1 receptor transcripts [P. Allavena and N. Polentarutti, unpublished results].

6.5   Dendritic cells

Recently we have observed that *in vitro* cultured dendritic cells (CD1a+, MHC class II L243+, CD14-, CD3- and CD20- migrate in response to MCP-3, RANTES and MIP-1α but not to MCP-1 and MCP-2, *in vitro*. Peak active concentrations and the percentage of input cells migrating in response to chemokines were comparable to those observed with monocytes. Active cytokines were also able to induce a significant increase of cytosolic calcium concentration [109A]. Dendritic cells exert a sentinel function by picking up antigens in nonlymphoid organs and triggering naive T cell-mediated immune responses. To accomplish this role, dendritic cells need to localize in tissues and subsequently to migrate to lymphoid organs. It is very likely that chemokines will play an important role in directing dendritic cells traffic. The effect of chemokines on other biological functions peculiar to these cells, such as macropinocitosis or antigen presentation are at the moment unknown.

Thus, the spectrum of action of MCPs, previously restricted to monocytes, encompasses T lymphocytes, NK cells and dendritic cells and chemokines are likely to play a role in regulating extravasation of these cells *in vivo*.

7   *In vivo* effects and significance

Most available information on the *in vivo* production and role of C–C chemokines refers to MCP-1. There is evidence that MCP-1 may play a role in neoplastic diseases, inflammatory reactions and atherosclerosis (Table 5). However, with a few notable exceptions, available information is indirect and correlative in nature.

7.1   Neoplasia

One of the pathways that lead to the identification of MCP-1 stems from analysis of mechanisms of recruitment of macrophages in tumors [6, 9, 13, 17, 110]. Several lines of evidence suggest that MCP-1 can represent an important determinant of the levels of TAM [9, 110]. In early studies with murine tumors or human tumors in nude mice a correlation was found between MCP-1 activity and percentage of TAM, a finding confirmed in subsequent analysis with the MCP-1 probe [111]. Subcutaneous inoculation of tumor-derived human MCP-1, MCP-2 and MCP-3 leads to macrophage infiltration [15,50]. Finally, and conclusively, transfer of the mouse or human MCP-1 gene was associated with augmented levels of macrophage infiltration [86,87]. High expression of MCP-1 was associated with abrogation of tumorigenicity of CHO cells [86] but not of malignant mouse tumors [87]. At low tumor inocula, MCP-1 gene transfer was associated with higher tumorigenicity and lung colonizing ability, in spite of a lower growth of resulting lesions [87, 112]. These findings were interpreted in the light of the dual influence that TAM can exert on tumor growth as discussed in detail elsewhere [9, 110].

Leukocyte infiltration is associated with administration of cytokine such as interferons, IL-2 or IL-4 by conventional routes or following gene transfer. Interferon and IL-2 have been shown to induce endogenous chemokines in a renal cancer model [113]. Thus secondary induction of chemokines may play a pivotal role in leukocyte recruitment in tumors treated with cytokines other than chemokine.

Various human tumor lines express MCP-1 *in vitro* spontaneously or after exposure to inflammatory signals and some of them do so *in vivo*. The latter include gliomas, histiocytomas, sarcomas, and melanoma [13, 15, 114, 115]. Expression of MCP-1 was recently found in Kaposi's sarcoma (KS) *in vivo* and in KS-derived spindle cell cultures [116]. For these studies, we used as novel anti-MCP-1 monoclonal antibody (5D3) and assays based on it [117]. Since KS is characterized by a conspicuous macrophage infiltrate and is believed to represent a cytokine-propelled disease, production of MCP-1 may turn out to be particularly significant in this disease.

Freshly isolated ovarian carcinoma cells, primary cultures and some established cell lines were shown in early studies to release TDCF activity [6–8]. These observations were recently revised [118]. It was found by immunohistochemistry and *in situ* hybridization that ovarian carcinoma cells and, in some tumors, also stromal elements express MCP-1. High levels of MCP-1 were measured in the ascites (but not in blood) of patients with ovarian cancer but not in the peritoneal fluid of patients with non malignant conditions. Production of MCP-1 and recruitment of TAM is likely to play an important role in progression of this disease because macrophage-derived cytokines promote the growth of ovarian carcinoma and its secondary implantation in peritoneal organs [for review see 119].

All in all the available information suggests that MCP-1 is an important determinant of macrophage infiltration in murine and, at least some, human tumors. Human tumor lines of epithelial origin [breast, colon, ovary, refs 6, 8] were shown to release small molecular weight chemoattractant(s). Only for ovarian carcinoma was the TDCF recently identified as MCP-1 (see above). It remains to be defined whether MCP-1 or a related chemokine explains these observations and is involved in macrophage recruitment in common epithelial cancers. Tumor-derived MCP-1 could downregulate important antitumor pathways (e.g. NO, ref [98]), induce production of growth stimulatory cytokines [e.g. IL-1 or IL-6 in ovarian cancer, refs 91, 96], stimulate the production of proteolytic enzymes which could promote a process of counter-current invasion [38, 50, 93, 94]. Thus, MCP-1 and related molecules produced by certain tumors may play a role in the immunobiology of neoplastic tissues which extends beyond the mere recruitment of mononuclear phagocytes.

Examination of macrophage function and inflammation in neoplastic disorders, as well as in other inflammatory conditions, reveals a paradoxical situation in which recruitment at the tumor site coexists with a systemic defect in the ability to mount local inflammatory reactions [9, 120]. We speculated that chemokines produced continuously in tumors may contribute also to the systemic impairment of macrophage function observed in advanced neoplasia [9]. In support of this hypothesis, chemoattractants were recently found to cause rapid release of the IL-1 decoy receptor and of the p75 TNF receptor [121, 122], which could buffer the action of these inflammatory mediators.

7.2   Atherosclerosis

Recruitment of monocytes is the first recognizable event in the natural history of atherosclerosis. Vessel wall elements (endothelial cells, smooth muscle cells) produce abundant amounts of MCP-1 in response to inflammatory cytokines and modified lipids. MCP-1 has been detected in arterial walls in animal models of atherosclerosis [123–125]. Moreover, MCP-1 has been detected in human atheromatous plaques [124–126]. Interestingly, in plaques, MCP-1 expression is most prominent in subendothelial macrophage and endothelial cells. Their relative expression is dependent on the progression level of atherosclerotic lesion [124].

7.3   Inflammatory and immune reactions

Expression of MCP-1 was detected in a variety of animal models of inflammatory and immune reactions, including cardiac allografts [127], allergic encephalomyelytis [128], bleomycin-induced pulmonary fibrosis [129, 130], pulmonary granuloma and immune complex alveolitis [131, 132] and renal

ischemia [133] and bacteremia [134]. In a rodent model of glomeruloneph-
ritis and in kidney biopsy from patients with inflammatory glomerulop-
athies, MCP-1 expression was upregulated and was associated to a prominent monocyte infiltrate [135]. More recently, increased levels of MCP-
1 were observed in urine samples of patients with lupus nephritis. MCP-1
was detected only in the active form of the disease and was decreased by
glucocorticoids administration [135A]. In human disease, *in situ* hybridization and polyclonal antisera have revealed MCP-1 mRNA and/or protein in idiopathic pulmonary fibrosis [136], chronic active hepatitis [137,
138], skin delayed-type hypersensitivity reactions [139], rheumatoid
arthritis [42, 140–142]. In relation to the latter disease, it is of interest that
MCP-1 expression could be induced in synovial fibroblasts while synovial
macrophages constitutively express the chemokine [140]. Blood levels of
MCP-1 in humans have been studied using sandwich ELISAs based on
polyclonal antisera and/or mAb with discrepant results as to its presence
in normal serum [143,144]. Free anti-MCP-1 IgG are present in normal
human donors and their levels decrease following i.v. inoculation of endotoxin, concomitantly with a rapid increase in MCP-1 levels [143]. These
findings raise the interesting possibility that anti-chemokine autoantibod-
ies represent a regulatory pathway for these mediators.

Although MCP-1 was found in a variety of inflammatory conditions,
there are only a few studies providing direct evidence of its *in vivo* importance. In a rat model of immune-complex-induced alveolitis, anti-MCP-
1 antibody administration reduced the severity of the disease [131]. In
another study it was found that an antiMCP-1 antiserum partially inhibits lung granuloma formation in rats [132]. In the same vein anti-MCP-
1 antiserum reduced the inflammatory reaction in Schistosoma egg gra-
nulomas [145].

8   Therapeutic strategies

Given the involvement of chemokines in a wide range of inflammatory
diseases, it is not surprising that considerable efforts are being made to
exploit these molecules therapeutically. The main strategies under evaluation are summarized in Table 6 and briefly discussed here.

8.1   Inhibition of synthesis

Classic immunosuppressive and antiinflammatory drugs are potent inhibitors of the production of at least certain chemokines, such as IL-8 and

MCP-1. Active molecules include glucocorticoid hormones, FK 506, Cyclosporine A [133, 146–150]. The identification of 5' regulatory sequences has allowed definition to some extent of the molecular targets. Given the promiscuity of transcription factors such as NFkB it is at present unclear whether this approach may eventually lead to development of selective anti-chemokine agents.

8.2   Antibodies

As illustrated above, C–C chemokines are invaluable in defining the role of molecules in pathophysiology. Monoclonal antibodies (mAb) directed against IL-8 have been more systematically explored for their potential to modify pathology in animal models. Anti-IL-8 mAb were found beneficial in a range of pathological conditions including ischemia reperfusion injury, inflammatory kidney diseases, septic shock and delayed-type hypersensitivity reactions [151, 152]. The latter observation is intriguing and surprising in view of the marginal role generally attributed to neutrophils in this type of reaction.

8.3   Antagonists

Considerable efforts have been made to develop chemokine antagonists, prompted also by the nature of the receptors which belong to a class of classical targets for pharmacological approaches. Chemokines with altered sequence can act as antagonists, as exemplified by N-terminally altered MCP-1 [153, 154]. Recently, based on the 3D structure of a peptide agonist, a first simple chemical with low but significant rapacity to compete for receptor binding of IL-8 was described [T. Wells, personal communication].
The identification of eotaxin (and its receptor) as a specific eosinophil attractant will probably generate further impetus to develop chemokine antagonists.

8.4   Hematopoiesis

Various chemokines affect hematopoietic precursors but this is a prominent property of MIP-1α [see above, refs 155, 156]. MIP-1α inhibits the proliferation of normal early hematopoietic precursors. It has therefore been suggested that it may be useful to protect normal stem cells from damage of cytotoxic chemotherapy.
MIP-1α, IL-8 and probably other chemokines cause the recruitment from the bone marrow into the blood of hematopoietic precursors [157]. They

may therefore represent an alternative to G-CSF in obtaining precursors from blood for transplantation.

8.5   Gene therapy

Transfer of chemokine (MCP-1, IP-10) genes into tumors caused growth retardation or regression [86, 87]. The effect was highly dependent upon the tumor system (unpublished). In the perspective of gene therapy, the recent identification of chemokines active on dendritic cells may provide a tool to direct dendritic cell traffic in immunization strategies.

9   Concluding remarks

Chemokines have emerged as central mediators of inflammation, immunity and allergy. As such they now represent a prime target for the development of novel therapeutic strategies. While chemical antagonists remain the holy grail for the future, it is likely that the first anti-chemokine strategy to undergo clinical evaluation is likely to be antibodies. Redundancy and promiscuity of receptor usage represent formidable stumbling blocks for the development of effective antichemokine strategies.

Table 1.
Cellular sources of MCPs

Producer cell type	Chemokine production MCP-1 MCP-2 MCP-3			Inducer
Epithelial cells	+			IL-1β, TNF-α, IFN-γ
Keratinocytes	+			TNF-α, IFN-γ
Melanocytes	+			IL-1α, TNF-α
Fibroblasts	+	+	+	IL-1α, IL-1β, TNF-α, IFN-γ, PDGF, IL-4, IL-10, virus, dsRNA
Monocytes/macrophages	+	+	+	IL-1β, TNF-α, IFN-γ, IFNβ, GM-CSF, LPS, ConA, PHA, virus, dsRNA
Granulocytes		(+)		LPS
Endothelial cells	+	(+)		IL-1β, TNF-α, IL-4, LDL, thrombin, LPS, PMA, shear stress
Smooth muscle cells	+			IL-1β, TNF, LPS, LDL
Mesathelial cells	+			IL-1β, TNF-α, IFN-γ
Mesangial cells	+			IL-1β, TNF-α, IFN-γ, IgG, thrombin, LPS
Chondrocytes	+			IL-1β, TNF-α, PDGF, TGF-β, LIP, LPS, retinoic acid
Osteoblasts	+			IL-1β, TNF-α
Lipocytes	+			IL-1β, TNF-α, IFN-γ
Astrocytes	+			TNF-α
Tumor cells:				
- carcinoma (Hep-2)	+	(+)		IL-1β, IFN-γ, PMA
- sarcoma (MG-63)	+	+		IL-1β, IFN-γ, virus
- melanoma (Bowes)	+	+	+	
- mielomonocytic leukemia (THP-1)	+	+	+	IFN-γ, LPS, PMA
- glioma (U-105MG)	+			

Table 2.
The spectrum of action of C–C chemokines

Family	Molecule	Neu	Eo	Ba	Mo	TLy	NK	DC	BLy	Other
Cys-X-Cys	IL-8	++	±	±	–	±	±	–	–	melanomas, keratinocytes, endothelium
Cys-Cys	MCP-1	–	–	++	+++	+++	++	–	–	nt
	MCP-2	–	+	+	+++	+++	++	–	nt	nt
	MCP-3	–	++	++	+++	+++	++	+++	nt	nt
	RANTES	–	++	++	+	++	++	+++	+	nt
	MIP-1α	±*	+	+	+	+	++	+++	+	hematopoietic precursors
	MIP-1β	–	–	–	+	++	nt	nt	nt	nt
	I309	–	nt	nt	+	?	nt	nt	nt	nt

By way of comparison the spectrum of action of IL-8 (C–X–C) is shown. The activity considered is migration.
Neo, neutrophils; Eo, eosinophils; Ba, basophils; Mo, monocytes; Ly, lymphocytes; NK, natural killer cells; DC, dendritic cells; nt, not tested. *Disputed.

Table 3.
Effects of MCPs on leukocyte functions other than chemotaxis

Chemokine	Cells	Function	References
MCP-1	Monocytes	Oxydative burst	[15, 74]
		Lysosomal enzyme release	[15, 82]
		Inhibition of NO synthase	[98]
		Gelatinase, uPA, uPA-R	[38, 50, 93]
		Adhesion molecules (CD11 b and c)	[91, 92]
		IL-1 and IL-6	[91, 96]
		Tumor cytostasis and/or lysis	[15, 96, 97]
	Basophils	Histamine release	[101, 158]
MCP-2	Monocytes	Gelatinase	[50]
		Lysosomal enzyme release	[82]
	Basophils	Histamine release	[105]
MCP-3	Monocytes	Gelatinase	[50]
		Lysosomal enzyme release	[82]
	Basophils	Histamine release	[50, 105]

Table 4.
Potency of MCP-1, -2 and -3 as chemotactic factors for various leukocyte cell types

Cell type	Minimum effective concentration (mM)		
	MCP-1	MCP-2	MCP-3
monocytes	0.1	0.1–0.3	0.1–0.3
T-lymphocytes	0.1	0.1	0.1
NK cells	3–6	3	3
basophils	3	10	3
eosinophils	>300	30	3
neutrophils	>100	>100	>100

Table 5.
Evidence for an *in vivo* role of MCPs

	Species	Molecule	Disease	Evidence	Selected ref.
Neoplasia	mouse	MCP-1	various histologies	correlations; gene transfer*	[86, 87]
	man	MCP-1	histocytoma	*in situ* expression	[115]
			glioma	*in situ* expression	[13, 159]
			sarcomas	*in situ* expression	[160]
			melanoma	*in situ* expression	[114]
			Kaposi's sarcoma	*in situ* expression	[116]
			ovarian carcinoma	*in situ* expression	[8, 118]
Atherosclerosis	primates	MCP-1	hypercholesterolemia	*in situ* expression	[123]
	rabbit	MCP-1	plaques	*in situ* expression	[125]
	man	MCP-1	plaques	*in situ* expression	[124–126]
Inflammatory/ immune reactions	mouse	MCP-1	encephalomyelitis	*in situ* expression	[128]
	rat	MCP-1	pulmonaryalveolitis	*in situ* expression; antibody blocking	[131]
			pulmonary granuloma	*in situ* expression; antibody blocking	[132]
			allograft	*in situ* expression	[127]
			kidney hischemia	*in situ* expression	[133]
	man	MCP-1	rheumatoidarthritis	*in situ* expression	[42, 141]
			idiopathic pulmonary fibrosis	*in situ* expression	[129, 130, 136]
			chronic active hepatitis	*in situ* expression	[137, 138]
			schistosoma egg granulomas	*in situ* expression; antibody blocking	[145]

* Underlined is direct evidence showing *in vivo* functions of MCPs.

Table 6.
Therapeutic strategies aimed at chemokines

Strategy	Molecules	Chemokine	Pathology	Selected ref.
Inhibition of synthesis	glucocorticoids, FK506	IL-8, MCP-1	various	[133, 146–150]
Blocking antibodies	mAb	IL-8 MCP-1	ischemia-reperfusion, kidney etc.	[151, 152] [131, 132, 145]
Antagonists, peptides	analogue	MCP-1	nt	[153, 154]
		IL-8		[161]
Antagonists: simple chemicals	?	IL-8	nt	[T. Wells, personal communication]
Hematopoietic precursor inhibition or recruitment	MIP-1α/LD78	MIP-1α/LD78	myelosuppression; blood precursor transplantation	[155] [157]
Gene therapy	MCP-1	MCP-1	neoplasia	[86, 87]

References

1   Oppenheim, J.J., Zachariae, C.O., Mukaida, N. and Matsushima, K.: Annu. Rev. Immunol. *9*, 617 (1991).
2   Baggiolini, M., Dewald, B. and Moser, B.: Adv. Immunol. *55*, 99 (1994).
3   Kelner, G.S., Kennedy, J., Bacon, K.B. et al.: Science *266*, 1395 (1994).
4   Ward, P.A., Remold, H.G. and David, J.R.: Cell Immunol. *1*, 162 (1970).
5   Meltzer, M.S., Stevenson, M.M. and Leonard, E.J.: Cancer Res. *37*, 721 (1977).
6   Bottazzi, B., Polentarutti, N., Acero, R. et al.: Science *220*, 210 (1983).
7   Bottazzi, B., Polentarutti, N., Balsari, A. et al.: Int. J. Cancer *31*, 55 (1983).
8   Bottazzi, B., Ghezz,i P., Taraboletti, G. et al.: Int. J. Cancer *36*, 167 (1985).
9   Mantovani, A., Bottazzi, B., Colotta, F., Sozzani, S. and Ruco, L.: Immunol. Today *13*, 265 (1992).
10 Valente, A.J., Fowler, S.R., Sprague, E.A., Kelley, J.L., Suenram C.A. and Schwartz C.J.: Am. J. Pathol. *117*, 409 (1984).
11 Zullo, J.N., Cochran, B.H., Huang, A.S. and Stiles, C.D.: Cell *43*, 793 (1985).
12 Rollins, B.J., Morrison, E.D. and Stiles, C.D.: Proc. Natl. Acad. Sci. USA *85*, 3738 (1988).
13 Yoshimura, T., Robinson, E.A., Tanaka, S., Appella, E., Kuratsu, J. and Leonard, E.J.: J. Exp. Med. *169*, 1449 (1989).
14 Matsushima, K., Larsen, C.G., DuBois, G.C. and Oppenheim, J.J.: J. Exp. Med. *169*, 1485 (1989).
15 Zachariae, C.O., Anderson, A.O., Thompson, H.L. et al.: J. Exp. Med. *171*, 2177 (1990).
16 Van Damme, J., Decock, B., Lenaerts, J.P. et al.: Eur. J. Immunol. *19*, 2367 (1989).
17 Graves, D.T., Jiang, Y.L., Williamson, M.J. and Valente, A.J.: Science *245*, 1490 (1989).
18 Furutani, Y., Nomura, H., Notake, M. et al.: Biochem. Biophys. Res. Commun. *159*, 248 (1989).
19 Yoshimura, T., Yuhki, N., Moore, S.K., Appella, E., Lerman, M.I. and Leonard, E.J.: FEBS Lett. *244*, 487 (1989).
20 Bottazzi, B., Colotta, F., Sica, A., Nobili, N. and Mantovani, A.: Int. J. Cancer *45*, 795 (1990).
21 Schall, T.J.: The cytokine handbook, edited by Thomson A. London: Academic Press, p. 419 (1994).
22 Van Damme, J.: The cytokine handbook, edited by Thomson A. London: Academic Press, p. 185 (1994).
23 Yoshimura, T., Robinson, E.A., Tanaka, S., Appella, E. and Leonard, E.J.: J. Immunol. *142*, 1956 (1989).
24 Van Damme, J., Proost, P., Put, W. et al.: J. Immunol. *152*, 5495 (1994).
25 Colotta, F., Borre, A., Wang, J.M. et al.: J. Immunol. *148*, 760 (1992).
26 Colotta, F., Sciacca, F.L., Sironi, M., Luini, W., Rabiet, M.J. and Mantovani, A.: Am. J. Pathol. *144*, 975 (1994).
27 Sica, A., Wang, J.M., Colotta, F. et al.: J. Immunol. *144*, 3034 (1990).
28 Larsen, C.G., Zachariae, C.O., Oppenheim, J.J. and Matsushima, K.: Biochem. Biophys. Res. Commun. *160*, 1403 (1989).
29 Zachariae, C.O., Thestrup Pedersen, K. and Matsushima, K.: J. Invest. Dermatol. *97*, 593 (1991).
30 Wang, J.M., Sica, A., Peri, G. et al.: Arterioscler. Thromb. *11*, 1166 (1991).
31 Elner, S.G., Strieter, R.M., Elner, V.M., Rollins, B.J., Del Monte, M.A. and Kunkel, S.L.: Lab. Invest. *64*, 819 (1991).

32   Jonjic, N., Peri, G., Bernasconi, S. et al.: J. Exp. Med. *176*, 1165 (1992).
33   Brown, Z., Strieter, R.M., Neild, G.H., Thompson, R.C., Kunkel, S.L. and Westwick, J.: Kidney. Int. *42*, 95 (1992).
34   Van Damme, J., Decock, B., Bertini, R. et al.: Eur. J. Biochem. *199*, 223 (1991).
35   Chang, H.C., Hsu, F., Freeman, G.J., Griffin, J.D. and Reinherz, E.L.: Int. Immunol. *1*, 388 (1989).
36   Minty, A., Chalon, P., Guillemot, J.C. et al.: Eur. Cytokine Netw. *4*, 99 (1993).
37   Kulmburg, P.A., Huber, N.E., Scheer, B.J., Wrann, M. and Baumruker, T. J.: Exp. Med. *176*, 1773 (1992).
38   Opdenakker, G., Froyen, G., Fiten, P., Proost, P. and Van Damme, J.: Biochem. Biophys. Res. Commun. *191*, 535 (1993).
39   Costa, J.J., Matossian, K., Resnick, M. B. et al.: J. Clin. Invest. *91*, 2673 (1993).
40   Colotta, F., Sironi, M., Borre, A., Luini, W., Maddalena, F. and Mantovani, A.: Cytokine. *4*, 24 (1992).
41   Sironi, M., Munoz, C., Pollicino, T. et al.: Eur. J. Immunol. *23*, 2692 (1993).
42   Villiger, P.M., Terkeltaub, R. and Lotz, M.: J. Clin. Invest. *90*, 488 (1992).
43   Robinson, E.A., Yoshimura, T., Leonard, E.J. et al.: Proc. Natl. Acad. Sci. USA *86*, 1850 (1989).
44   Decock, B., Coning, R., Lenaerts, J.P., Billiau, A. and Van Damme, J.: Biochem. Biophys. Res. Commun. *167*, 904 (1990).
45   Woldemar Carr, M., Roth, S.J., Luther, E., Rose, S.S. and Springer, T.A.: Proc. Natl. Acad. Sci. USA *91*, 3652 (1994).
46   Jiang, Y., Valente, A.J., Williamson, M.J., Zhang, L. and Graves, D.T.: J. Biol. Chem. *265*, 18318 (1990).
47   Gronenborn, A.M. and Clore, G.M.: Protein. Eng. *4*, 263 (1991).
48   Lodi, P.J., Garrett, D.S., Kuszewski, J. et al.: Science *263*, 1762 (1994).
49   Paolini, J.F., Willard, D., Consler, T., Luther, M. and Krangel, M.S.: J. Immunol. *153*, 2704 (1994).
50   Van Damme, J., Proost, P., Lenaerts, J.P. and Opdenakker, G.: J. Exp. Med. *176*, 59 (1992).
51   Proost, P., Van Leuven, P., Wuyts, A., Ebberink, R., Opdenakker, G. and Van Damme, J.: Cytokine *7*, 97 (1995).
52   Opdenakker, G., Rudd, P., Wormald, M., Dwek, R.A. and Van Damme, J.: FASEB. J. *9*, 453 (1995).
53   Mehrabian, M., Sparkes, R.S., Mohandas, T., Fogelman, A.M. and Lusis, A.J.: Genomics *9*, 200 (1991).
54   Rollins, B.J., Morton, C.C., Ledbetter, D.H., Eddy, R.L.J. and Shows, T.B.: Genomics *10*, 489 (1991).
55   Opdenakker, G., Fiten, P., Nys, G. et al.: Genomics *21*, 403 (1994).
56   Shyy, Y.J., Li, Y.S. and Kolattukudy, P.E.: Biochem. Biophys. Res. Commun. *169*, 346 (1990).
57   Ueda, A., Okuda, K., Ohno, S. et al.: J. Immunol. *153*, 2052 (1994).
58   Rollins, B.J., Stier, P., Ernst, T. and Wong, G.G.: Mol. Cell Biol. *9*, 4687 (1989).
59   Thirion, S., Nys, G., Fiten, P., Masure, S., Van Damme, J. and Opdenakker, G.: Biochem. Biophys. Res. Commun. *201*, 493 (1994).
60   Heinrich, J.N., Ryseck, R.P., Macdonald-Bravo, H. and Bravo, R.: Mol. Cell Biol. *13*, 2020 (1993).
61   Sozzani, S., Locati, M., Zhou, D. et al.: J. Leukoc. Biol. *57*, 788 (1995).
62   Sozzani, S., Zhou, D., Locati, M. et al.: J. Immunol. *152*, 3615 (1994).

63   Van Riper, G., Siciliano, S., Fischer, P.A., Meurer, R., Springer, M.S. and Rosen, H.:
      J. Exp. Med. *177*, 851 (1993).
64   Wang, J.M., McVicar, D.W., Oppenheim, J.J. and Kelvin, D.J.: J. Exp. Med. *177*, 699
      (1993).
65   McColl, S.R., Hachicha, M., Levasseur, S., Neote, K. and Schall, T.J.: J. Immunol. *150*,
      4550 (1993).
66   Rot, A., Krieger, M., Brunner, T., Bischoff, S.C., Schall, T.J. and Dahinden, C.A.: J.
      Exp. Med. *176*, 1489 (1992).
67   Bischoff, S.C., Krieger, M., Brunner, T. and Dahinden, C.A.: J. Exp. Med. *175*, 1271
      (1992).
68   Dahinden, C.A., Geiser, T., Brunner, T. et al.: J. Exp. Med. *179*, 751 (1994).
69   Sozzani, S., Molino, M., Locati, M. et al.: J. Immunol. *150*, 1544 (1993).
70   Neote, K., DiGregorio, D., Mak, J.Y., Horuk, R. and Schall, T.J.: Cell *72*, 415 (1993).
71   Gao, J.L., Kuhns, D.B., Tiffany, H.L. et al.: J. Exp. Med. *177*, 1421 (1993).
72   Sozzani, S., Luini, W., Molino, M. et al.: J. Immunol. *147*, 2215 (1991).
73   Miller, M.D. and Krangel, M.S.: Proc. Natl. Acad. Sci. USA *89*, 2950 (1992).
74   Rollins, B.J., Walz, A. and Baggiolini, M.: Blood *78*, 1112 (1991).
75   Vaddi, K. and Newton, R.C.: J. Leukoc. Biol. *55*, 756 (1994).
76   Charo, I.F., Myers, S.J., Herman, A., Franci, C., Connolly, A.J. and Coughlin, S.R.:
      Proc. Natl. Acad. Sci. USA *91*, 2752 (1994).
77   Myers, S.J., Wong, L.M. and Charo, I.F.: J. Biol. Chem. *270*, 5786 (1995).
78   Maghazachi, A.A., Alaoukaty, A. and Schall, T.J.: J. Immunol. *153*, 4969 (1994).
79   Bizzarri, C., Bertini, R., Sozzani, S. et al.: Blood *86*, 2388 (1995).
80   Locati, M., Zhou, D., Luini, W., Evangelista, V., Mantovani, A. and Sozzani, S.: J. Biol.
      Chem. *269*, 4746 (1994).
81   Sozzani, S., Rieppi, M., Locati, M. et al.: Biochem. Biophys. Res. Commun. *199*, 761
      (1994).
81A   Franci, W., Wong, L.M., Van Damme, J., Proost, P. and Charo, I.F.: J. Immunol. *154*,
      6511 (1995).
82   Uguccioni, M., Dapuzzo, M., Loetscher, M., Dewald, B. and Baggiolini, M.: Eur. J.
      Immunol. *25*, 64 (1995).
83   Luini, W., Sozzani, S., Van Damme, J. and Mantovani, A.: Cytokine *6*, 28 (1994).
84   Schall, T.J., Simpson, N.J. and Mak, J.Y.: Eur. J. Immunol. *22*, 1477 (1992).
85   Yoshimura, T. and Yuhki, N.: J. Immunol. *146*, 3483 (1991).
86   Rollins, B.J. and Sunday, M.E.: Mol. Cell Biol. *11*, 3125 (1993).
87   Bottazzi, B., Walter, S., Govoni, D., Colotta, F. and Mantovani, A.: J. Immunol. *148*,
      1280 (1992).
88   Miller, M.D. and Krangel, M.S.: Crit. Rev. Immunol. *12*, 17 (1992).
89   Beall, C.J., Mahajan, S. and Kolattukudy, P.E.: J. Biol. Chem. *267*, 3455 (1992).
90   Lustinarasimhan, M., Power, C.A., Allet, B. et al.: J. Biol. Chem. *270*, 2716 (1995).
91   Jiang, Y., Beller, D.I., Frendl, G. and Graves, D.T.: J. Immunol. *148*, 2423 (1992).
92   Vaddi, K. and Newton, R.C.: J. Immunol. *153*, 4721 (1994).
93   Mantovani, A., Sozzani, S., Bottazzi, B. et al.: The Chemokines. Biology of the Inflam-
      matory Peptide Supergene Family II, edited by Lindley, I.J.D., Westwick, J. and Kun-
      kel, S. New York, Plenum Press, p. 47 (1993).
94   Opdenakker, G. and Van Damme, J.: Cytokine *4*, 251 (1992).
95   Giavazzi, R., Garofalo, A., Bani, M.R. et al.: Cancer Res. *50*, 4771 (1990).
96   Yano, S., Sone, S., Nishioka, Y., Mukaida, N., Matsushima, K. and Ogura, T.: J. Leu-
      koc. Biol. *57*, 303 (1995).

97   Singh, R.K., Berry, K., Matsushima, K., Yasumoto, K. and Fidler, I.J.: J. Immunol.
        151, 2786 (1993).
98   Rojas, A., Delgado, R., Glaria, L. and Palacios, M.: Biochem. Biophys. Res. Com-
        mun. *196*, 274 (1993).
99   Leonard, E.J. and Yoshimura, T.: Immunol. Today. *11*, 97 (1990).
100   Bischoff, S.C., Krieger, M., Brunner, T. et al.: Eur. J. Immunol. *23*, 761 (1993).
101   Alam, R., Forsythe, P.A., Lett Brown, M.A. and Grant, J.A.: Am. J. Respir.Cell Mol.
        Biol. *7*, 427 (1992).
102   Alam, R., Lett Brown, M.A., Forsythe, P.A. et al.: J. Clin. Invest. *89*, 723 (1992).
103   Kuna, P., Reddigari, S.R., Rucinski, D., Oppenheim, J.J. and Kaplan, A.P.: J. Exp. Med.
        175, 489 (1992).
104   Noso, N., Proost, P., Van Damme, J. and Schroder, J.M.: Biochem. Biophys. Res. Com-
        mun. *200*, 1470 (1994).
105   Alam, R., Forsythe, P., Stafford, S. et al.: J. Immunol. *153*, 3155 (1994).
106   Loetscher, P., Seitz, M., Clarklewis, I., Baggiolini, M. and Moser, B.: FASEB J. *8*, 1055
        (1994).
107   Taub, D.D., Proost, P., Murphy, W.J. et al.: J. Clin. Invest. *95*, 1370 (1995).
108   Carr, M.W., Roth, S.J., Luther, E., Rose, S.S. and Springer, T.A.: Proc. Natl. Acad. Sci.
        USA *91*, 3652 (1994).
109   Allavena, P., Bianchi, G., Zhou, D. et al.: Eur. J. Immunol. *24*, 3233 (1994).
109A   Sozzani, S., Sallusto, F., Luini, W., Zhou, D., Piemonti, L., Allavena, P., van Damme,
        J., Valitutti, S., Lanzavecchia, A. and Mantovani, A.: J. Immunol. *155*, 3292 (1995).
110   Opdenakker, G. and Van Damme, J.: Immunol. Today. *13*, 463 (1992).
111   Walter, S., Bottazzi, B., Govoni, D., Colotta, F. and Mantovani, A.: Int. J. Cancer *49*,
        431 (1991).
112   Mantovani, A., Bottazzi, B., Sozzani, S. et al.: Res. Immunol. *144*, 280 (1993).
113   Sonouchi, K., Hamilton, T.A., Tannenbaum, C.S., Tubbs, R.R., Bukowski, R. and Finke,
        J.H.: Am. J. Pathol. *144*, 747 (1994).
114   Graves, D.T., Barnhill, R., Galanopoulos, T. and Antoniades, H.N.: Am. J. Pathol. *140*,
        9 (1992).
115   Takeya, M., Yoshimura, T., Leonard, E.J., Kato, T., Okabe, H. and Takahashi, K.: Exp.
        Mol. Pathol. *54*, 61 (1991).
116   Sciacca, F.L., Stürzl, M., Bussolino, F. et al.: J. Immunol. *153*, 4816 (1994).
117   Peri, G., Milancse, C., Mattcucci, C. et al.: J. Immunol. Methods *174*, 249 (1994).
118   Negus, R.P.M., Stamp, G.W.H., Relf, M.G. et al.: J. Clin. Invest. *95*, 2391 (1995).
119   Mantovani, A.: Lab. Invest. *71*, 5 (1994).
120   Snyderman, R. and Cianciolo, G.: Immunol. Today. *5*, 240 (1984).
121   Colotta, F., Orlando, S., Fadlon, E.J., Sozzani, S., Matteucci, C. and Mantovani, A.: J.
        Exp. Med. *181*, 2181 (1995).
122   Porteu, F. and Nathan, C.: J. Exp. Med. *172*, 599 (1990).
123   Yu, X., Dluz, S., Graves, D.T. et al.: Proc. Natl. Acad. Sci. USA *89*, 6953 (1992).
124   Takeya, M., Yoshimura, T., Leonard, E.J. and Takahashi, K.: Hum. Pathol. *24*, 534
        (1993).
125   Yla Herttuala, S., Lipton, B.A., Rosenfeld, M.E. et al.: Proc. Natl. Acad. Sci. USA
        88, 5252 (1991).
126   Nelken, N.A., Coughlin, S.R., Gordon, D. and Wilcox, J.N.: J. Clin. Invest. *88*, 1121 (1991).
127   Russell, M.E., Adams, D.H., Wyner, L.R., Yamashita, Y., Halnon, N.J. and Karnov-
        sky, M.J.: Proc. Natl. Acad. Sci. USA *90*, 6086 (1993).
128   Ransohoff, R.M., Hamilton, T.A., Tani, M. et al.: FASEB J. *7*, 592 (1993).

129   Zhang, K., Gharaeekermani, M., Jones, M.L., Warren, J.S. and Phan, S.H.: J. Immunol. *153*, 4733 (1994).

130   Sakanashi, Y., Takeya, M., Yoshimura, T., Feng, L., Morioka, T. and Takahashi, K.: J. Leukoc. Biol. *56*, 741 (1994).

131   Jones, M.L., Mulligan, M.S., Flory, C.M., Ward, P.A. and Warren, J.S.: J. Immunol. *149*, 2147 (1992).

132   Flory, C.M., Jones, M.L. and Warren, J.S.: Lab. Invest. *69*, 396 (1993).

133   Poon, M., Megyesi, J., Green, R.S. et al.: J. Biol. Chem. *266*, 22375 (1991).

134   Jansen, P.M., Van Damme, J., Put, W., De Jong, I.W., Taylor, F.B.Jr. and Hack, E.C.: J. Infect. Dis. *171*, 1640 (1995).

135   Rovin, B.H., Rumancik, M., Tan, L. and Dickerson, J.: Lab. Invest. *71*, 536 (1994).

135A Noris, M., Bernasconi, S., Casiraghi, F., Sozzani, S., Gotti, E., Remuzzi, G. and Mantovani, A.: Lab. Invest. *73*, 804 (1995).

136   Antoniades, H.N., Neville Golden, J., Galanopoulos, T., Kradin, R.L., Valente, A.J. and Graves, D.T.: Proc. Natl. Acad. Sci. USA *89*, 5371 (1992).

137   Marra, F., Valente, A.J., Pinzani, M. and Abboud, H.E.: J. Clin. Invest. *92*, 1674 (1993).

138   Czaja, M.J., Geerts, A., Xu, J., Schmiedeberg, P. and Ju, Y.: J. Leukoc. Biol. *55*, 120 (1994).

139   Yu, X., Barnhill, R.L. and Graves, D.T.: Lab. Invest. *71*, 226 (1994).

140   Koch, A.E., Kunkel, S.L., Harlow, L.A. et al.: J. Clin. Invest. *90*, 772 (1992).

141   Villiger, P.M., Terkeltaub, R. and Lotz, M.: J. Immunol. *149*, 722 (1992).

142   Hachicha, M., Rathanaswami, P., Schall, T.J. and McColl, S.R.: Arthritis Rheum. *36*, 26 (1993).

143   Sylvester, I., Suffredini, A.F., Boujoukos, A.J. et al.: J. Immunol. *151*, 3292 (1993).

144   Yoshimura, T., Takeya, M., Takahashi, K., Kuratsu, J. and Leonard, E.J.: J. Immunol. *147*, 2229 (1991).

145   Chensue, S.W., Warmington, K.S., Lukacs, N.W. et al.: Am. J. Pathol. *146*, 130 (1995).

146   Zipfel, P.F., Bialonski, A. and Skerka, C.: Biochem. Biophys. Res. Commun. *181*, 179 (1991).

147   Mukaida, N., Gussella, G.L., Kasahara, T. et al.: Immunology *75*, 674 (1992).

148   Wertheim, W.A., Kunkel, S.L., Standiford, T.J. et al.: J. Immunol. *151*, 2166 (1993).

149   Mukaida, N., Morita, M., Ishikawa, Y. et al.: J. Biol. Chem. *269*, 13289 (1994).

150   Loetscher, P., Dewald, B., Baggiolini, M. and Seitz, M.: Cytokine *6*, 162 (1994).

151   Sekido, N., Mukaida, N., Harada, A., Nakanishi, I., Watanabe, Y. and Matsushima, K.: Nature *365*, 654 (1993).

152   Broaddus, C.V., Boylan, A.M., Hoeffel, J.K. et al.: J. Immunol. *152*, 2960 (1994).

153   Zhang, Y.J., Rutledge, B.J. and Rollins, B.J.: J. Biol. Chem. *269*, 15918 (1994).

154   Gong, J.H. and Clarklewis, I.: J. Exp. Med. *181*, 631 (1995).

155   Maze, R., Sherry, B., Kwon, B.S., Cerami, A. and Broxmeyer, H.E.: J. Immunol. *149*, 1004 (1992).

156   Dunlop, D.J., Wright, E.G., Lorimore, S. et al.: Blood *79*, 2221 (1992).

157   Lord, B. I., Woolford, L.B., Wood, L.M. et al.: Blood *85*, 3412 (1995).

158   Alam, R., Forsythe, P.A., Stafford, S., Lett Brown, M.A. and Grant, J.A.: J. Exp. Med. *176*, 781 (1992).

159   Morita, M., Kasahara, T., Mukaida, N. et al.: Eur. Cytokine Netw. *4*, 351 (1993).

160   Iyonaga, K., Takeya, M., Saita, N. et al.: Hum. Pathol. *25*, 455 (1994).

161   Moser, B., Dewald, B., Barella, L., Schumacher, C., Baggiolini, M. and Clark Lewis, I.: J. Biol. Chem. *268*, 7125 (1993).

Progress in Drug Research, Vol. 47 (E. Jucker, Ed.)
© 1996 Birkhäuser Verlag, Basel (Switzerland)

Subclassification and nomenclature of α_1- and α_2-adrenoceptors

By J. Paul Hieble and Robert R. Ruffolo, Jr

Division of Pharmacological Sciences, SmithKline Beecham Pharmaceuticals, King of
Prussia, Pennsylvania 19406, USA
Address correspondence to: Robert R. Ruffolo, Jr, Ph.D., Pharmacological Sciences,
UW2523, 709 Swedeland Road, P.O. Box 1539, King of Prussia, PA 19406-0939, USA

1   Introduction

It has been nearly ten years since the first suggestion that both α_1- [1, 2] and α_2- [3, 4] adrenoceptors could be further subdivided into additional subtypes. Shortly after this time, the first α-adrenoceptors were cloned [5–7], providing definitive evidence for multiple subtypes of both the α_1- and α_2-adrenoceptors. Six distinct α-adrenoceptors have now been cloned from both human and rat, and several of these subtypes have been cloned from several other species, including mouse, hamster, cow and opossum. Functional responses have been assigned to most of the known α-adrenoceptor subtypes, and correspondence has been established between recombinant α-adrenoceptors and native α-adrenoceptors found in cells, tissues and organs. Furthermore, subtype-selective antagonists for many of the α-adrenoceptors are now becoming available. α-Adrenoceptor subtype selectivity is now being widely used as an approach to tissue-targeting of drug action, although clinical evidence indicating that this approach will reduce side-effects is still sparse. Development of subtype selective α-adrenoceptor agonists and antagonists as therapeutic agents will undoubtedly continue as more selective drugs are identified and techniques for localizing α-adrenoceptor subtypes are refined. Although no additional α-adrenoceptor subtypes have been cloned in the past several years, there is functional evidence to suggest that additional subtypes of both α_1- and α_2-adrenoceptors remain to be cloned.

2   Nomenclature of the α_1-adrenoceptors

The nomenclature of the α_1-adrenoceptors has been a subject of controversy over the past several years. Recently, however, most, if not all, of this controversy has been resolved. A consensus statement from the IUPHAR Adrenoceptor Nomenclature Subcommittee has been published [8] which supports the proposal of Ford et al. [9] that the three α_1-adrenoceptor subtypes be designated as α_{1A}, α_{1B}, and α_{1D} (the term α_{1C} should not be used and has only historical significance; see below). Consistent with the practice used for several other neurotransmitter receptors, upper case subscripts will be used to refer to receptors found in native tissues, and lower case subscripts for their corresponding recombinant counterparts. As such, an α_{1A}-adrenoceptor would refer to a native receptor found in a cell, tissue and organ, and an α_{1a}-adrenoceptor denotes the recombinant form of the same receptor.

A brief review of the events leading to the cloning of the α_1-adrenoceptors illustrates the initial confusion in nomenclature that occurred, and how this confusion was ultimately resolved. Initially, α_1-adrenoceptors in native tissues were classified as α_{1A} or α_{1B}, based on sensitivity to chloroethylclonidine or WB-4101 (see Section 3.1). The first α_1-adrenoceptor to be cloned was from a hamster smooth muscle cell line [7], displayed an affinity profile for a series of drugs that was in excellent agreement with that observed for the α_{1B}-adrenoceptor, and as such, this cloned receptor was designated as the α_{1b}-adrenoceptor. Subsequently, a different clone was identified from bovine brain [10]. This recombinant receptor differed from both the native α_{1A}- and α_{1B}-adrenoceptors, based on sensitivity to chloroethylclonidine as well as several other selective antagonists, and had a tissue distribution that was thought to be different from either of these α_1-adrenoceptors. As such, this receptor was designated as the α_{1c}-adrenoceptor to distinguish it from the α_{1A}- and α_{1B}-adrenoceptors. In retrospect, it now appears certain that most of the differences in antagonist affinity and sensitivity observed between this recombinant receptor and the native α_{1A}-adrenoceptor resulted from minor species differences and/or differences in experimental technique between laboratories. Extensive correlation studies of antagonist affinity between α_1-adrenoceptors in native tissues and cells expressing the putative α_{1c}-adrenoceptor have clearly shown the latter receptor to correspond to the α_{1A}-adrenoceptor [9, 11]. Furthermore, more sensitive assays used to map the distribution of α_1-adrenoceptors, such as the RNase protection assay, have demonstrated the presence of the α_{1c}-adrenoceptors in tissues known to possess the α_{1A}-adrenoceptor and in which responses corresponding to the α_{1A}-adrenoceptor have been observed [11, 12]. Hence, the recombinant adrenoceptor formerly designated as the α_{1c}-adrenoceptor has now been clearly shown to represent the α_{1a}-adrenoceptor. To avoid further confusion, it has been recommended by the IUPHAR Subcommittee on Adrenoceptor Nomenclature that the term α_{1c}-adrenoceptor no longer be used to refer to any α_1-adrenoceptor identified in the past or future, and as such, this term is of only historical significance [8].

The last α_1-adrenoceptor to be cloned, from rat brain [13], had some of the characteristics of the α_{1A}-adrenoceptor, and was initially designated as the α_{1a}-adrenoceptor. However, through more extensive evaluation using additional α_1-adrenoceptor antagonists, it was subsequently shown that an identical α_1-adrenoceptor clone having pharmacological characteristics that were distinct from all native α_1-adrenoceptors known at the time, including the α_{1A}-adrenoceptor, made it clear that this receptor represented a novel α_1-adrenoceptor subtype; hence it was subsequently designated as the α_{1d}-adrenoceptor [14]. Since its original identification, this recombinant α_1-adrenoceptor has been referred to as the α_{1a}-adrenoceptor, α_{1d}-adrenoceptor and $\alpha_{1a/d}$-adrenoceptor. It is now agreed that this receptor will be referred to only as the α_{1d}-adrenoceptor, and native receptors found in intact tissues that produce pharmacological effects corresponding to the α_{1D}-adrenoceptor have now been identified [15].

3   Subclassification of the α_1-adrenoceptors

3.1   Subclassification based on radioligand binding characteristics

Although several previous investigators had proposed the possibility of multiple α_1-adrenoceptor subtypes [16, 17], the subdivision of α_1-adrenoceptors into the α_{1A} and α_{1B} subtypes was first proposed by Morrow and Creese [1], who demonstrated that the α_1-adrenoceptor antagonist, WB-4101, produced biphasic displacement of [^{3}H] prazosin binding to rat brain homogenates. They proposed that prazosin could bind to two distinct α_1-adrenoceptor subtypes having differential affinity for WB-4101, and designated the sites having higher affinity for WB-4101 as α_{1A}-adrenoceptors, and the lower affinity sites as α_{1B}-adrenoceptors. Analysis of the biphasic displacement of [^{3}H] prazosin by WB-4101 showed a nearly equal percentage of high and low affinity sites, which was in agreement with the observation that the density for high affinity binding sites for [^{3}H] WB-4101 approximately half of that observed for [^{3}H] prazosin.

Biphasic inhibition of the binding of [^{3}H]-Prazosin or [^{125}I]-IBE-2254 ([^{125}I]-HEAT) by WB-4101 has been observed in several other tissues, such as kidney [18], lung [19] and heart [20, 21], confirming the existence of α_{1A}- and α_{1B}-adrenoceptors. Some tissues show only monophasic inhibition curves, with dissociation constants that were consistent with those obtained for the high affinity (i.e., α_{1A}; rat submaxillary gland [22, 23]), or low affinity (i.e., α_{1B}; rat liver or spleen [19, 20, 24, 25]) binding sites in rat brain. A homogeneous population of α_{1B}-adrenoceptors has also been observed in certain cell culture lines, such as the DDT$_1$MF-2, derived from the smooth muscle cells of hamster vas deferens [26].

WB-4101 is approximately 10–20 fold selective for the α_{1A}-adrenoceptor compared to the α_{1B}-adrenoceptor, as assessed either through analysis of its biphasic inhibition curves in tissues containing both subtypes, or by comparison of affinity constants in tissues thought to have relatively pure α_1-adrenoceptor subtype populations. Other antagonists, such as 5-methylurapidil and (+)niguldipine, show up to 100-fold selectivity for the α_{1A}-

adrenoceptor in these assays [18, 27, 28]. Radioligand binding affinities for these subtype selective antagonists in representative α_{1A}- and α_{1B}-adrenoceptor models and test systems are shown in Table 1.

The subdivision of α_1-adrenoceptors into the α_{1A}- and α_{1B}-adrenoceptor subtypes was supported by Johnson and Minneman [29] who showed that the alkylating agent, chloroethylclonidine, regardless of concentration, would only inactivate approximately 60% of the [^{125}I]-HEAT binding sites in rat cortex. As such, chloroethylclonidine has become a useful tool for the differentiation of α_{1A}- and α_{1B}-adrenoceptors, both in radioligand binding assays and in the functional experiments described below. Other irreversible α-adrenoceptor antagonists, including phenoxybenzamine [30], dibenamine, benextramine and EEDQ [29], alkylate the entire receptor population of α_1-adrenoceptor subtypes, with no evidence for selective interaction with any particular subtype. α_1-Adrenoceptors in different brain regions differ in their sensitivities to receptor inactivation by chloroethylclonidine, with the hippocampus showing nearly complete resistance. Accordingly, WB-4101 and phentolamine were slightly more potent inhibitors of [^{125}I]-HEAT binding in hippocampus compared to cortex. Following treatment of cortical membranes with chloroethylclonidine, the potency of WB-4101 was observed to increase, becoming equivalent to that observed in the hippocampus. These data suggested that chloroethylclonidine selectively alkylated that α_1-adrenoceptor population that was less sensitive to inhibition by WB4101, which corresponded to the α_{1B}-adrenoceptor of Morrow and Creese [1]. Rat hippocampus pretreated with chloroethylclonidine to eliminate the α_{1B}-adrenoceptor population has become a standard tissue preparation for the study of α_{1A}-adrenoceptors [28, 31].

Although α_{1A}- and α_{1B}-adrenoceptors could be readily identified in many native tissues, either through radioligand binding studies or analyses of function responses, the instance of α_{1D}-adrenoceptors in native tissues was more difficult to establish. Recently, a functional response, namely contraction of the rat aorta, has been shown to be mediated by the α_{1D}-adrenoceptor [15]. Radioligand binding assays using a cell line derived from rat thoracic aorta show the α_1-adrenoceptor population present in these cells to have characteristics consistent with the α_{1D}-adrenoceptor, based on the potency of a novel antagonist, (–)-discretamine, which shows moderate selectivity for the α_{1D}-adrenoceptor versus either the α_{1A}- or α_{1B}-adrenoceptor subtypes [32]. In addition, the binding characteristics of [^{125}I] HEAT to SK-N-MC neuroepithelioma cells is best explained by assuming the presence of three α_1-adrenoceptor subtypes, including the α_{1D}-adrenoceptor, in these cells [33]. It is likely that more detailed analyses of the effects of the subtype-selective antagonists on the binding of non-selective α_1-adrenoceptor radioligands will show the presence of the α_{1D}-adrenoceptor in other tissues as well.

Analysis of the subtype selectivity of α_1-adrenoceptor agonists and antagonists has been greatly simplified by the availability of cell lines expressing the recombinant α_1-adrenoceptors, since pure populations of a particular α_1-adrenoceptor subtype can rarely be guaranteed in native tissues or cells. All three known α_1-adrenoceptor subtypes have now been cloned from human sources [31, 34, 35, 37], allowing for these receptors to be investigated without the potential for species differences (although only minor differences in affinity are typically observed between the human subtypes and their corresponding animal clones).

Detailed studies using recombinant α_1-adrenoceptors have confirmed the antagonist selectivities observed previously between α_1-adrenoceptor subtypes determined using radioligand binding assays in native tissues (Table 2). Although the relative affinities of a particular antagonist for different α_1-adrenoceptor subtypes are reasonably consistent between the various reported studies, the data presented in Table 2 illustrate that the absolute affinities of an antagonist for a given receptor subtype can vary over a large range between different laboratories. This variability is surprising, considering that the identical receptor protein is being studied, which in many cases was expressed in the same cell line and competing for the same radioligand. The dependence of the binding affinity of the highly lipophilic antagonist, (+)-niguldipine, on assay volume has been reported [36]; however, the inter-study variability observed with (+)-niguldipine does not appear to be different from the variability observed with the other antagonists. As such, it is now thought to be critical to evaluate the relative affinities of a variety of compounds when characterizing or classifying α_1-adrenoceptors.

The availability of recombinant α_1-adrenoceptors had led to the discovery of many new antagonists showing greater selectivity profiles. Many structural analogs of (+)-niguldipine have been found to be highly selective antagonists of the α_{1a}-adrenoceptor, and without having the calcium channel blocking activity associated with (+)-niguldipine [38, 39]. One of the most selective analogs observed to date is SNAP-5089 (Table 3). The (–)-enantiomer of this dihydropyridine shows even greater α_{1a}-adrenoceptor selectivity, having at least 1000-fold higher affinity for the α_{1a}-adrenoceptor (K_i = 0.18 nM) than for either α_{1b} (K_i = 180 nM) or α_{1d} (K_i = 630 nM) adrenoceptors [38]. Other structural classes also show selectivity for the α_{1a}-adrenoceptor versus the other two α_1-adrenoceptor subtypes, although not of the magnitude observed with the dihydropyridines (Table 3).

The modest α_{1B} versus α_{1A}-adrenoceptor selectivity observed for spipe-rone in radioligand binding assays using native tissue homogenates (Table 1) is observed in some, but not all, studies with recombinant α_1-adreno-ceptors (Table 2). AH11110A (Table 4), was recently reported to be selec-tive for the α_{1B}-adrenoceptor [40]; however another report examining the affinity of this compound for recombinant α_1-adrenoceptors [41] showed only marginal selectivity for the α_{1B}-adrenoceptor.

Although the α_{1D}-adrenoceptor was identified only recently, and its func-tional role is still unclear, several antagonists showing selectivity for the α_{1d}-adrenoceptor versus the other two α_1-adrenoceptor subtypes have been identified (Table 4), although the compounds identified thus far also have high affinity for other (non α_1) neurotransmitter receptors, such as the α_2-adrenoceptor (SK&F 104856, SK&F 105854) or $5HT_{1A}$ receptor (BMY 7378). Other furo- and thieno-benzazepines structurally related to SK&F 104856 and SK&F 105854 also show some degree of selectivity for the α_{1d}-adrenoceptor [42].

Inhibition of binding of an antagonist radioligand by α_1-adrenoceptor ago-nists often yields shallow displacement curves indicative of an interaction with multiple sites.

However this biphasic interaction does not necessarily imply agonist selec-tivity between subtypes, inasmuch as agonists can bind to high and low affinity "states" of a single receptor. Analysis of the inhibition of [^{3}H] praz-osin binding to rat cortex by epinephrine, norepinephrine and phenyleph-rine suggests that the two catecholamines do not discriminate between α_{1A}- and α_{1B}-adrenoceptors, whereas phenylephrine has apparent selec-tivity for the α_{1A}-adrenoceptor subtype [1]. However, it is not clear whether the relatively moderate selectivities observed in this study rep-resent real or reliable estimates in view of the caveats discussed above. Norepinephrine, phenylephrine and other phenethylamine agonists of α_1-adrenoceptors show consistently low potencies as inhibitors of the bind-ing of several antagonist radioligands for the α_1-adrenoceptor, including [^{3}H] WB-4101, [^{3}H] prazosin, [^{125}I] HEAT and [^{3}H] Tamsulosin [22, 43–47]. When affinity for these agonists is compared in tissues possessing rela-tively pure populations of α_{1A} and α_{1B}-adrenoceptors, neither norepineph-rine or phenylephrine show any substantial α_1-adrenoceptor subtype selec-tivity. In contrast, the imidazoline partial agonist, oxymetazoline, shows substantially higher affinity and selectivity for the α_{1A}-adrenoceptor sub-type [22, 44].

When the affinities of α_1-adrenoceptor agonists for recombinant α_1-adrenoceptors is determined, the low affinity of the phenethylamines for both α_{1a} and α_{1b}-adrenoceptors is confirmed. Interestingly, nearly all studies comparing the affinities of these agonists for the three recombinant α_1-adrenoceptors show substantially higher affinity. for the α_{1d}-adrenoceptor subtype (Table 5). The selectivity of oxymetazoline for α_{1a}- versus α_{1b}-adrenoceptors is confirmed, and α_{1a}- versus α_{1d}-adrenoceptor selectivity is demonstrated. Another imidazoline agonist, A-61603, has recently been shown to have even greater selectivity for the α_{1a}-adrenoceptor [48].

3.2   Subclassification based on functional antagonist sensitivity

3.2.1   Functional significance of α_1-adrenoceptor subtypes identified via molecular biology and radioligand binding techniques

At the time that the α_1-adrenoceptors were being subclassified based upon radioligand binding criteria, functional evidence to support this subclassification was already available. Morrow and Creese [1] summarized literature data comparing the relative potencies of phentolamine and prazosin against a variety of α_1-adrenoceptor mediated responses. Those responses showing a prazosin/phentolamine potency ratio between 3 and 12 were predicted to be mediated by the α_{1A}-adrenoceptor, and those where prazosin was > 50-fold more potent than phentolamine were predicted to be mediated by the α_{1B}-adrenoceptor. While there were some inconsistencies, the overall pattern observed was, in general, consistent with current knowledge of α_{1A}- and α_{1B}-adrenoceptor subtype distribution.

WB-4101 has a moderate degree of functional selectivity, blocking norepinephrine-induced contraction in rat vas deferens ($K_B = 0.3$ nM) with higher affinity than in rat spleen ($K_B = 5.4$ nM) [2]. These observations were consistent with the affinity of WB-4101 for α_{1A}- and α_{1B}-adrenoceptors predicted by radioligand binding assays. 5-Methylurapidil also demonstrated the predicted selectivity in these tissues, with dissociation constants of 6 and 110 nM in rat vas deferens and spleen, respectively [49]. Several other α-adrenoceptor antagonists, such as BE 2254, yohimbine and phentolamine, are equipotent in rat vas deferens and spleen, suggesting that the selectivity observed with WB-4101 and 5-methylurapidil is indeed based on selective interactions of these antagonists with distinct α_1-adrenoceptor subtypes.

5-Methylurapidil has proven to be a useful tool for functional subclassification of α_1-adrenoceptor mediated responses. In addition to classification of the contractile responses in rat vas deferens and spleen as being mediated by the α_{1A}- and α_{1B}-adrenoceptors, respectively, dissociation constants of ≤ 1.0 nM for 5-methylurapidil obtained in rat mesenteric microvessels [50], perfused rat kidney [51], and perfused rat mesenteric circulation [52] suggest that these responses are also mediated by the α_{1A}-adrenoceptor subtype. In contrast, the α_1-adrenoceptor mediated inotropic response to epinephrine in rat heart was found to be less sensitive to inhibition by 5-methylurapidil (K_B = 22 nM [27]), suggesting that this tissue, like the rat spleen, responds to α_1-adrenoceptor stimulation primarily through the α_{1B}-adrenoceptor.

As observed in radioligand binding assays, chloroethylclonidine shows α_1-adrenoceptor subtype selectivity in its ability to produce irreversible blockade of the contractile response to α-adrenoceptor agonists in functional studies. The selectivity of this alkylating agent for the α_{1B}-adrenoceptor observed in radioligand binding assays has been confirmed in functional assays, inasmuch as no effect of chloroethylclonidine is observed on norepinephrine-induced contraction in the rat vas deferens, whereas significant inhibition is observed in the rat spleen [2]. Sensitivity to chloroethylclonidine has been used to classify α_1-adrenoceptors mediating contraction of several rat blood vessels [53]. The ability of chloroethylclonidine to suppress the maximum response to norepinephrine in blood vessels correlates inversely with the potency of WB-4101 to inhibit norepinephrine-induced responses, suggesting that in these blood vessels, the sensitivity to chloroethylclonidine is related to the activation of α_{1B}-adrenoceptors in the contractile response.

However, there are some inconsistencies in the use of chloroethylclonidine for functional subclassification of α_1-adrenoceptors. In aortae from several species, the tissue showing greatest sensitivity to chloroethylclonidine (rat aorta) was also found to be the most sensitive to competitive blockade by WB-4101 [54], which is inconsistent with the α_{1A}- and α_{1B}-adrenoceptor classification schemes described above. Divergent effects of chloroethylclonidine are observed in the rat aorta, ranging from apparently parallel rightward shifts in the norepinephrine concentration-response curve, with no effect on maximum response [54], to a large parallel rightward shift with a small (30%) reduction in maximum response [31, 37] to a nearly complete abolition of the norepinephrine induced response [53]. Wenham and Marshall [55] observe a concentration-related reduction in the response to norepinephrine at concentrations up to 300 μM, with a secondary response occurring that reaches the original maximum, at concentrations of norepinephrine above 1 mM.

Even before the identification of α_1-adrenoceptor subtypes, the rat aorta was known to have distinct pharmacological characteristics from other blood vessels [56]. When the α_{1A} and α_{1B}-adrenoceptor subtypes were first identified, it became clear that the α_1-adrenoceptor of the rat aorta did not fit clearly into either class, and it was proposed that this tissue either represented an atypical α_1-adrenoceptor [57, 58], or that the functional contractile response resulted from the contribution of multiple receptors [55, 59, 60]. The response to α_1-adrenoceptor stimulation in the rat aorta is sensitive to inhibition by 5-methylurapidil, but with a potency that is intermediate between that observed in the rat vas deferens and rat spleen (Table 5). This intermediate potency of 5-methylurapidil between that expected for the α_{1A}- and α_{1B}-adrenoceptors is also observed with the cloned α_{1d}-adrenoceptor, suggesting that the rat aorta contains the α_{1D}-adrenoceptor (Table 2). Comparison of the functional potency of an extensive series of antagonists with their affinity for the three recombinant α_1-adrenoceptors in radioligand binding assays yields the best correlation of the results obtained in rat aorta with the α_{1d}-adrenoceptor [15, 61, 62]. The sensitivity of the contractile response in the rat aorta to chloroethylclonidine [54] is also consistent with the relatively high sensitivity of the recombinant α_{1d}-adrenoceptor to irreversible alkylation by this agent [11]. Hence it is likely that activation of the α_{1D}-adrenoceptor is responsible for the major component of the contractile response to an α_1-adrenoceptor agonist in the rat aorta, although it is possible that another subtype may also contribute to the response [59, 60]. Most studies examining the α_1-adrenoceptor subtype responsible for contraction of individual blood vessels have only considered the α_{1A}- and α_{1B}-adrenoceptor subtypes, evaluating their relative contributions via sensitivity to chloroethylclonidine and one of the selective α_{1A}-adrenoceptor antagonists. Because mRNA for the α_{1D}-adrenoceptor has been detected in a variety of blood vessels [63, 64], it is possible that this subtype plays a role in α_1-adrenoceptor mediated contraction of other blood vessels as well. The newly identified α_{1D}-adrenoceptor antagonists should facilitate the evaluation of the role of α_{1D}-adrenoceptors in vasoconstriction.

The formation of inositol phosphates can also be used as an index of functional activity of α_1-adrenoceptor agonists in cells transfected with recombinant α_1-adrenoceptors [65]. In these systems, norepinephrine and epinephrine are observed to have nearly equivalent potencies and identical intrinsic activities at the three α_1-adrenoceptor subtypes. 6-Fluoronorepinephrine, which can selectively stimulate α- versus β-adrenoceptors, also has equal potencies and intrinsic activities for the three α_1-adrenoceptors. Phenylephrine has lower potency, and reduced intrinsic activity, at the α_{1b}-adrenoceptor compared to either the α_{1a}- or α_{1d}-adrenoceptor. Methoxamine shows over 10-fold selectivity for the α_{1a}-adrenoceptor, with reduced intrinsic activity at the α_{1b}-adrenoceptor. A variety of other agonists, including imidazolines (oxymetazoline, cirazoline), iminoimidazolidines (clonidine, St-587), aminotetralins (SK&F 89748), and a phenethylamine (amidephrine) show marked functional selectivity for the α_{1a}-adrenoceptor. Although their intrinsic activities at the α_{1a}-adrenoceptor are reduced, relative to the catecholamines, activity at the α_{1b}- and α_{1d}-adrenoceptors is dramatically reduced, and is essentially abolished in the case of oxymetazoline, St-587 and amidephrine. Although oxymetazoline also shows selectivity for α_{1a}-adrenoceptors based on the ability to inhibit [125I] HEAT binding to cells expressing the receptors, the other agonists show little or no α_{1a}-adrenoceptor selectivity in radioligand binding studies. Hence, the effects of structural changes on the ability of agonists to bind to the α_1-adrenoceptor subtypes are independent from their effect on the ability of these compounds to activate the receptor. It has been observed that A-61063, an imidazoline agonist showing selectivity for the recombinant and native α_{1a}-adrenoceptor based on radioligand binding assays, to produce potent activation of phosphoinositide hydrolysis in cells transfected with the α_{1a}-adrenoceptor, but not in those expressing the α_{1b}- or α_{1d}-adrenoceptor subtypes [48]. A-61063 produces a maximal response of equivalent magnitude to norepinephrine in the cells expressing the recombinant α_{1a}-adrenoceptor, and also shows selectivity as an α_{1A}-adrenoceptor agonist in functional assays using native tissues [48].

3.2.2   Evidence for additional α_1-adrenoceptor subtypes

While the functional and radioligand binding data presented above provide consistent evidence for the division of α_1-adrenoceptors into the three subclasses that are now designated as α_{1A}-, α_{1B}- and α_{1D}-adrenoceptors, there are additional data suggesting that these three α_1-adrenoceptor subtypes alone are not sufficient to explain all the pharmacological actions resulting from α_1-adrenoceptor activation.

As observed by Morrow and Creese [1] in their initial subclassification of the α_1-adrenoceptors in rat brain, Jagadeesh and Deth [66] found biphasic displacement of [3H] prazosin binding to bovine aorta by WB-4101 and phentolamine. However, the affinities of these antagonists were substantially different from those determined by Morrow and Creese [1] in the brain. Jagadeesh and Deth [66] interpreted their [3H] prazosin binding data as showing two distinct binding sites for prazosin. Other investigators [67–73] have suggested the presence of multiple [3H] prazosin binding sites in a variety of tissues. However, the affinity of prazosin for the two postulated sites often differs by less than one order of magnitude [66–206], and/or one site represents only a relatively low percentage (<15%) of the total binding [66, 72], and hence the heterogeneity in praz-

osin binding observed in these studies may not have functional significance. Many other studies have detected only a single [^{3}H] prazosin binding site in these tissues, and as such the biphasic binding of this radiolig-
and cannot always be reproduced in the tissues where it has been previously observed [74].

Several studies [70–72, 75] have detected [^{3}H] prazosin binding sites with
dissociation constants of 3–10 nM, which are substantially lower than those
commonly observed for this radioligand, suggesting the presence of functional α_1-adrenoceptors having lower affinity for prazosin. Also consistent with these functional experiments is the relative insensitivity of the
low affinity [^{3}H] prazosin binding sites to irreversible alkylation by phenoxybenzamine [75, 76].

Although prazosin is a potent and highly selective α_1-adrenoceptor antagonist, many investigators have noted differences in the ability of prazosin to antagonize α_1-adrenoceptor-mediated responses in functional assays.
Comparison of dissociation constants for prazosin against norepinephrine-induced contraction in a variety of smooth muscle tissues, both vascular and non-vascular, shows a range of at least 100-fold [77–79]. While
at least some of this variation can be explained by differences in experimental conditions, consistent and reproducible differences in the potency
of prazosin have been observed, and are highly suggestive of α_1-adreno-
ceptor heterogeneity.

The ability of prazosin to inhibit norepinephrine-induced responses has
been used to subclassify α_1-adrenoceptors by Muramatsu and coworkers
[71–73, 80–84], building upon a postulate originally presented by Flavahan and Vanhoutte [85]. When the affinity of prazosin is determined in a
series of blood vessels from several species, α_1-adrenoceptors can be
divided into three subtypes, the α_{1H}-adrenoceptor having high affinity (K_B
< 1 nM) for prazosin, the α_{1L}-adrenoceptor having lower affinity for both
prazosin (K_B > 2 nM) and yohimbine (K_B > 300 nM), and the α_{1N}-adren-
oceptor, which has an affinity for prazosin that is comparable to the α_{1L}-
adrenoceptor, but a higher affinity for yohimbine (K_B < 100 nM). The prazosin-insensitive α_1-adrenoceptors can also be differentiated by their affinity for HV-723, which has higher affinity for the α_{1N}-adrenoceptor (K_B =
0.4–1 nM) than for the α_{1L}-adrenoceptor (K_B = 2–7 nM) [81]. These α_1-
adrenoceptor subtypes appear to make differential contributions to the
responses of different blood vessels to both exogenous agonists and to
sympathetic nerve stimulation [80].

Schild analysis of the antagonism by prazosin of norepinephrine-induced
contraction in the rabbit aorta and rabbit carotid artery can detect two
distinct dissociation constants, differing by approximately one order of

magnitude [73,81,83,84]. Other α_1-adrenoceptor antagonists did not produce a biphasic Schild plot against norepinephrine, and blockade by prazosin of methoxamine-induced contraction in the aorta resulted in only one dissociation constant that corresponds to the low affinity component observed against norepinephrine. In the rat spleen, prazosin produces a biphasic Schild plot, suggesting the presence of two α_1-adrenoceptor populations, with receptor dissociation constants of 0.6 nM and 25 nM [49]. Treatment of the tissue with phenoxybenzamine eliminates that component of the contractile response showing high affinity for prazosin. These data suggest that norepinephrine can activate both α_{1H}- and α_{1L}-adrenoceptors, with methoxamine having selectivity for the α_{1L}-adrenoceptor, and phenoxybenzamine being able to selectively inactivate the α_{1H}-adrenoceptor. The potential selectivity observed for methoxamine is consistent with the findings of Flavahan and Vanhoutte [85] who compared the dissociation constants of prazosin against clonidine and methoxamine in the rabbit pulmonary artery (also implying that clonidine has selectivity for the α_{1H}-adrenoceptor). The insensitivity of the α_{1L}-adrenoceptors in the rat spleen to alkylation by phenoxybenzamine is consistent with radioligand binding studies showing relative insensitivity of the low affinity [3H] prazosin binding sites to irreversible alkylation by phenoxybenzamine [75, 76].

This subclassification scheme based on affinity to prazosin may explain the earlier results in canine splenic artery [86] where both prazosin (K_B = 9 nM) and rauwolscine (K_B = 91 nM) produced competitive blockade of the constrictor response to norepinephrine.

Prazosin-insensitive α_1-adrenoceptors may also be involved in the contraction of prostatic smooth muscle. There is much current interest in the design of α_1-adrenoceptor antagonists showing selectivity for the prostate versus vascular smooth muscle; as such agents would be useful in the treatment of the obstructive symptoms associated with benign prostatic hypertrophy [31,37,38,42,87]. Selectivity between α_1-adrenoceptor subtypes has been postulated as a useful route to achieve this goal [38, 39]. Several radioligand binding assays, as well as receptor localization studies using α_1-adrenoceptor subtype specific probes, suggest that the predominant α_1-adrenoceptor subtype present in prostates from several species, including humans, is the α_{1A}-adrenoceptor [25, 43, 88].

However, several radioligand binding studies in canine and human prostate [70–72, 76, 89] have detected [3H] prazosin binding sites with dissociation constants of 1–10 nM, which are substantially lower than is commonly observed for this radioligand, and which potentially correlate with the functional α_1-adrenoceptors discussed above having lower affinity for prazosin, namely the α_{1L}-adrenoceptors. The dissociation constant obtained by Sulpizio et al. [89] for [^{3}H] prazosin in canine prostate (1.5 nM) shows this tissue to have nearly 10-fold lower affinity for this radioligand compared to similar studies performed with canine aorta (K_D = 0.17 nM; J.P. Hieble, unpublished data).

Although there is substantial variability in the reported data, prazosin also appears to be relatively weak as a functional antagonist at α_1-adrenoceptors in prostatic tissue (Table 7). Correlation of the functional potency of α_1-adrenoceptor antagonists with their affinity for the three recombinant α_1-adrenoceptor subtypes suggests that the α_{1a}-adrenoceptor is responsible for the contractile activity of norepinephrine in the prostate [34,35,90]. Correlation between dissociation constants obtained in human prostate with affinity for the human recombinant α_{1a}-adrenoceptor is observed even for antagonists showing a high degree of subtype selectivity [35]. However, several antagonists have been identified which have high affinity and selectivity for the α_{1a}-adrenoceptor, but which are weak functional antagonists in human prostate [39,91]. One of these compounds, RS 17053, has a dissociation constant below 1 nM at both native α_{1A}-adrenoceptors (Table 1) and recombinant α_{1a}-adrenoceptors (Table 3), and yet this compound has a dissociation constant of > 50 nM against norepinephrine-induced contraction in human prostate or prostatic urethra [91]. These data are consistent with the premise that a novel α_1-adrenoceptor, perhaps the α_{1L}-adrenoceptor described above, is responsible for mediating, at least in part, the contractile response in prostatic tissue. Agents such as RS 17053 may be examples of compounds which block the α_{1a}-adrenoceptors, but not the α_{1L}-adrenoceptor. Confirmation of this hypothesis will require the identification of suitable functional and radioligand binding assays for the characterization of the α_{1L}-adrenoceptor, followed by a systematic comparison of structurally diverse series of α_1-adrenoceptor antagonists for the α_{1A}- and α_{1L}-adrenoceptors.

4   Nomenclature of the α_2-adrenoceptors

As with the α_1-adrenoceptors, there has been some controversy regarding the nomenclature of the α_2-adrenoceptor subtypes. Four α_2-adrenoceptor subtypes have been defined by radioligand binding assays in native tissues, although functional responses have not unequivocally been attributed to all of these subtypes. These four subtypes have been designated as the α_{2A}-, α_{2B}-, α_{2C}- and α_{2D}-adrenoceptors, and their pharmacological profiles correspond well with four recombinant α_2-adrenoceptors, designated as the α_{2a}-, α_{2b}-, α_{2c}- and α_{2d}-adrenoceptors [92]. These particular recombinant receptors have been cloned from several species, and have been given several different designations (Table 8). However, four distinct recombinant α_2-adrenoceptors have not yet been found in a single species, and it is commonly believed that the α_{2a}- and α_{2d}-adrenoceptors should be considered as species homologs of the same receptor [93]. Any given species appears to have either α_{2A}-, α_{2B}- and α_{2C}-adrenoceptors (human, pig, chicken) or α_{2B}-, α_{2C}- and α_{2D}-adrenoceptors (rat, mouse, cow) [93]. This subclassification is based in many cases on the radiolig- and binding properties of native α_2-adrenoceptors, since most of the individual α_2-adrenoceptor subtypes have not been cloned from species other than humans, rats and mice. The α_{2A}- and α_{2D}-adrenoceptors can be distinguished pharmacologically based on their affinities for yohimbine, rauwolscine and analogous alkaloids (see below).

Previously, the recombinant human α_2-adrenoceptors have been designated based on the chromosomal location of the gene coding for the particular subtype (α_2C 10, α_2C2, α_2C4; Table 8). This nomenclature is no longer necessary, inasmuch as each of these receptors clearly corresponds to one of the previously identified native α_2-adrenoceptors. However, a question remains regarding nomenclature of the recombinant α_2-adrenoceptors of rat and mouse. Two of the three subtypes cloned from these species correspond well to the recombinant human α_2-adrenoceptors and to the native receptors of human or rodent origin, and can clearly be designated as α_{2b}- and α_{2c}-adrenoceptors. The third subtype from these species, namely that having the pharmacological profile of the α_{2D}-adrenoceptor, has close homology (approximately 90% amino acid identity) to the human α_{2a}-adrenoceptor, and to a porcine α_2-adrenoceptor [94] having an identical pharmacological profile to the human α_{2a}-adrenoceptor. Therefore, some feel that is most appropriate to designate this receptor as the α_{2a}- (rodent) adrenoceptor. On the other hand, at least one non-rodent species (cow) appears to have receptors with similar pharmacological characteristics to the rodent clones, and pharmacological profiles characteristic of the α_{2D}-adrenoceptor are well established in several native tissue assays as being distinct from those of the α_{2A}-adrenoceptor [95, 96]. This would support the designation of this recombinant receptor as either α_{2a}- or α_{2d}-adrenoceptor, depending on its pharmacological profile which, at present, appears to be determined by the species from which the receptor is cloned. Further cloning of α_2-adrenoceptors from additional species, and the characterization of their pharmacological profiles, is likely to determine which of these nomenclature schemes will prevail.

5   Subclassification of the α_2-adrenoceptors

5.1   Subclassification based on radioligand binding characteristics

The first suggestion that α_2-adrenoceptors could be subdivided was provided by the finding that prazosin, previously thought to interact only with
the α_1-adrenoceptor, could produce relatively potent inhibition ($K_i < 100$
nM) of the binding of [^{3}H] rauwolscine in certain tissues, such as neonatal rat lung and rat kidney, as well as in some cell lines, such as NG-108.
In other tissues, such as human platelet, or in the HT-29 cell line, the dissociation constant of prazosin against [^{3}H] rauwolscine binding was > 1000
nM. The prazosin insensitive α_2-adrenoceptor was designated as the α_{2A}-
adrenoceptor, whereas the prazosin sensitive receptor was referred to as
the α_{2B}-adrenoceptor (see review by Bylund, 1992). Analysis of competition data for prazosin inhibition of [^{3}H] rauwolscine binding demonstrated that other tissues, such as rat [97] and human cortex [98], had mixed
populations of α_{2A}-and α_{2B}-adrenoceptors, showing that this α_2-adreno-
ceptor subclassification scheme did not simply represent a species differ-
ence in α_2-adrenoceptor characteristics. Other antagonists have been identified having a selective action at α_{2B}-adrenoceptors (ARC 239, spiroxa-
trine, SK&F 104856). Interestingly, most α_{2B}-adrenoceptor selective
antagonists are also potent α_1-adrenoceptor antagonists, the only currently
known exception being imiloxan [99]. We have recently reported [42, 100]
that doxazosin, a close structural analog of prazosin, has virtually no affinity for the α_{2B}-adrenoceptor, suggesting that different structural elements
of these molecules are required for interaction with α_1- and α_{2B}-adreno-
ceptors.
In the initial subclassification of α_2-adrenoceptors, it was noted that the
partial agonist, oxymetazoline, had the opposite selectivity profile to prazosin, interacting preferentially with the α_{2A}-adrenoceptor. Another imidazoline containing molecule, BRL 44408, has been shown to be a selective α_{2A}-adrenoceptor antagonist [101,102]. BRL 48962, the R-enantiomer
of BRL 44408, shows even greater selectivity for the α_{2A}-adrenoceptor
[103].
Because a variety of antagonists having α_2-adrenoceptor subtype selectivity are now available, a more precise mode of receptor characterization is possible, based on correlation of inhibitory potency against α_2-
adrenoceptor binding for a series of antagonists between different receptor sources. This type of analysis has been used to demonstrate the presence
of two additional α_2-adrenoceptor subtypes. The α_{2C}-adrenoceptor was
initially shown to be present in a cell line derived from the opossum kid-

ney [104], and has now also been found in native opossum kidney [105] and a human retinoblastoma cell line [102]. Studies using another α_2-adrenoceptor radioligand, [^{3}H] MK 912, have demonstrated a mixed α_2-adrenoceptor population in rat cortex and spinal cord, with one component representing the α_{2C}-adrenoceptor subtype [106]. Interestingly, this radioligand, like rauwolscine, appears to have 10-fold greater affinity for the α_{2C}-adrenoceptor compared to the α_{2B}-adrenoceptor. The differences between α_{2C}- and α_{2B}-adrenoceptors are subtle, with no one antagonist showing clear selectivity. The principal distinguishing characteristics of the α_{2C}-adrenoceptor is a very high affinity for rauwolscine, and a higher prazosin/oxymetazoline affinity ratio (Table 3). As can be seen from Table 3, the characteristics of these two subtypes are sufficiently close to make assignment ambiguous based only on the affinity of yohimbine, rauwolscine, prazosin and oxymetazoline. However when the affinities of a more extensive series of antagonists are correlated, the differences between these subtypes become more apparent.

A fourth subtype, designated α_{2D}-adrenoceptor, has been found in bovine pineal and rat submaxillary gland [95]. The α_{2D}-adrenoceptor has characteristics similar to the α_{2A}-adrenoceptor, but has lower affinity for rauwolscine and yohimbine than the other α_2-adrenoceptor subtypes, resulting in a decreased prazosin/yohimbine potency ratio (Table 3). The α_{2D}-adrenoceptor also has lower affinity for other alkaloids structurally analogous to yohimbine [107, 108]; however, other α-adrenoceptor antagonists, such as RX 821002 and phentolamine, affinity for α_{1D}-adrenoceptors that is comparable to the other α_2-adrenoceptor subtypes. The dissociation constants for the binding of [^{3}H] RS-15385-197 to α_{2A}-, α_{2B}- and α_{2D}-adrenoceptors do not differ from one another [109]. The low affinity of the α_{2D}-adrenoceptor for yohimbine and rauwolscine, relative to other α_2-adrenoceptor subtypes, is also reflected as a decreased inhibitory potency of these alkaloids against other radioligands binding to the α_2-adrenoceptor [106, 109].

Several other tissues possess an α_2-adrenoceptor having low affinity for yohimbine and rauwolscine, including adipocytes from several species, and rabbit jejunal enterocytes. Based on the data shown in Table 3, it is likely that these tissues represent additional examples of the α_{2D}-adrenoceptor. Studies in the rat brain using two highly potent and selective α_2-adrenoceptor radioligands, [^{3}H] RS-15385-197 [109] and [^{3}H] MK-912 [106], show the presence of a site having low affiffity for yohimbine and rauwolscine, consistent with an α_{2D}-adrenoceptor. Other than yohimbine and rauwolscine, only BAM 1303 can discriminate between α_{2A}- and α_{2D}-adrenoceptors; however, these two subtypes can be distinguished when the potency ratios for several antagonist pairs are compared [95].

Considering adipocyte α_2-adrenoceptors, it appears that there are species-dependent differences in α_2-adrenoceptor subtypes, with human and dog having α_{2A}-adrenoceptors, and rat, rabbit and hamster having α_{2D}-adrenoceptors (Table 9). Species-dependent assignment of pineal tissue between α_{2A}- (chicken) and α_{2D}- (bovine) adrenoceptors has also been made, based on a 10-fold difference observed in the affinity of yohimbine and rauwolscine [95]. The possibility that these two α_2-adrenoceptor subtypes represent species homologs is consistent with both functional and molecular data presented below.

The subdivision of α_2-adrenoceptors into the four subtypes noted above, based primarily on radioligand binding characteristics of the receptors in native tissue homogenates, is consistent with the subclassification using the recombinant α_2-adrenoceptors. The α_2-adrenoceptors which have been cloned from various species fit well into the tissue-defined subtypes (Table 9), with the three subtypes cloned from human sources having characteristics of α_{2A}-, α_{2B}- and α_{2C}-adrenoceptors, and those of rat and mouse having characteristics of α_{2B}-, α_{2C}- and α_{2D}-adrenoceptors. The individual recombinant receptors obtained from porcine and opossum also can be classified using this scheme. As is the case with the α_1-adrenoceptors (see Tables 2 and 5), there is a substantial variability between the affinity values determined for agonists (Table 10) and antagonists (Table 11) of the recombinant α_2-adrenoceptors. The endogenous catecholamines, norepinephrine and epinephrine, generally show relatively low potency for inhibition of the commonly used radioligands (Table 10), although affinity is apparently dependent on the buffer utilized [110]. The catecholamines are potent inhibitors of the binding of [^{3}H] clonidine to the recombinant α_{2a}-adrenoceptor [111] and direct determination of the dissociation constant for [^{3}H] norepinephrine at the α_{2a}-adrenoceptor shows high affinity (K_i = 13 nM; Hieble and Naselsky, unpublished data).

In contrast to the α_1-adrenoceptor, few α_2-adrenoceptor subtype selective antagonists have been identified to date. Consistent with observations in native tissues, prazosin and ARC-239 show selectivity for the α_{2b}- versus α_{2a}-adrenoceptor, while SK&F 104856 shows moderate selectivity for the α_{2b}-adrenoceptors versus either of the other two α_2-adrenoceptor subtypes. All of the above antagonists also have high affinity for the α_1-adrenoceptors. Imiloxan, the only antagonist reported to have selectivity for α_{2B}-adrenoceptors without affinity for the α_1-adrenoceptor, based on radioligand binding assays in native tissues [99], has apparently not been examined for affinity to the recombinant α_2-adrenoceptor subtypes.

It has been suggested that the α_{2A}- or α_{2B}-adrenoceptors in rat kidney and spleen can be subdivided into two populations, based on differential affinity of guanoxabenz [112–114]. However, it was recently shown that these results were probably a consequence of conversion of guanoxabenz to a metabolite having higher affinity for the α_2-adrenoceptor [115].

5.2   Subclassification based on functional antagonist sensitivity

5.2.1   *Functional significance of α_2-adrenoceptor subtypes identified via molecular biology and radioligand binding techniques*

Although the subdivision of α_2-adrenoceptors into the α_{2A}-, α_{2B}, α_{2C}- and α_{2D}-adrenoceptors has been based primarily on radioligand binding studies, there is some support for this classification scheme from functional studies. Clearly, most „classical" α_2-adrenoceptor mediated responses fall into the α_{2A}- or α_{2D}-adrenoceptor groups, since they are usually defined as being „α_2-adrenoceptors" as a result of their lack of sensitivity to prazosin.

The ability of prazosin and ARC-239 to produce functional blockade of UK-14304 mediated inhibition of adenylate cyclase in cells containing homogenous populations of α_{2A}- (HT-29) or α_{2B}- (NG-108) adrenoceptors, correlates with its ability to inhibit [^{3}H] rauwolscine binding [116]. ARC-239 was 100-fold more potent in the NG-108 cells, with a dissociation constant of 10 nM, while yohimbine and phentolamine were equipotent in the two cell lines. Hence, inhibition of the actions of this α_2-adrenoceptor agonist on adenylate cyclase in the NG-108 cell appear to be mediated by α_{2B}-adrenoceptors.

In a similar experiment, prazosin was shown to be effective in blocking UK 14,304 induced inhibition of adenylate cyclase in OK cells, a response presumably mediated by the α_{2C}-adrenoceptor [104]. Although a dissociation constant was not calculated in these experiments, prazosin appeared to be a less potent antagonist of the action of UK 14,304, compared to yohimbine, than in the NG-108 cells, consistent with binding affinity ratios at α_{2B}- and α_{2C}-adrenoceptors.

The functional characteristics of presynaptic α_2-adrenoceptors at a variety of sites have been studied extensively. Most prejunctional receptors show a low sensitivity to prazosin, and therefore appear to be either α_{2A}- or α_{2D}-adrenoceptors, depending on the species [117]. Presynaptic α_2-adrenoceptors of rat cerebral cortex [117], kidney [156] and submaxillary gland [119] appear to be α_{2D}-adrenoceptors. Although the prejunctional α_2-adrenoceptors of the rat vas deferens were assigned to the α_{2A}-adrenoceptor subtype [120], the data are, in fact, more consistent with the α_{2D}-

adrenoceptor [119]. Several reports initially suggested that the presynaptic α_2-adrenoceptor of the rat atrium might represent the α_{2B}-adrenoceptor subtype [120, 122], comparison of functional dissociation constants for a series of antagonists as inhibitors of UK 14,304 induced inhibition with radioligand binding affinities for the four α_2-adrenoceptor subtypes shows closest similarity to the α_{2D}-adrenoceptor, although subtle differences exist, suggesting the possibility of a mixed receptor population. Hence it has been postulated [117] that most presynaptic receptors in the rat are of the α_{2D}-adrenoceptor subtype.

In contrast to these results, presynaptic α_2-adrenoceptors in the rabbit are thought to be of the α_{2A}-adrenoceptor subtype, based on studies in cortex [117] and pulmonary artery [123]. The differences in subtype of presynaptic α_2-adrenoceptors between rat and rabbit is based primarily on the higher relative potency of phentolamine versus rauwolscine in rat tissues. The use of this ratio to differentiate α_{2A}- and α_{2D}-adrenoceptors is consistent with the low potency of rauwolscine for the α_{2D}-adrenoceptor (see above).

It has recently been suggested that the prejunctional α_2-adrenoceptor in the human kidney may represent an example of the α_{2C}-adrenoceptor subtype, based on the correlation of the potency of a series of α_2-adrenoceptor antagonists for potentiation of stimulation-induced norepinephrine overflow with their binding affinities at α_2-adrenoceptor subtypes [118]. However, both prazosin and ARC-239 have relatively low potency, and the antagonist potencies correlate very well ($r = 0.96$) with corresponding values for these antagonists [119] in the rat atrium. Hence, like the rat atrium, the presynaptic α_2-adrenoceptor of the human kidney may not correspond precisely to any of the α_2-adrenoceptor subtypes identified via radioligand binding techniques.

Different presynaptic α_2-adrenoceptors in a single tissue, modulating the release of different neurotransmitters, may occur. Prazosin appears to block those receptors controlling stimulation-evoked release of norepinephrine in guinea pig ileum, while having no effect on α_2-adrenoceptors controlling acetylcholine release from the same tissue. Conversely, oxymetazoline activated only those α_2-adrenoceptors controlling acetylcholine release [124]. However, additional studies in this system with other subtype selective antagonists will be required to establish firmly whether these differences result from differences in α_2-adrenoceptor subtype populations on adrenergic and cholinergic neurons.

Little data are available regarding the functional assignment of postjunctional α_2-adrenoceptors to the subtypes identified using radioligand binding techniques. Although it has been suggested that the postjunctional α_2-adrenoceptor of the human saphenous vein has α_{2B}-adrenoceptor characteristics, based on the correlation of dissociation constants for a series of antagonists against norepinephrine-induced contraction with their radioligand binding affinities [121], most studies in this tissue show prazosin to be a weak antagonist of norepinephrine-induced contraction [125]. Furthermore, some contribution of α_1-adrenoceptor blockade to the antagonist action of prazosin and ARC-239 in this tissue cannot be eliminated. A recent report [126] assigns the contractile action of UK 14,304 in the rat caudal artery to the α_{2c}-adrenoceptor, based on correlation of the EC_{50} values for agonists and KB values for antagonists with their affinities for the recombinant α_2-adrenoceptor subtypes.

Functional responses to α_2-adrenoceptor activation can be determined in cells transfected with recombinant α_2-adrenoceptors. Norepinephrine and other agonists will inhibit forskolin-induced activation of adenylate cyclase in cells transfected with human [127, 128] or rat [129, 130] α_2-adrenoceptors. Subtype-dependent differences were observed in both the potency of several agonists as inhibitors of adenylate cyclase and in the maximum inhibition observed [127]. However, the functional agonist potency did not necessarily relate to receptor affinity, as determined by inhibition of [^{3}H] rauwolscine binding to these cells. Consistent with its selectivity profile in binding assays using both tissue homogenates and recombinant α_2-adrenoceptors, oxymetazoline was most potent as an inhibitor of adenylate cyclase in cells expressing the α_{2a}-adrenoceptor [127]. However, other agonists, including norepinephrine, showed functional selectivity that was not reflected in their binding affinity. Furthermore, both the absolute affinity and relative subtype selectivity of clonidine showed marked differences between the two studies thus far reported [127, 128], suggesting that these assays may be dependent on either differences in experimental conditions or differences related to cellular expression, such as receptor density or characteristics of the cells in which the recombinant receptor is expressed.

Recently, the gene expressing the α_{2c}-adrenoceptor has been inactivated in mice [131]. The resulting animals show the expected reduction in α_2-adrenoceptor density in areas of the brain known to possess a high density of the α_{2c}-adrenoceptor subtype, but show no apparent defects in their behavior or reproductive capability. Further evaluation of these animals should provide evidence for functional roles for this α_2-adrenoceptor subtype.

5.2.2   Functional evidence for additional α_2-adrenoceptor subtypes

Some novel α_2-adrenoceptor antagonists, including SK&F 104078, SK&F 104856 and several related compounds [8], are capable of blocking some α_2-adrenoceptor-mediated responses, such as constriction of peripheral blood vessels, while having no effect on the neuroinhibitory effect of α_2-adrenoceptor agonists in atria from several species or in guinea pig ileum [132–134]. In several *in vivo* models, neither SK&F 104078 or SK&F 104856 produce evidence of prejunctional α_2-adrenoceptor blockade. It was initially suggested that these compounds could differentiate between pre- and postjunctional α_2-adrenoceptors. However, in the field-stimulated rat vas deferens, SK&F 104078 can produce relatively potent blockade of the neuroinhibitory actions of some, but not all, α_2-adrenoceptor agonists [57, 135]. Hence, it is more appropriate to assume that these antagonists can discriminate between α_2-adrenoceptors on a functional, rather than an anatomical basis. SK&F 104078 and SK&F 104856 are also differentiated from other α_2-adrenoceptor antagonists by their failure to blunt the hyper-glycemic response to oral glucose challenge in the conscious rat [133,134], and SK&F 104856 does not potentiate epinephrine-induced lipolysis in the anesthetized rat (Hieble and Kolpak, unpublished data). Hence these two antagonists do not appear to interact with the α_2-adrenoceptors on pancreatic islet cells or on adipocytes.

The functional selectivity of these antagonists cannot be explained by their affinity for known α_2-adrenoceptor subtypes. Thus, SK&F 104078 has equal affinity for α_{2A}- and α_{2B}-adrenoceptors, as well as relatively high affinity for the three recombinant human [136, 137] and rat [138] α_2-adrenocep-tors. SK&F 104856 shows a moderate degree of selectivity for the α_{2B}-adrenoceptor in radioligand binding assays [96] and for the recombinant human α_{2b}-adrenoceptor [8, 39]. It has been suggested, therefore, that the prejunctional α_2-adrenoceptor may represent the α_{2D}-adrenoceptor sub-type, since SK&F 104078 has relatively low affinity against [^{3}H] rauwol-scine binding in the bovine pineal gland, a tissue known to contain the α_{2D}-adrenoceptor [139]. However, SK&F 104078 has higher affinity in other test systems assigned to the α_{2D}-adrenoceptor subtype, and the other functionally selective α_2-adrenoceptor antagonist, SK&F 104856, has rel-atively high affinity for the α_{2D}-adrenoceptor in the bovine pineal or rat submaxillary gland [95].

Because there are several functional α_2-adrenoceptor models, both *in vitro* and *in vivo*, where these antagonists are inactive or extremely weak, it is likely that additional α_2-adrenoceptor subtypes remain to be cloned. As in the case of the prazosin-insensitive α_1-adrenoceptors, which have also not yet been cloned, those α_2-adrenoceptors that are insensitive to SK&F 104078 and SK&F 104856 may represent a distinct class of α_2-adrenocep-tors, having a lower degree of sequence similarity to the known α_2-adren-oceptors to be detected by homology screening using probes prepared from the known α_2-adrenoceptors.

6 Application of α-adrenoceptor subtype selectivity to the design of novel therapeutic agents

An important consequence of the subclassification of α-adrenoceptors is the identification of subtype-selective agonists and antagonists. In addition to their utility as pharmacologic tools, these agents may offer therapeutic advantages over currently available drugs that have little or no subtype selectivity.

Efforts to design subtype selective α_1-adrenoceptor antagonists are now focused on the design of selective α_{1A}-adrenoceptor antagonists for the treatment of benign prostatic hypertrophy. The goal is to identify a drug that can block the α_1-adrenoceptor on prostatic smooth muscle without blocking vascular α_1-adrenoceptors. Such agents would reduce cardiovascular side effects, such as dizziness, orthostatic hypotension and syncope, which are associated with the α_1-adrenoceptor antagonists currently utilized in the treatment of benign prostatic hypertrophy. Several highly selective α_{1a}-adrenoceptor antagonists have been shown to produce potent blockade of phenylephrine-induced contraction of human prostate [35], and one of these agents, SNAP-5150, while being 5-fold more potent than terazosin as a functional antagonist in isolated human prostatic strips [35], is 100-fold less potent than terazosin in an anesthetized rat model of orthostatic hypotension [140]. Despite this and other evidence suggesting an important role of the α_{1A}-adrenoceptor in prostatic smooth muscle contraction, one must remain cautious inasmuch as other highly potent and selective α_{1A}-adrenoceptor antagonists, such as RS-17043 [91], are only weak antagonists of the α_1-adrenoceptors in human prostate. It is likely, therefore, that another α_1-adrenoceptor subtype, as yet uncharacterized using molecular biology techniques, is also involved in the adrenoceptor- mediated contractile response of prostatic smooth muscle.

While there is currently less interest in α_1-adrenoceptor antagonists as antihypertensive drugs, this pharmacological class offers one highly desirable therapeutic advantage, namely the reduction in low-density plasma lipoproteins [141]. The particular α_1-adrenoceptor subtype(s) involved in the control of vascular resistance is not known with certainty, and may vary between species and/or vascular beds. Furthermore, little is known regarding the α_1-adrenoceptor subtype involved in modulation of plasma lipoproteins. However, it is possible that an α_1-adrenoceptor antagonist having a specific subtype selectivity profile, perhaps combining affinities for several α_1-adrenoceptor subtypes, could offer a useful profile as an antihypertensive/ antihyperlipidemic drug.

In addition to its activity as a centrally acting antihypertensive drug, the α_2-adrenoceptor agonist, clonidine, is utilized clinically for a variety of other indications, such as the suppression of the symptoms of opiate withdrawal [142], analgesia or preanesthetic medication [143], and attention deficit hyperactivity disorder [144]. Other α_2-adrenoceptor agonists, such as guanfacine and dexmedetomidine, are being utilized or evaluated for several of these indications [143, 144]. Although radioligand binding studies show clonidine to have some selectivity for the α_{2a}-adrenoceptor (Table 10; [145]), functional studies in cells expressing human α_2-adrenoceptors show nearly equal potency at all three α_2-adrenoceptor subtypes [127]. α_2-Adrenoceptor activation produces a wide variety of effects, and it is possible that at least some of these could be mediated by different α_2-adrenoceptor subtypes. The α_2-adrenoceptor subtype responsible for centrally mediated blood pressure reduction has not been determined; indeed, at least in some models, there is evidence that a non-adrenergic imidazoline receptor may be involved in this action [146]. The sedative/hypnotic action of medetomidine appears to be mediated by the α_{2A}-adrenoceptor [143]. An agonist having selectivity for the α_{2A}-adrenoceptor may therefore have advantages over clonidine or medetomidine for this indication.

α_2-Adrenoceptor antagonists have not yet been successfully developed as therapeutic agents, despite pharmacological evidence that such compounds could be effective for a variety of indications, including as hypertension [147, 148], depression [149], impotence, non-insulin dependent diabetes and obesity [150]. It is also possible that combined blockade of α_1- and α_2-adrenoceptors may offer advantages over selective α_1-adrenoceptor blockade in the treatment of benign prostatic hypertrophy [151, 152]. Many α_2-adrenoceptor antagonists elevate plasma norepinephrine levels through the blockade of the prejunctional α_2-adrenoceptors that inhibit neuronal neurotransmitter release [153]. This prejunctional blockade may give rise to a variety of cardiovascular side effects when α_2-adrenoceptor blockade at other sites is desired. Recent evidence suggests that vascular α_2-adrenoceptors on a rat blood vessel, the caudal artery, may be of a different subtype (i.e., α_{2c} [126]), than the prejunctional α_2-adrenoceptor in this species (i.e., α_{2d} [154]). This difference may offer the possibility for selective targeting of α_2-adrenoceptor blockade. In addition, the possibility of blocking some, but not all, α_2-adrenoceptor mediated responses has been demonstrated with novel antagonists, such as SK&F 104856 [155]. The therapeutic implications of this functional selectivity remain to be explored.

Table 1.
Affinity of subtype selective α_1-adrenoceptor agonists and antagonists as determined by inhibition of radioligand binding to native tissue homogenates

Compound (Subtype)	Rat Submaxillary Gland[a] α_{1A}	Rat Hippocampus[b] α_{1A}	Rat Liver[c] α_{1B}	Rat Spleen[d] α_{1B}	MDCK-DI Cells[e] α_{1B}
Oxymetazoline	3.2	4.5, 21	193 ± 7.3 (3)	245	380
WB-4101	0.1	0.61 ± 0.25 (3)	7.6 ± 3.4 (6)	5.9 ± 2.9 (4)	6.3
5-Methylurapidil	0.7, 0.6	1.0, 0.53	80 ± 40 (4)	63 ± 28 (3)	676
(+) Niguldipine	0.25	2.1, 0.1	113 ± 77 (4)	267, 12	11
RS-17053	0.7		16		
Spiperone	7.2, 7.9		1.0 ± 0.4 (3)		

[a] Data from Michel et al., 1989; Ford et al., 1994; Ford et al., 1995; Ward et al., 1995 [9, 22, 23, 91].

[b] Data from Han et al., 1987; Michel et al., 1995; Hanft and Gross, 1989; Han and Mineman, 1991; Minneman et al., 1988. Although the predominant α_1-adrenoceptor subtype in this tissue is the α_{1A}-adrenoceptor, binding to α_{1B}-adrenoceptors is also observed by most investigators, as evidenced by biphasic inhibition of the binding of a non-selective radioligand. The values shown here represent the high affinity component of this binding interaction [2, 20, 27, 28, 157].

[c] Data from Minneman et al., 1988; Han and Minneman, 1991; Garcia-Sainz et al., 1992; Michel et al., 1989; Hiramatsu et al., 1994; Testa et al., 1994; Testa et al., 1993; Hanft and Gross, 1989; Michel et al., 1995; Han et al., 1987 [2, 19, 20, 22, 24, 25, 27, 28, 44, 157].

[d] Data from Han et al., 1987; Minneman et al., 1988; Han and Minneman, 1991; Michel et al., 1995; Tsuchihashi et al., 1991; Hieble and Naselsky, unpublished data [2, 18, 20, 28, 75, 157].

[e] Data from Klijn et al., 1991 [18]. MDCK-D1 cells are derived from canine renal distal tubule/collecting duct.

Table 2.
Affinities of α_1-adrenoceptor antagonists for recombinant receptor subtypes

Compound	α_{1A} (human)	α_{1A} (bovine)	α_{1B} (human)	α_{1B} (hamster)	α_{1D} (human)	α_{1D} (rat)	Reference	Notes
Prazosin	0.2			0.19	0.16	0.16	[158]	COS, [^{125}I] HEAT
	0.39		0.07		0.04	0.08	[159]	COS, [^{125}I] HEAT
	0.13	0.50	0.32	0.13		0.3	[12]	Rat-1, [^{125}I] HEAT
					0.33		[11]	L-Cells, [^{3}H] Prazosin
	0.58		0.55	0.037			[34, 35]	L-Cells, [^{3}H] Prazosin
			0.035	0.25			[160]	COS, [^{3}H] Prazosin
				0.11		0.31	[14]	COS, [^{3}H] Prazosin
		0.06		0.066			[161]	HeLa, [^{125}I] HEAT
		0.18		0.56		0.19	[162]	HeLa, [^{3}H] Prazosin
		0.37		0.14		0.33	[13, 136]	COS, [^{125}I] HEAT
				0.38		0.39	[163]	CHO, [^{125}I] HEAT
	0.57	2.19		0.46		1.94	[164]	Rat-1, [^{125}I] HEAT
	0.22	0.60	0.28	0.05	0.29	0.10	[44]	CHO, [^{3}H] Prazosin
		0.19				0.32	[165]	LTK-, [^{3}H] Prazosin
				0.19		0.20	[166]	Rat-1, [^{3}H] Prazosin
	2.4	0.60		0.15			[166]	Rat-1, [^{125}I] HEAT
							[167]	Sf9 (Insect), [^{125}I] HEAT
					0.27		[33]	293, [^{125}I] HEAT
Terazosin	7.1			2.7	4.6	2.5	[158]	
	8.2		0.89		4.0		[159]	
	25	32	4.0	3.2	3.5	5.0	[12]	
	6.9		1.9				[34, 35]	
		3.0		0.7		1.8	[161]	
		39.8		2.4		3.5	[163]	
	6.9	26	2.2	30	2.4	35	[37]	
	2.0	3.3		0.7		1.1	[164]	
	15						[166]	
Phentolamine	1.4		200	22	31.6	11	[158]	
	20	12.5		79		20	[12]	

Compound							Ref	Preparation
Phentolamine (continued)	10	26		70	10	43	[61]	COS, [125I] HEAT
			0.95				[159]	
		31	15.3	39		138	[11]	
			2.0	82		12.9	[160]	
			33.8	15		111	[14]	
			1.3	340		16	[162]	
						55	[13,136]	COS, [3H] Prazosin
	2.9			52	24	4.6	[168]	
				6.8			[164]	
							[165]	
				40		6.1	[33]	
	20			88		35	[166]	
			18				[166]	
	4.9	25	3.2	89	14.6	68	[167]	
							[37]	
WB-4101	0.23	10		4.5	1.25	0.31	[158]	
	1.25	1.6		7.9	0.59	1.25	[12]	
	0.4		0.63				[159]	
				6.2	0.91	2	[61]	
	0.39	4.6		7.0			[11]	
		7.0		5.9			[34,35]	
			0.70	12		1.9	[160]	
			0.08	3.7		0.42	[14]	
			0.68	28.6		2.1	[161]	
				5.2			[162]	
				6.9			[13,136]	
	0.33	3.2	1.38	57.5	0.63	1.34	[163]	
	0.10		0.62	0.63		6.3	[164]	
			0.04	16		0.12	[37]	
						0.67	[165]	
						0.71	[166]	
							[166]	
							[167]	
	4.9		0.55	4.8	0.66		[33]	

Table 2. (Continued).

Compound	α_{1A} (human)	α_{1A} (bovine)	α_{1B} (human)	α_{1B} (hamster)	α_{1D} (human)	α_{1D} (rat)	Reference	Notes
5-Methylurapidil	4.1			160		32	[158]	
	2						[159]	
	3.2	2.0	23	316	30	79	[12]	
			251	430	63		[61]	
						40	[11]	COS, [3H] Prazosin
	2.1				12.3		[34, 35]	
			174	70		15	[160]	
			64	41			[14]	
		6.8		340		18	[161]	
		1.3		62			[162]	
				180			[163]	
		3.1		51		630	[207]	
		0.63		91		14	[165]	
		2.6				62	[164]	
		2.0		1047		501	[37]	
	2.8		81	57	18	9.8	[166]	[3H] Prazosin
		2.9		145		5.5	[166]	[125I] HEAT
							[167]	
	11				16		[33]	
Spiperone	158	32	40	32	25	40	[12]	
						14	[11]	
		2.2		0.9		5.0	[162]	
		68		11.2		29	[164]	
						7.9	[62]	[125I] HEAT
	15.4	18	0.97	13	4.9	41	[166]	
		13		7.1		22	[37]	
(+) Niguldipine	7.9	10	790	500	500	500	[12]	
						209	[11]	
	1.8		85		190		[34, 35]	

Drug							Ref.
(+) Niguldipine (continued)	0.1	55	44	41	430	46	[159]
		0.38		776		831	[14]
				25	200	83	[164]
							[37]
							[33]
Indoramin	13	29	41	21	182	69	[158]
		5.0	12	226	38	611	[13, 136]
	4.5			58		446	[34, 35]
	2.8	1.5		25		275	[164]
	2.8			4.8		63	[37]
						0.4	[62]
							[165]
Abanoquil	0.04	0.08		0.07	0.04		[61]
		0.08			0.05		[34, 35]
				0.13		0.06	Hieble, unreported data
							[37]
							CHO, [³H] Prazosin
Tamsulosin	0.035	0.03	0.63	0.7	0.09	0.11	[158]
		0.15	0.29	8.5	0.06	0.08	[61]
	0.05	0.03		0.88		1.8	[163]
	0.83			6.8		0.07	[207]
	0.03			0.21			[37]
	0.02						[167]
							[165]
							[168]
Yohimbine	770	1562		680	289	440	[158]
	1057	334		1003	165		[160]
				670			[163]
							Hieble, unreported data
							[33]

Table 3.
Selective α_{1a}-adrenoceptor antagonists, as characterized by affinity for recombinant α_1-adrenoceptors

Compound	Structure	α_{1a}	α_{1b}	α_{1d}	Reference
SNAP-5089		1.5	111	315	Hieble and Naselsky, unpublished data
		0.35	220	540	[138]
Indoramin		2.8	12	38	Hieble and Naselsky, unpublished data
		4.5	41	182	[34, 35]
RS-17053		0.6	14	17	[91]
SB 216469 (Rec 15/2739)		0.74	19	6.4	[37]
		4.4	72	154	[39]

Table 4.
Subtype selective α_1-adrenoceptor antagonists, as characterized by affinity for reombinant α_1-adrenoceptors

Compound	Structure	α_{1a}	α_{1b}	α_{1d}	Reference
AH 11110A		2500	76	2750	[40]

		161	40	382	[41]
BMY 7378		251	63	0.4	[169]

| SK&F 104856 | | 36 | 23 | 1.6 | [8] |

| SK&F 105854 | | 3300 | 783 | 72 | [8] |

Table 5.
Affinity of α-adrenoceptor agonists for recombinant receptors as determined by radioligand binding assay

Compound	α_{1A} (human)	α_{1A} (bovine)	α_{1B} (human)	α_{1B} (hamster)	α_{1D} (human)	α_{1D} (rat)	Reference	Notes
Norepinephrine	1700						[158]	COS, [^{125}I] HEAT
	20,000	20,000	4000	1300	200	51	[12]	Rat-1, [^{125}I] HEAT
				2000		125	[11]	L, [^{3}H] Prazosin
	7940				1550	254	[34, 35]	L, [^{3}H] Prazosin
			13,800	1900			[160]	COS, [^{3}H] Prazosin
			1800	13,500		1400	[61]	COS, [^{3}H] Prazosin
	17,200			2900			[161]	HeLa, [^{125}I] HEAT
		40,700		10,000		500	[65]	HEK 293 [^{125}I] HEAT
		9730				100	[13,136]	COS, [^{125}I] HEAT
				920			[163]	CHO, [^{125}I] HEAT
		38,900		3200		234	[164]	Rat-1, [^{125}I] HEAT
		4600		17,400		776	Testa, unpublished data	COS, [^{3}H] Prazosin
				3200		40	[7]	COS, [^{125}I] HEAT
		316				320	[207]	
				1210			[14]	COS, [^{3}H] Prazosin
	7500						[170]	
	557		1046		167		Hieble, unpublished data	CHO, [^{3}H] Prazosin
					269		1995 [33]	HEK 293, [^{125}I] HEAT
		436		288		20	[165]	LTK-, [^{3}H] Prazosin
Phenylephrine	2900		1150	23,000	1030	260	[158]	
	14,900		18,600		3200		[159]	
	8320						[34, 35]	
		2100		6200		426	[162]	
		72,400		6200		1620	[161]	
		28,200		93,300		3600	Testa, unpublished data	

Compound										Ref.	
Phenylephrine (continued)		12,600				13,400				[161]	
						6500				[7]	
						12,000				[163]	
		47,800				13,500		1440		[13, 136]	
		20,000				27,700		1380		[65]	
								24,600		[61]	
								1808		[11]	
	3061	933	3860	1260	1585			162		[165] Hieble, unpublished data	
[-]-Epinephrine	2000	7940	3200	840	250		56		[158]	
	10,000			1580			250		[12]	
				7100	970		130		[61]	COS, [125I] HEAT
	6600		360						[159]	
				230			393		[11]	
							239		[14]	
		6250		650			546		[13, 136]	
									[163]	
		14,800		1510			251		[168]	
		6400		1800					[164]	
				2000					[161]	
				9800					[7]	
	2570	14,500	4370	141	489		512		[65]	COS, [3H] Prazosin
	2500	295					32		[34, 35]	
									[165]	
									[170]	
Methoxamine	17,000	250,000	2,000,000	170,000	79,400		9900		[158]	
	79,400		664,000	500,000	29,700		63,000		[12]	
	73,600		2,119,000						[159]	
							661,000		[61]	
							5422		[11]	
		85,300	495,000	619,000					[160]	
				527,000					[161]	

Compound	α_{1A} (human)	α_{1A} (bovine)	α_{1B} (human)	α_{1B} (hamster)	α_{1D} (human)	α_{1D} (rat)	Reference	Notes
Methoxamine (continued)		6160		123,000		15,100	[162]	
		203,000				110,000	[13, 136]	
							[163]	COS, [^{3}H] Prazosin
		741,000		160,000		151,000	[164]	
		3,200		1,000,000		12,580	[168]	
		148,000		417,000		31,600	[65]	
		5,500		44,700		5,800	[165]	
	19,000						[170]	
Oxymetazoline	23			390		490	[158]	
	15					610	[159]	
	16	25	110	158	794	794	[12]	
			398	4,400		37,000	[61]	
						1099	[11]	
				120			[34, 35]	
			110				[160]	
		13					[14]	
		15		190			[161]	
				223			[162]	
				380		954	[207]	
				229			[164]	
		102		2700		1780	Testa, unpublished data	
		66				2800	[7]	
		114		140			[13, 136]	
		32		173		2140	[65]	
						602	[170]	
	28	13		204		338	[165]	
			356		1124		Hieble, unpublished data	
	14.8				346		[33]	

Table 6.
Functional antagonist potency of 5-methylurapidil in rat vas deferens, aorta and spleen

K_B (Vas Deferens)	K_B(Aorta)	K_B (Spleen)	Reference
1.9	10	65	[32]
0.8	93		[171]
3.7	7.6	240	[58]
	18		[172]
	53		[59]
	8.5		[60]
4.1	15	68	[165]
	23		[37]
6.0		110	[49]
2.0		79	[173]
	16		[62]
	24		[57]
3.1 ± 0.7	27 ± 8.0	112 ± 29	

Table 7.
Functional potency of prazosin in prostatic tissue

Species	K_B (nM)[a]	Reference
Human	4.0	[174]
	5.1	[175]
	11	[176]
	2.0	[177]
	2.0	[178]
	3.0	[179]
	1.3*	[180]
	0.7	[34, 35]
Dog	18	[153]
	13	[181]
	12	[72]
	3.5	[165]
Rabbit	10	[181]
	10	Hieble, unpublished data

[a]K_B versus norepinephrine or phenylephrine-induced contraction
*Prostatic Urethra

Table 8.
Correspondence between the characteristics of recombinant and pharmacologically defined α_2-adrenoceptors

Clone	Species	Name	Pharmacology
α_{2a}	human	α_2-C10	α_{2A}
	pig		α_{2A}
	rat	RG20	α_{2D}
	mouse	$M\alpha_2$-l0H	α_{2D}
α_{2b}	human	α_2-C2	α_{2B}
	rat	RNG	α_{2B}
	mouse	$M\alpha_2$-2H	α_{2B}
α_{2c}	human	α_2-C4	α_{2C}
	rat	RG10 (pA2d, RBα_{2B}	α_{2C}
	mouse	$M\alpha_2$-4H	α_{2C}
	opossum		α_{2C}

Table 9.
Radioligand binding affinities of antagonists to α_2-adrenoceptor subtypes

Source	K_i (nM)[*]				affinity ratio			
	YOH	RAU	PRZ	OXY	PRZ/ OXY	OXY/ YOH	PRZ/ YOH	
human platelet	0.9	1.3	540	3.5	154	3.8	600	a
HT-29 cell	1.8	1.2	2000	2.2	923	1.2	1128	b
human adipocyte	3	4	2200	16	137	5	733	[183]
canine adipocyte	4		2700	16	158	4	675	[183]
α_{2a}-(human)	3.8	4.7	1600	10.5	153	2.8	423	c
α_{2a}-(porcine)	4.4		4100	21	197	5	941	[94]
neonatal rat lung	1	0.4	5	52	0.1	52	5	[22]
rat kidney	5	2.5	51	220	0.2	44	10	[4]
NG-108 cell	0.6	0.8	13	132	0.1	220	22	d
α_{2b}-(human)	4.1	3.9	108	1000	0.1	245	26	e
α_{2b}-(rat)	8.7	9.6	46	610	0.1	70	5.3	f
α_{2b}-(mouse)	12	73	59	1200	0 1	100	5	[184]

Table 9. (Continued).

| Source | K_i (nM)* | | | | affinity ratio | | | |
	YOH	RAU	PRZ	OXY	PRZ/ OXY	OXY/ YOH	PRZ/ YOH	
opossum kidney	0.4	0.1	36	73	0.5	182	90	[105]
OK cell	0.6	0.3	34	26	1.3	43	57	g
Y-79 cell		0.4	123	14	8.8	35**	307**	[102]
α_{2c}-(human)	0.6	0.8	40	73	0.5	122	67	h
α_{2c}-(mouse)	3.8	0.8	97	109	0.9	29	26	[185]
α_{2c}-(rat)	2.4	0.9	53	140	0.4	58	22	i
α_{2c}-(opossum)	0.1	0.2		29			263	[186]
hamster adipocyte	33		2260	3	753	0.1	68	[187]
rabbit adipocyte	35		10000	14	642	0.4	285	[182]
rat adipocyte	70		1800	54	34	0.7	27	[188]
rat enterocyte	54	45	1900	10	190	0.2	35	[189]
rat submaxillary		18	457	8	57**	0.4**	25**	j
RINm5F cell	104	83	1900	121	16	1.2	18	[190]
bovine pineal	3.6	3.4	106	1.5	71	0.4	29	[95]
α_{2d}-(rat)	52	51	2065	28	74	0.5	40	k
α_{2d}-(mouse)	54	53	2150	33	65	0.6	40	[185]

* K_i for inhibition of the binding of [^{3}H] yohimbine, [^{3}H] rauwolscine, [^{3}H] RX 821002 or [^{3}H] MK-912 to membrane homogenates.

** oxymetazoline/rauwolscine or prazosin/rauwolscine

a Mean values from data reported by Bylund, 1990; Hieble and Naselsky, 1993; Brown et al., 1990; Daiguji et al., 1982 [100, 191–193].

b Mean values from data reported by Gleason and Hieble, 1991; Bylund et al., 1992; Langin et al., 1989 [96, 194, 195].

c Mean values from data reported by Lanier et al., 1991, Lomasney et al., 1991a; Bylund et al., 1992 and unpublished data from our laboratory [13, 120, 194].

d Mean values from Murphy and Bylund, 1988 and Gleason and Hieble, 1991 [96, 104].

e Mean values from Lomasney et al., 1991b; Bylund et al., 1992; Weinshank et al., 1990 and unpublished data from our laboratory [136, 194, 196].

f Mean values from Harrison et al., 1991 and Xia et al., 1993 [113, 114, 138].

g Mean values from Bylund et al., 1992 and Gleason and Hieble, 1992 [102, 194].

h Mean values from Lomasney et al., 1991; Lomasney et al., 1990 and Bylund et al., 1992 [13, 194, 197].

i Mean values from Harrison et al., 1991; Lanier et al., 1991; Flordellis et al., 1990; Voigt et al., 1991 and Uhlen et al., 1992 [106, 129, 130, 138, 198].

j Mean values from Simonneaux et al., 1992 and Gleason and Hieble, 1992 [102, 199].

k Mean values from Harrison et al., 1991 and Lanier et al., 1991 [129, 138].

Table 10.
Affinity of agonists for the recombinant α_2-adrenoceptors, as determined by radioligand binding assays

Compound	α_{2a} (human)	α_{2b} (human)	α_{2c} (human)	α_{2d} (rat)	Reference	Notes
Norepinephrine	3677	1265	606		[197]	COS, [3H] Yohimbine
	2471		342		[185]	COS, [3H] Yohimbine
	3456			5759*	[185]	COS, [3H] Atipamezole
				3576	[129]	COS, [3H] Rauwolscine
				633	[138]	COS, [3H] Rauwolscine
	515			3007*	[202]	COS, [3H] RX821002
				3190	[202]	COS, [3H] RX821002
				19,000	[115]	[3H] RX821002
	7500				[5]	Xenopus, [3H] Yohimbine
		370			[200]	Yeast, [3H] Rauwolscine
		1146			[200]	S 115, [3H] Rauwolscine
		965			[200]	Sf-9, [3H] Rauwolscine
	5740				Hieble, unpublished	COS, [3H] Rauwolscine
	933				Hieble, unpublished	CHO, [3H] Rauwolscine
	44	284	85		[110]	S 115, [3H] RX821002
	88	475	191		[127]	S115, [3H] Rauwolscine
Epinephrine	1671	1851	318		[197]	COS, [3H] Yohimbine
		255			[198]	L, [3H] Rauwolscine
	1170		218		[185]	COS, [3H] Yohimbine
	1434			2512*	[185]	COS, [3H] Atipamezole
				2100	[129]	
				5900	[115]	
	1900				[5]	
	3756				Hieble, unpublished	COS, [3H] Rauwolscine
	357				Hieble, unpublished	CHO, [3H] Rauwolscine

Oxymetazoline	13	1506	125		[197]	COS, [³H] Yohimbine
	13	213	206		[196]	COS, [³H] Atipamezole
	15			33*	[185]	
				43	[185]	
				12.3	[129]	
	13	1435	180		[138]	COS, [³H] RX821002
				17	[201]	
				38	[202]	
	11	1558			[115]	
		889			Hieble, unpublished	COS, [³H] Rauwolscine
		2986			[200]	Yeast, [³H] Rauwolscine
		2407			[200]	S115, [³H] Rauwolscine
	3.3	754	31		[200]	Sf-9, [³H] Rauwolscine
	4.0	40	20		[194]	COS, [³H] Rauwolscine
	2.0	1406	52		[126]	
	2.8	1798	220		[110]	S115, [³H] RX821002
					[127]	S115, [³H] Rauwolscine
p-NH₂-Clonidine	31	120	97		[197]	COS, [³H] Yohimbine
		4.5			[196]	COS, [³H] Atipamezole
	77		204	77*	[185]	
					[185]	
	140				[5]	Xenopus, [³H] Yohimbine
Clonidine		7.2		16	[196]	
	7.9	6.2	56		[138]	L, [³H] Rauwolscine
	10.7	40	134		[128]	
					[127]	S115, [³H] Rauwolscine

* Mouse α_{2d} adrenoceptor

Table 11.
Affinities of antagonists for the recombinant α_2-adrenoceptors, as determined by radioligand binding assays

Compound	α_{2a} (human)	α_{2b} (human)	α_{2c} (human)	α_{2d} (rat)	Reference	Notes
Rauwolscine	0.32	0.37	0.13		[194]	COS, [3H] Rauwolscine
				19	[107]	COS, [3H] RX821002
		5.5			[200]	Yeast, K_d
		5.6			[200]	S115, K_d
		5.7			[200]	Sf-9, K_d
	2.1		0.43		[203]	COS, K_d
	3.5				[5]	Xenopus, [3H] Yohimbine
	5.0	5.0	1.0		[137]	S115, [3H] Rauwolscine
	0.62				[108]	CHO, [3H] RX821002
				28.3	[138]	COS, K_d
	9			51	[129]	COS, [3H] Rauwolscine
	4.6		1.7		[185]	COS, [3H] Yohimbine
				53*	[185]	COS, [3H] Atipamezole
		0.32			[196]	L, [3H] Rauwolscine
	7.1	11	2.1		[197]	COS, [3H] Yohimbine
	1.7	2.2		16*	[204]	CHO, [3H] Rauwolscine
	0.76			19	[202]	COS, [3H] RX821002
				62	[202]	COS, [3H] RX821002
					[115]	
				4.0	[126]	L, [3H] Rauwolscine
Yohimbine	0.50	1.18	0.30		[194]	COS, [3H] Rauwolscine
	1.6		0.93		[203]	
	4.4				[5]	
	23	4.3	0.8		[137]	COS, [3H] RX821002
	3.51	6.27	2.03		[201]	COS, [3H] Rauwolscine
				42.6	[138]	
	7			61	[129]	
			3.1		[185]	COS, [3H] Yohimbine
	3.4			53.6*	[185]	COS, [3H] Atipamezole

Compound					Reference	Preparation
Yohimbine (continued)	0.77	1.2			[196]	
	1.6	6.3			[204]	
	0.9	7.2	1.1		Hieble, unpublished data	
				22*	[202]	CHO, [3H] Rauwolscine
				72	[115]	
RX821002				0.54	[107]	K_d
	2.2	11.3			[200]	Yeast, [3H] Rauwolscine
	0.29	9.3			[200]	S115, [3H] Rauwolscine
	1.46	12.5			[200]	Sf-9, [3H] Rauwolscine
	0.4	4.6	2.5		[137]	
		9.82	6.77	2.5*	[108]	CHO, K_d
					[201]	
					[202]	
Phentolamine	4.1	6.8	12.7	4.9	[194]	
	10		33		[107, 108]	
	27				[203]	
	18	3.1	52		[5]	
	4.9	6.9	26.1	3.2	[137]	
					[201]	
	11		14.4	14	[138]	
	6.2	9.2	8.4		[129]	
	2.6	7.6			[197]	
					Hieble, unpublished data	
Prazosin	302	30.6	10.7	890	[194]	
					[107]	
	1800	376	41		[200]	Yeast, [3H] Rauwolscine
	880	310	98		[200]	S115, [3H] Rauwolscine
	2750	374			[200]	Sf-9, [3H] Rauwolscine
		108			[203]	
					[5]	
					[137]	

Table 11. (Continued).

Compound	α_{2a} (human)	α_{2b} (human)	α_{2c} (human)	α_{2d} (rat)	Reference	Notes
Prazosin (continued)	560				[108]	
	4687	366	199		[201]	
				2530	[138]	
	2790			1586	[129]	
	2034		121		[185]	COS, [3H] Yohimbine
				2157*	[185]	COS, [3H] Atipamezole
		23	68		[196]	
			95		[197]	
	2237	293			Hieble, unpublished data	
	2133	365	22		[205]	L, [3H] Rauwolscine
	174	23			[202]	
	1371			3007	[126]	
				251	[110]	
	769	67	19	930	[115]	S115, [3H] RX821002 [3H] RX821002
ARC-239	131	2.67	3.82		[194]	
				365	[107]	
	219	176	219		[108]	
	2914	12.5			[201]	
	602	10	21		[204]	
	373				Hieble, unpublished data	
				810	[115]	
SK&F 104856	24	3.4	21		[8]	CHO, [3H] Rauwolscine
	50	3.2	25		[39]	L, [3H] Rauwolscine
Corynanthine	710		73		[203]	
	2200				[5]	
	1246	469	113		[201]	
				1250	[138]	
		77	182		[196]	
	1188	1002			[197]	

* Mouse α_{2d} adrenoceptor

References

1   Morrow, A.L. and I. Creese: Mol. Pharmacol. *29*, 321 (1986).

2   Han, C., P.W. Abel and K.P. Minneman: *329*, 333 (1987).

3   Bylund, D.B.: Pharmacol. Biochem. Behav. *22*, 835 (1985).

4   Bylund, D.B., C. Ray-Prenger and T.J. Murphy: J. Pharmacol. Exp. Ther. *245*, 600 (1988).

5   Kobilka, B.K., T. Frielle, S. Collins, T. Yang-Feng, T.S. Kobilka, U. Francke, R.J. Lefkowitz and M.G. Caron: Nature *329*, 75 (1987).

6   Kobilka, B.K., H. Matsui, T.S. Kobilka, T.L. Yang-Feng, U. Francke, M.G. Caron, R.J. Lefkowitz and J.W. Regan: Science *238*, 650 (1987).

7   Cotecchia, S., D.A. Schwinn, R.R. Randall, R.J. Lefkowitz, M.G. Caron and B.K. Kobilka: Proc. Natl. Acad. Sci. USA *85*, 7159 (1988).

8   Hieble, J.P., Bylund, D.B., Clarke, D.E., Eikenberg, D.C., Langer, S.Z., Lefkowitz, R.J., Minneman, K.P. and R.R. Ruffolo, Jr.: Pharmacol. Rev. *47*, 267 (1995).

9   Ford, A.P.D.W., T.J. Williams, D.R. Blue and D.E. Clarke: Trends in Pharmacol. Sci. *15*, 167 (1994).

10   Schwinn, D.A., Lomasney, J.W., Lorenz, W., Szklut, P.J., Fremeau, R.T., Jr., Yang-Feng, T.L., Caron, M.G., Lefkowitz, R.J. and Cotecchia, S.: J. Biol. Chem. *265*, 8183 (1990).

11   Laz, T.M., C. Forray, K.E. Smith, J.A. Bard, P.J.-J. Vaysse, T.A. Branchek and R.L. Weinshank: Mol. Pharmacol. *46*, 414 (1994).

12   Schwinn, D.A., G.I. Johnson, S.O. Page, M.J. Mosley, K.H. Wilson, N.P. Worman, S. Campbell, M.D. Fidock, L.M. Furness, D.J. Parry-Smith, B. Peter and D.S. Baily: J. Pharmacol. Exp. Ther. *272*, 134 (1995).

13   Lomasney, J.W., S. Cotecchia, R.J. Lefkowitz and M.G. Caron: Biochim. et Biophys. Acta *1095*, 127 (1991).

14   Perez, D.M., M.T. Piascik and R.M. Graham: Mol. Pharmacol. *40*, 876 (1991).

15   Saussy, D.L., A.S. Goetz, H.K. King and T.A. True: Can. J. Physiol. Pharmacol. *72* (Suppl. 1), 323 (1994).

16   Ruffolo, R.R., Jr., Turowski, B.S. and Patil, P.N.: J. Pharm. Pharmacol. *29*, 378 (1977).

17   McGrath, J.C.: Biochem. Pharmacol. *31*, 467 (1982).

18   Klijn, K., S.R. Slivka, K. Bell and P.A. Insel: Mol. Pharmacol. *39*, 407 (1991).

19   Hiramatsu, Y., R. Muraoka, S. Kigoshi and I. Muramatsu: J. Recep. Res. *14*, 75 (1994).

20   Minneman, K.P., C. Han and P.W. Abel: Mol. Pharmacol. *33*, 509 (1988).

21   Noguchi, H., R. Muraoka, S. Kigoshi and I. Muramatsu: Brit. J. Pharmacol. *114*, 1026 (1995).

22   Michel, A.D., Loury, D.N. and Whiting, R.L.: Brit. J. Pharmacol. *98*, 883 (1989).

23   Ward, S.D.C., A.S. Goetz, H.K. King, T.A. True and D.L. Saussy: Can. J. Physiol. Pharmacol. *72* (Suppl. 1), 323 (1994).

24   Garcia-Sainz, J.A., Romero-Avila, M.A., Alcantara-Hernandez, R., Macias-Silva, M., Olivares-Reyes, J.A. and Gonzales-Espinosa, C.: Biochem. Biophys. Res. Commun. *186*, 760 (1992).

25   Testa, R., L. Guarneri, M. Ibba, G. Strada, E. Poggesi, C. Taddei, I. Simonazzi and A. Leonardi: Eur. J. Pharmacol. *249*, 307 (1993).

26   Han, C., T.A. Esbenshade and K.P. Minneman: Eur. J. Pharmacol. (Mol. Pharmacol.) *226*, 141 (1992).

27   Hanft, G. and G. Gross: Brit. J. Pharmacol. *97*, 691 (1989).

28   Han, C. and K.P. Minneman: Mol. Pharmacol. *40*, 531 (1991).

29   Johnson, R.D. and K.P. Minneman: Mol. Pharmacol. *31*, 239 (1987).

30   Minneman, K.P.: Eur. J. Pharmacol. *94*, 171 (1983).

31   Testa, R., L. Guarneri, E. Poggesi, I. Simonazzi, C. Taddei and A. Leonardi: Brit. J. Pharmacol. *114*, 745 (1995).

32   Ko, F.-N., J.-H. Guh, S.-M. Yu, Y.-S. Hou, Y.-C. Wu and C.-M. Teng: Brit. J. Pharmacol. *112*, 1174 (1994).

33   Esbenshade, T.A., A. Hirasawa, G. Tsujimoto, T. Tanaka, J. Yano, K.P. Minneman and T.J. Murphy: Mol. Pharmacol. *47*, 977 (1995).

34   Forray, C., J.A. Bard, T.M. Laz, K.E. Smith, P.J.J. Vaysse, R.L. Weinshank, C. Gluchowski and T.A. Branchek: FASEB J. *8*, A353 (1994).

35   Forray, C., J.A. Bard, R.L. Weinshank, T.A. Branchek and C. Gluchowski: J. Urol. *151* (5), 267A (1994).

36   Boer, R., A. Grassegger, C. Schudt and H. Glossman: Eur. J. Pharmacol. (Mol. Pharmacol.) *172*, 131 (1989).

37   Testa, R., C. Taddei, E. Poggesi, C. Destefani, S. Cotecchia, J.P. Hieble, A.C. Sulpizio, D.P. Naselsky, D.J. Bergsma, C. Ellis, A. Swift, S. Ganguly, R.R. Ruffolo, Jr. and A. Leonardi: Pharmacol. Comm. *6*, 79 (1995).

38   Wetzel, J.M. and S.W. Miao, C. Forray, L.A. Borden, T.A. Branchek and C. Gluchowski: J. Med. Chem. *38*, 1579 (1995).

39   Gluchowski, C., Wetzel, J.M., Chiu, G., Marzabadi, M., Wong, W.C., Nagarathnam, D.: International Patent Application No. WO 94/22829, October 13, 1994.

40   King, H.K., A.S. Goetz, S.D.C. Ward and D.L. Saussy, Jr.: Soc. for Neuroscience Abstracts *20*, 526 (1994).

41   Leonardi, A., R. Testa, G. Motta, P.G. DeBenedetti, P. Hieble and D. Giardina: In: D. Giardina, A. Piergentili and M. Pigini (Eds.): Perspectives in Receptor Research, Proceedings of the Tenth Camerino-Noordwijkerhout Symposium, September 1995.

42   Ruffolo, R.R., Jr., Bondinell, W., Ku, T., Naselsky, D.P. and Hieble, J.P.: Proc. West. Pharmacol. Soc. *38*, 121, (1995).

43   Yazawa, H. and Honda, K.: Japan J. Pharmacol. *62*, 297 (1993).

44   Testa, R., E. Poggesi, C. Taddei, L. Guarneri, M. Ibba and A. Leonardi: Neurology and Urodynamics *13*, 473 (1994).

45   Garcia-Sainz, J.A., M.-T. Romero-Avila and M.E. Torres-Marquez, M.E.: Eur. J. Pharmacol. (Mol. Pharmacol.) *289*, 81 (1995).

46   Garcia-Sainz, J.A., M.-T. Romero-Avila and C. Gonzales-Espinosa: Eur. J. Pharmacol. *272*, 139 (1995).

47   Starke, K., Rev. Physiol. Biochem. Pharmacol. *88*, 199 (1981).

48   Knepper, S.M., S.A. Buckner, M.E. Brune, J.F. DeBernardis, M.D. Meyer and A.A. Hancock: J. Pharmacol. Exp. Ther. *274*, 97 (1995).

49   Sulpizio, A.C. and J.P. Hieble: Pharmacologist *35*, 166 (1993).

50   Ipsen, M., N. Dragsted and M.J. Mulvany: Pharmacol. Res. *31* (Suppl.) 192 (1995).

51   Blue, D.R., Jr., A.P.D.W. Ford, M.S. Kava, J.R. Pfister, R.L. Vimont, Q.M. Zhu and D.E. Clarke: FASEB J. *9*, A105 (1995).

52   Williams, T.J. and D.E. Clarke: Brit. J. Pharmacol. *114*, 531 (1995).

53   Han, C., J. Li and K.P. Minneman: Eur. J. Pharmacol. *190*, 97 (1990).

54   Oriowo, M.A. and Ruffolo, R.R., Jr.: J. Vasc. Res. *29*, 33 (1992).

55   Wenham, D. and I. Marshall: Br. J. Pharmacol. *107*, 375 (1992).

56   Ruffolo, R.R., Jr., Waddell, J.E. and Yaden, E.L.: J. Pharmacol. Exp. Ther. *221*, 309 (1982).

57   Oriowo, M.A., J.P. Hieble and R.R. Ruffolo, Jr.: Pharmacology *43*, 1 (1991).

58   Aboud, R., M. Shafii and J.R. Docherty: Brit. J. Pharmacol. *109*, 80 (1993).

59 van der Graaf, P.H., N.J. Welsh, N.P. Shankley and J.W. Black: Br. J. Pharmacol. *110*, (1993).

60 van der Graaf, P.H., N.J. Welsh, N.P. Shankley and J.W. Black: Br. J. Pharmacol. *112*, (1994).

61 Perez, D.M., J.L. Chen, N. Malik and R.M. Graham: FASEB J. *8*, A353 (1994).

62 Kenny, B.A., D.H. Chalmers and A.M. Naylor: Brit. J. Pharmacol. *115*, 25P (1995)

63 Price, D.T., R.J. Lefkowitz, M.G. Caron, D. Berkowitz and D.A. Schwinn: Mol. Pharmacol. *45*, 171 (1994).

64 Piascik, M.T., E.E. Soltis and D.M. Perez: Circulation *90*, 144 (1994).

65 Minneman, K.P., T.L. Theroux, S. Hollinger, C. Han and T.A. Esbenshade: Mol. Pharmacol. *46*, 929 (1994).

66 Jagadeesh, G. and R.C. Deth: J. Pharmacol. Exp. Ther. *243*, 430 (1987).

67 Babich, M., N.W. Pedigo, B.T. Butler and M.T. Piascik: Life Sci. *41*, 663 (1987).

68 Mignot, E., S.S. Bowersox, J. Maddaluno, W. Dement and R. Ciaranello: Brain Res. *486*, 56 (1989).

69 Piascik, M.T., J.W. Kusiak, J. Pitha, B.T. Butler, H.T. Le and M. Babich: J. Pharmacol. Exp. Ther. *246*, 1001 (1988).

70 Maruyama, K., H. Tsuchihashi, S. Baba, F. Mano and T. Nagatomo: J. Pharm. Pharmacol. *44*, 727 (1992).

71 Oshita, M., M. Takita, S. Kigoshi and L. Muramatsu: Japan J. Pharmacol. *58* (Suppl. II), 276 (1992).

72 Ohmura, T., S. Sakamoto, H. Hayashi, S. Kogoshi and I. Muramatsu: Japan J. Pharmacol. *58* (Suppl. II), 174 (1992).

73 Oshita, M., S. Kigoshi and I. Muramatsu: Br. J. Pharmacol. *108*, 1071 (1993).

74 Esbenshade, T.A., C. Han and K.P. Minneman: Pharmacol. Comm. *3*, 323 (1993).

75 Tsuchihashi, H., K. Maruyama, S. Baba, F. Mano, J. Kinami and T. Nagatomo: Japan J. Pharmacol. *56*, 523 (1991).

76 Takeda, T., Hatano, A., Takahashi, H., Tamaki, M., Koneyama, T., Mizusawa, T., Koizumi, T., Tsutsui, T., Sato, S., Maruyama, K. and Nagatomo, T.: J. Urol. *149*, 241A (1993).

77 Agrawal, D.K., C.R. Triggle and E.E. Daniel: J. Pharmacol. Exp. Ther. *229*, 831 (1984).

78 Drew, G.M.: Clin. Sci. *68* (Suppl. 10), 15s (1985).

79 Wilson, V.G., C.M. Brown and J.C. McGrath: Exp. Physiol. *76*, 317 (1991).

80 Muramatsu, I.: Br. J. Pharmacol. *102*, 210 (1991).

81 Muramatsu, I., S. Kigoshi and M. Oshita: Br. J. Pharmacol. *101*, 662 (1990).

82 Muramatsu, I., T. Ohmura, S. Kigoshi, S. Hashimoto and M. Oshita: Brit. J. Pharmacol. *99*, 197 (1990).

83 Muramatsu, I., S. Kigoshi and T. Ohmura: Japan J. Pharmacol. *57*, 535 (1991).

84 Muramatsu, I., K. Yamanaka and S. Kigoshi: Japan J. Pharmacol. *55*, 391 (1991).

85 Flavahan, N.A. and Vanhoutte, P.M.: Trends in Pharmacol. Sci. 7, 347 (1986).

86 Hieble, J.P. and D.F. Woodward: Naunyn-Schmiedeberg's Arch. Pharmacol. *328*, 44 (1984).

87 George, P., F. Borg, S. O'Conner, J. Lechaire, S. Arbilla, C. Pimoule, D. Graham, T. Wedzikowsky and S.Z. Langer: Eur. J. Med. Chem. *30*, 299s (1995).

88 Price, D.T., D.A. Schwinn, J.W. Lomasney, L.F. Allen, M.G. Caron and R.J. Lefkowitz: J. Urology *150*, 546 (1993).

89 Sulpizio, A.C., D.P. Naselsky and J.P. Hieble: FASEB J. *6*, A1021 (1992).

90 Marshall, I., R.P. Burt and C.R. Chapple: Brit. J. Pharmacol. *115*, 781 (1995).

91 Ford, A.P.D.W., N.F. Arredondo, D.R. Blue, D.W. Bonhaus, M.S. Kava, T.J. Williams, R.L. Vimont, Q.M. Zhu, J.R. Pfister and D.E. Clarke: Brit. J. Pharmacol. *114*, 24P (1995).

92   Bylund, D.B., D.C. Eikenberg, J.P. Hieble, S.Z. Langer, R.J. Lefkowitz, K.P. Minneman, P.B. Molinoff, R.R. Ruffolo,Jr. and U. Trendelenburg: Pharmacol. Rev. 46, 121 (1994).

93   Bylund, D.B., J.W. Regan, J.E. Faber, J.P. Hieble, C.R. Triggle and R.R. Ruffolo, Jr.: Can. J. Physiol. Pharmacol. 73, 533 (1995).

94   Guyer, C.A., D.A. Horstman, A.L. Wilson, J.D. Clark, E.J. Cragoe and L.E. Limbird: J. Biol. Chem. 265, 17307 (1990).

95   Simonneaux, V., M. Ebadi and D.B. Bylund: Mol. Pharmacol. 40, 235 (1991).

96   Gleason, M.M. and J.P. Hieble: J. Pharmacol. Exp. Ther. 259, 1124 (1991).

97   Kawahara, R.S. and D.B. Bylund: J. Pharmacol. Exp. Ther. 233, 603 (1985).

98   Petrash, A.C. and D.B. Bylund: Life Sci. 38, 2129 (1986).

99   Michel, A.D., D.N. Loury and R.L. Whiting: Br. J. Pharmacol. 99, 560 (1990).

100   Hieble, J.P. and D.P. Naselsky: Pharmacologist 35, 166 (1993).

101   Young, P., J. Berge, H. Chapman and M.A. Cawthorne: Eur. J. Pharmacol. 168, 381 (1989).

102   Gleason, M.M. and J.P. Hieble: Br. J. Pharmacol. 107, 222 (1992).

103   Beeley, L.J., J.M. Berge, H. Chapman, P. Hieble, J. Kelly, D.P. Naselsky, C.M. Rockell and P.W. Young: Reports in Bio-organic and Medicinal Chemistry 3, 1693–1698 (1995).

104   Murphy, T.J. and D.B. Bylund: J. Pharmacol. Exp. Ther. 244, 571 (1988).

105   Blaxall, H.S., T.J. Murphy, J.C. Baker, C. Ray and D.B. Bylund: J. Pharmacol. Exp. Ther. 259, 323 (1991).

106   Uhlen, S., Y. Xia, V. Chhajlani, C.C. Felder and J.E.S. Wikberg: Br. J. Pharmacol. 106, 986 (1992).

107   O'Rourke, M.F., H.S. Blaxall, L.J. Iversen and D.B. Bylund: J. Pharmacol. Exp. Ther. 268, 1362 (1994).

108   O'Rourke, M.F., L.J. Iversen, J.W. Lomasney and D.B. Bylund: J. Pharmacol. Exp. Ther. 271, 735 (1994).

109   MacKinnon, A.C., A.T. Kilpatrick, B.A. Kenny, M. Spedding and C.M. Brown: Br. J. Pharmacol. 106, 1011 (1992).

110   Halme, M., B. Sjoholm, J.M. Savbola and M. Scheinin: Biochem. Biophys. Acta 1266, 207 (1995).

111   Li, Y.O., J.P. Hieble, D.J. Bergsma, A.M. Swift, S. Ganguly and R.R. Ruffolo, Jr.: Pharmacol. Comm. 6, 125 (1995).

112   Uhlen, S. and J.E.S. Wikberg: Br. J. Pharmacol. 104, 657 (1991).

113   Xia, Y., V. Chhajlani and J.E.S. Wikberg: Eur. J. Pharmacol. (Mol. Pharmacol.) 246, 129 (1993).

114   Xia, Y., S. Uhlen, V. Chhajlani, E.J. Lien and J.E.S. Wikberg: Pharmacol. Toxicol. 72, 40 (1993).

115   Wikberg, J.E.S., G. Tiger, Y. Xia, V. Chhajlani and S. Uhlen: Pharmacol. Comm. 6, 109 (1995).

116   Bylund, D.B. and C. Ray-Prenger: J. Pharmacol. Exp. Ther. 251, 640 (1989).

117   Trendelenburg, A., N. Limberger and L.C. Rump: Naunyn-Schmiedeberg's Arch. Pharmacol. 347 (Suppl.), 482 (1993).

118   Trendelenburg, A., N. Limberger and K. Starke: Naunyn-Schmiedeberg's Arch. Pharmacol. 348, 35 (1993).

119   Limberger, N., A. Trendelenburg and K. Starke: Br. J. Pharmacol. 107, 246 (1992).

120   Smith, K., S. Connaughton and J.R. Docherty: Eur. J. Pharmacol. 211, 251 (1992).

121   Smith, K., D. Moore, G. Shanik and J.R. Docherty: J. Physiol. 446, 435 (1992).

122   Connaughton, S. and J.R. Docherty: Br. J. Pharmacol. 101, 285 (1990).

123   Molderings, G. and M. Gothert: Naunyn-Schmiedeberg's Arch. Pharmacol. *346*, R64 (1992).

124   Blandizzi, C., M. Del Tacca, G. Natale and E.S. Vizi: Pharmacol. Res. *25* (Suppl. 2), 273 (1992).

125   Docherty, J.R.: Trends in Pharmacol. Sci. *8*, 358 (1987).

126   Craig, D., M. Iacolina and C. Forray: FASEB J. *9*, A106 (1995).

127   Janssen, C.C., A. Marjamaki, K. Luomala, J.M. Savola, M. Scheinin and K.E.O. Akerman: Eur. J. Pharmacol. (Mol. Pharmacol.) *266*, 165 (1994).

128   Wong, W.C., D. Wang, C. Forray, P.J.J. Vaysse, T.A. Branchek and C. Gluchowski: Bioorganic & Med. Chem. Letters *4*, 2317 (1994).

129   Lanier, S.M., S. Downing, E. Duzic and C.J. Homcy: J. Biol. Chem. *266*, 10470 (1991).

130   Voigt, M.M., S.K. McCune, R.Y. Kanterman and C.C. Felder: FEBS Letters *278*, 45 (1991).

131   Link, R.E., M.S. Stevens, M. Kulatunga, M. Scheinin, G.S. Barsh and B.K. Kobilka: Mol. Pharmacol. *48*, 48 (1995).

132   Ruffolo, R.R., Jr., A.C. Sulpizio, A.J. Nichols, R.M. DeMarinis and J.P. Hieble: Naunyn-Schmiedeberg's Arch. Pharmacol. *336*, 415 (1987).

133   Hieble, J.P., A.C. Sulpizio, D.A. Ashton, D.P. Naselsky, G.P. McCafferty and C. Gluchowski: Pharmacologist *33*, 214 (1991).

134   Hieble, J.P., A.C. Sulpizio, R. Edwards, H. Chapman, P. Toung, S.P. Roberts, T.P. Blackburn, M.D. Wood, D.H. Shah, R.M. DeMarinis and R.R. Ruffolo, Jr.: J. Pharmacol. Exp. Ther. *259*, 643 (1991).

135   Akers, I., J. Coates, G.M. Drew and A.T. Sullivan: Br. J. Pharmacol. *102*, 943 (1991).

136   Lomasney, J.W., S. Cotecchia, W. Lorenz, W.Y. Leung, D.A. Schwinn, T.L. Yang-Feng, M. Brownstein, R.J. Lefkowitz and M.G. Caron: J. Biol. Chem. *266*, 6365 (1991).

137   Marjamaki, A., K. Luomala, S. Ala-Uotila and M. Scheinin: Eur. J. Pharmacol. (Mol. Pharmacol.) *246*, 219 (1993).

138   Harrison, J.K., D.D. D'Angelo, D. Zeng and K.R. Lynch: Mol. Pharmacol. *40*, 407 (1991).

139   Bylund, D.B. and L. Iversen: Pharmacologist *32*, 144 (1990).

140   Gong, G., G. Chiu, C. Gluchowski, T.A. Branchek, P.R. Hartig, W.A. Pettinger and C. Forray: FASEB J. *8*, A353 (1994).

141   Hieble, J.P. and R.R. Ruffolo, Jr.: In: Antilipidemic Drugs: Medicinal Chemical and Biochemical Aspects, Ed. by D.T. Witiak, H.A.I. Newman and D.R. Feller, Elsevier, Amsterdam, pp 301–344 (1991).

142   Hughes, P.L. and R.M. Morse: Mayo Clin. Proc. *60*, 47 (1985).

143   Maze, M., L. Poree and B.C. Rabin: Pharmacol. Comm. *6*, 175 (1995).

144   Hunt, R.D., Capper, L. and O'Connell, P.: J. Child and Adolesc. Psychopharmacol. *109*, 831 (1990).

145   Uhlen, S., R. Muceniece, N. Rangel, G. Tiger and J.E.S. Wikberg: Pharmacol. and Toxicol. *76*, 353 (1995).

146   Hieble, J.P. and R.R. Ruffolo, Jr.: Ann. N.Y. Acad. Sci. 1995 (in press).

147   McCafferty, J.P., J.P. Hieble, J.M. Roesler and L.J. Kopaciewicz: Fed. Proc. *41*, 1668 (1982).

148   Sawyer, R., P. Warnock and J.R. Docherty: J. Cardiovasc. Pharmacol. *7*, 809 (1985).

149   Pinder, R.M. and J.H. Wieringa: Medicinal Res. Rev. *13*, 259 (1993).

150   LaFontan, M., M. Berlan, J. Galitzky and J.L. Montastruc: Am. J. Clin. Nutr. *55*, 219S (1992).

151   Contantinou, C.E., S. Omata, B. Jin, W. Liu and I. Perkash: J. Urol. *151*, 510A (1994).

152   Yamada, S., M. Suzuki, Y. Kato, R. Kimura, R. Mori, K. Matsumoto, M. Maruyama and K. Kawabe: Life Sci. *50*, 127 (1991).

153   Hieble, J.P., R.M. DeMarinis, P.J. Fowler and W.D. Matthews: J. Pharmacol. Exp. Ther. *236*, 90 (1986).

154   Trendelenberg, A., N. Limberger and K. Starke: Naunyn-Schmiedeberg's Arch. Pharmacol. *348*, 35 (1993).

155   Hieble, J.P., Sulpizio, A.C., Edwards, R., Chapman, H., Young, P., Roberts, S.P., Blackburn, T.P., Wood, M.D., Shah, D.H., DeMarinis, R.M. and Ruffolo, R.R. Jr.: J. Pharmacol. Exp. Ther. *259*, 643 (1991).

156   Bohmann, C., U. Schaible, P. Schollmeyer and L.C. Rump: Eur. J. Pharmacol. *271*, 283 (1994).

157   Michel, M.C., Hanft, G. and Gross, G.: Brit. J. Pharmacol. *111*, 533 (1994).

158   Foglar, R., Shibata, K., Horie, K., Hirasawa, A. and Tsujimoto, G.: Europ. J. Pharmacol. (Mol. Pharmacol.) *288*, 201 (1995).

159   Weinberg, D.H., P. Trivedi, C.P. Tan, S. Mitra, A. Perkins-Barrow, D. Borkowski, C.D. Strader and M. Bayne: Biochem. and Biophysical Res. Communications *20*, 1296 (1994).

160   Ramarao, C.S., J.M.C. Denker, D.M. Perez, R.J. Gaivin, R.P. Rick and R.M. Graham: J. Biol. Chem. *267*, 21936 (1992).

161   Schwinn, D.A., S.O. Page, J.P. Middleton, W. Lorenz, S.B. Liggett, K. Yamamoto, E.G. Lapetina, M.G. Caron, R.J. Lefkowitz and S. Cotecchia: Mol. Pharmacol. *40*, 619 (1991).

162   Faure, C., C. Pimoule, G. Vallancien, S.Z. Langer and D. Graham: Life Sci. *54*, 1595 (1994).

163   Horie, K., A. Hirasawa and G. Tsujimoto: Europ. J. Pharmacol. (Mol. Pharmacol.) *268*, 399 (1994).

164   Goetz, A.S., Lutz, M.W., Rimele, T.J. and Saussy, D.L., Jr.: J. Pharmacol. Exp. Ther. *271*, 1228 (1994).

165   Buckner, S.A., K. Oheim, P. Morse, S. Knepper, A.A. Hancock and J.F. Kerwin, Jr.: FASEB J. *9*, A105 (1995).

166   Kenny, B.A., Naylor, A.M., Greengrass, P.M., Russell, M.J., Friend, S.J., Read, A.M. and Wyllie, M.G.: Brit. J. Pharmacol. *111*, 1003 (1994).

167   True, T, A.S. Goetz, S. Kadwell, H. King, T. Kost, M. James, J. Tseng Crank and D.L. Saussy, Jr.: Society for Neuroscience Abstracts *20*, 526 (1994).

168   Shibata, K., R. Foglar, K. Horie, K. Obika, A. Sakamoto, S. Ogawa and G. Tsujimoto: Mol. Pharmacol. *48*, 250 (1995).

169   Goetz, A.S., H.K. King, S.D.C. Ward, T.A. True, T.J. Rimele and D.L. Saussy: Eur. J. Pharmacol. *272*, R5 (1995).

170   Hirasawa, A., K. Horie, T. Tanaka, K. Takagaki, M. Murai, J. Yano and G. Tsujimoto: Biochem. Biophys. Res. Comm. *195*, 902 (1993).

171   Eltze, M. and R. Boer: Europ. J. Pharmacol. *224*, 125 (1992).

172   Fujimoto, S.: Brit. J. Pharmacol . *110*, 192P (1993).

173   Burt, R.P., C.R. Chapple and I. Marshall: Brit. J. Pharmacol. *115*, 467 (1995).

174   Hieble, J.P., Caine, M. and Zalaznik, E. Europ. J. Pharmacol. *107*, 111 (1985).

175   Muramatsu, I., M. Oshita, T. Ohmura, S. Kigoshi, H. Akino, M. Gobara and K. Okada: Brit J. Urol. *74*, 572 (1994).

176   Miranda, H.F., H. Ramierez, O. Castillo, K.P. Minneman and G. Pinardi: Pharmacol. Commun. *4*, 181 (1994).

177   Yamanaka, N., O. Yamaguchi, H. Kameoka, Y. Fukaya, T. Yokota, Y. Shiraiwa, J.

Yokoyama, K. Kumakawa, K. Itou, Y. Kuma, M. Kobayashi and M. Takaiwa: Acta Urol. Japan *37*, 1759 (1991).

178   Yu, S.M., F.N. Ko, S.C. Chueh, J. Chen, S.C. Chen, C.C. Chen and C.M. Teng: Europ. J. Pharmacol. *252*, 29 (1994).

179   Marshall, I., R.P. Burt, P.O. Andersson, C.R. Chapple, P.M. Greengrass, G.I. Johnson and M.G. Wyllie: Brit. J. Pharmacol. *112*, 59P (1992).

180   Kunisawa, Y., K. Kawabe, T. Nijima, K. Honda and T. Takenaka: J. Urol. *134*, 396 (1985).

181   Muramatsu, I., T. Ohmura, S. Hashimoto and M. Oshita: Pharmacol. Commun. *6*, 23 (1995).

182   Langin, D., H. Paris, M. Dauzats and M. Lafontan: Eur. J. Pharmacol. (Mol. Pharmacology Sec.) *188*, 261 (1990).

183   Taouis, M., M. Berlan, P. Mantastruc and M. Lafontan: J. Pharmacol. Exp. Ther. *242*, 1041 (1987).

184   Chruscinski, A.J., R.E. Link, D.A. Daunt, G.S. Barsh and B.K. Kobilka: Biochem. Biophys. Res. Com. *186*, 1280 (1992).

185   Link, R., D. Daunt, G. Barsh, A. Chruscinski and B. Kobilka: Mol. Pharmacol. *42*, 16 (1992).

186   Blaxall, H.S., D.R. Cerutis, N.A. Hass, L.J. Iversen and D.B. Bylund: Mol. Pharmacol. *45*, 176 (1994).

187   Saulnier-Blache, J., C. Carpene, D. Langin and M. Lafontan: Eur. J. Pharmacol. *171*, 145 (1989).

188   Carpene, C., J. Galitzky, D. Larrouy, D. Langin and M. Lafontan: Biochem. Pharmacol. *40*, 437 (1990).

189   Paris, H., T. Voisin, A. Remaury, C. Rouyer-Fessard, D. Daviaud and D. Langin: J. Pharmacol. Exp. Ther. *254*, 888 (1990).

190   Remaury, A. and H. Paris: J. Pharmacol. Exp. Ther. *260*, 417 (1992).

191   Bylund, D.B.: FASEB J. *6*, 832 (1992).

192   Brown, C.M., A.C. MacKinnon, J.C. McGrath, M. Spedding and A.T. Kilpatrick: Br. J. Pharmacol. *99*, 481 (1990).

193   Daiguji, M., H.Y. Meltzer and D.C. U'Prichard: Life Sci. *28*, 2705 (1982).

194   Bylund, D.B., H.S. Blaxall, L.J. Iversen, M.G. Caron, R.J. Lefkowitz and J.W. Lomasney: Mol. Pharmacol. *42*, 1 (1992).

195   Langin, D., M. Lafontan, M.R. Stillings and S. Paris: Eur. J. Pharmacol. *167*, 95 (1989).

196   Weinshank, R.L., J.M. Zgombick, M. Macchi, N. Adham, H. Lichtblau, T.A. Branchek and P.A. Hartig: Mol. Pharmacol. *38*, 681 (1990).

197   Lomasney, J.W., W. Lorenz, L.F. Allen, K. Kling, J.W. Regan, T.L. Yang-Feng, M.G. Caron and R.J. Lefkowitz: Proc. Natl. Acad. Sci. *87*, 5094 (1990).

198   Flordellis, C.S., D.E. Handy, M.R. Bresnahan, V.I. Zannis and H. Gavras: Proc. Natl. Acad. Sci. USA *88*, 1019 (1991).

199   Simonneaux, V., M. Ebadi and D.B. Bylund: Mol. Pharmacol. *40*, 235 (1991).

200   Pohjanoksa, K., Marjamaki, A., Ala-Uotilla, S., Oker-Blom, D., Sizman, H., Kurose, H. and Scheinin, M.: Soc. For Neuroscience Abstracts *19*, 1789 (1993).

201   Devedjian, J.C., F. Esclapez, C. Denis-Pouxviel and H. Paris: Europ. J. Pharmacol. *252*, 43 (1994).

202   Blaxall, H.S., M.F. O'Rourke, B. Kobilka, J. Lomasney, L.J. Iversen, D.A. Heck and D.B. Bylund: Can. J. Physiol. Pharmacol. *72* (Suppl. 1), 542 (1994).

203   Regan, J.W., T.S. Kobilka, T.L. Yang-Feng, M.G. Caron, R.J. Lefkowitz and B.K. Kobilka: Proc. Natl. Acad. Sci. *85*, 6301 (1988).

204   Pimoule, C., Graham, D., Arbilla, S. and Langer, S.Z.: Brit. J. Pharmacol. *107*, 378P (1992).
205   Chiu, G., Gluchowski, C., Fang, J., Forray, C., Borden, L.A., Adham, N., Branchek, T.A., Bard, J.A., Weinshank, R.A. and Hartig, P.: Presentation at 206th ACS National Meeting, Chicago, Illinois (1993).
206   Piascik, M.T., B.T. Butler, T.A. Pruitt and J.W. Kusiak: J. Pharmacol. Exp. Ther. *254*, 982 (1990).
207   Michel, M.C. and P.A. Insel: Brit. J. Pharmacol. *112*, 59P (1994).

Progress in Drug Research, Vol. 47 (E. Jucker, Ed.)
© 1996 Birkhäuser Verlag, Basel (Switzerland)

Perspective and overview of Chinese traditional medicine and contemporary pharmacology*

By E. Leong Way[1], Yong Qing Liu[2] and Chieh-Fu Chen[3]

[1]Departments of Pharmacology & Pharmaceutical Chemistry, School of Medicine and Pharmacy, University of California, San Francisco, CA 94143, USA, and Academica Sinica, Taipei, Taiwan, ROC; [2]Department of Pharmaceutical Services, San Francisco General Hospital and School of Pharmacy, University of California, San Francisco, CA 94110, USA; [3]National Research Institute of Chinese Medicine, Taipei Hsien, Taiwan, ROC 23172

*   This study was supported by generous grants from the Chiang Ching-Kuo Foundation for International Scholarly Exchange (USA) and the Soo Foundation Taiwan (ROC). The helpful critique and comments of Drs Frederick Meyers and Louis Lasagna are much appreciated.

1   Introduction

In addition to paper, the mariner's compass, gunpowder, silk, porcelain and many other things, the Chinese developed a system of medicine for treating sickness and disease that is still widely used by millions of people. Over a period of over millenia, by trial error and serendipity, the Chinese recorded the biologic actions of thousands of products derived from plants, animals and minerals. They thought about and tried to explain their pharmacologic effects. In so doing, there evolved a rationalization process relating man's relationship with the universe and laws of nature, and these ideas were coupled with the empirical findings to formulate a system of medicine that is still extant. The efforts culminated in the emergence of proto-disciplines related to botany, physiology, biochemistry and psychology as well as drug-related fields such as pharmacognosy, pharmacy, endocrinology, toxicology, immunology and forensic medicine. Such notions led to the use of a vast number of agents to prevent, diagnose, cure and alleviate illness. In the process, amazing insight and perspicacity were displayed with respect to factors that may alter drug action including host facets concerned with age, sex, mood, pathologic states, as well as environmental conditions related to daily and seasonal alterations on circadian rhythm. Medicinal agents were understood to act not by creating new functions but by correcting an underlying pathologic process. Especially intuitive were the concepts evolved concerning drug interactions that could result in synergism or antagonism.

Similar to many early civilizations, the first application of a plant, animal or mineral product for the treatment of illness in China must have resulted from a chance discovery and the armamentarium of remedies became further enlarged by serendipity as well as repeated trial and error. Mysticism prevailed in many of the proto-sciences but it was a far more complicating factor in traditional medicine which even today remains more an art that has not been incorporated into contemporary science. In the attempt to systematize the ever-increasing amounts of data that accumulated the Chinese coupled their empirical findings to a rationalization process.

Although initially rituals, symbolism and shamanism were combined with folkloric medicines in the treatment process, in time the mystic aspects were largely separated. A large body of information about herbal remedies was incorporated philosophically into cosmic principles enunciated to define man's relation with the universe [1–7].

2   The doctrine of *Yin* and *Yang*

According to ancient Chinese philosophy in *I Jing*, the Classic Book of Changes, the beginning started with *Qi* (*Chi*), a difficult to define form of ethereal energy. *Qi* gave birth to heaven and earth from which emanated *yin* and *yang*, two vital forces whose interactions were responsible for all matters related to life. The positive force, *yang*, stemmed from heaven and the negative *yin* from earth (Fig. 1). From their interactions, five elements were spawned, wood, fire, metal, earth and water which could be embodied in many things such as seasons, directions, color, taste, etc., and corresponded as well to five body organs, namely liver, heart, spleen, lung and kidney (Table 1). A harmonious relationship between these organs is considered essential to good health; any disruption results in illness. When an imbalance occurs the cure is to restore harmony. The emphasis on man is holistic with the focus being on prevention rather than treatment. The cause of a febrile state, for example, may be ascribed to excessive *yang* from liver (wood) blockage with consequential effects on the heart (fire). Prior to treatment, therefore, the type of ailment needs to be identified with the functional mechanism interrupted. Aberrations in *yin* deficiency in the kidney (water) should be excluded before appropriate cooling remedies are applied, taking into consideration also external factors such as the season, the time of day, weather, etc. Thus man's existence and well-being are intimately linked to the universe and nature and a complex system for diagnosis and treatment was elaborated from such relationships. Conceptualizations about life were built on cosmic principles and although the supernatural could be invoked, the Chinese deities gradually played lesser roles than those of the Greeks and Romans. In health matters, specific afflictions to the Chinese could be attributed to certain evil spirits (*xie*) but such functionaries were poorly defined and lacked personality. In time, as medicine became separated from shamanism, the term more or less lost its association with demons and came to mean an idiopathic state that is not easily definable. Other symptoms such as *Qi* (air, humor, energy) and *Feng* (wind, which may be associated with an ill-wind or a pathocondition) fall into this category [6–8]. If what the Chinese conjured is translated into contemporary parlance, one might say that the physiological state can be considered in terms of homeostatic theory that is, when the balanced state of interaction between the various body organs becomes altered, such as those concerned with feedback inhibition, pathologic consequences are likely to occur [6, 7, 51].

Much of the thought expounded by the Chinese about medication was several centuries in advance of Western ideas. Moreover, the principles

Basis of Chinese medicine

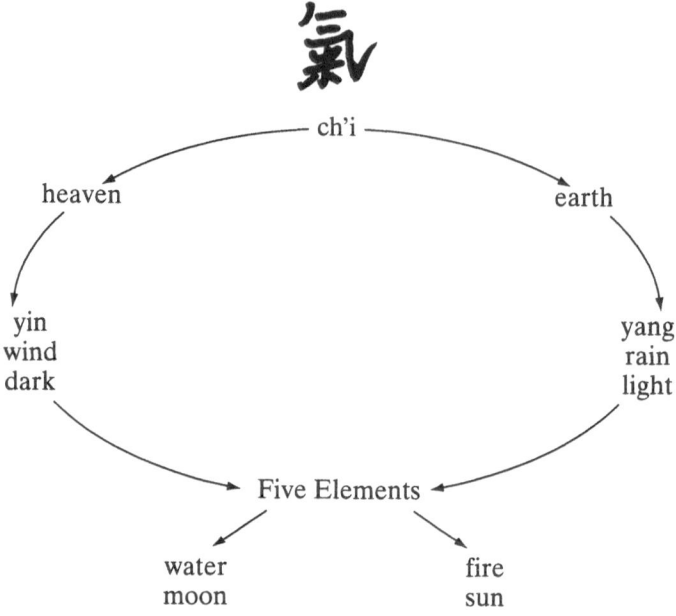

Fig. 1

they enunciated with respect to drug action transcend the thousands of remedies they discovered for treating the ills of their population. What they conjured and anticipated parallels in many respects the modern concepts of the West. Their theories, however, have been dated because of a lack of flexibility to incorporate the rapid advances made in modern science. In contrast to the Western approach, wherein the new findings can be applied to modify or correct existing theories, with traditional Chinese medicine, new data must be incorporated into existing dogma that is immutable. As a consequence, a curious dichotomy exists today in traditional medicine between its basic and practical facets. While pharmaceutical chemists and pharmacologists strive to isolate and characterize active plant principles, herbalists throughout the world, including Europe, the United States in addition to Asia, continue to ply their trade applying outmoded ancient theories and methodologies. Even the current communist regime in China appears to recognize this paradox without explicitly stat-

Five element categories

Category	Wood 木	Fire 火	Earth 土	Metal 金	Water 水
Season	spring	summer	between summer and fall	autumn	winter
Direction	East	South	center	West	North
Color	virid	red	yellow	white	black
Taste	sour	bitter	sweet	salt	acrid
Organ	liver	heart	spleen	lung	kidney

Table 1.

ing so, since early in their regime they ordered the practitioners at the institutions of Chincsc traditional medicine to learn the Western approach to validate herbal remedies. However, it was not a one-sided demand since Western trained physicians had to learn traditional medicine. I had the opportunity to analyze the program in 1958 [8, 9] and then make personal observations in 1974 [10].

3   Traditional Chinese medicine in the People's Republic of China

In 1974 shortly after the People's Republic of China and the United States had resumed diplomatic relationships, I was privileged to be appointed to a U.S. scientific delegation by the National Academy of Sciences to learn about the program of traditional medicine that had been initiated in China.

Following Chairman Mao's pronouncement that "Chinese medicine is a great national treasure; we must strive to improve and elevate its status", the Ministry of Health issued the edict in 1955 urging intensification of studies on traditional medicine. Physicians trained in Western medicine were directed to give greater attention to ancient methods of treatment and to cooperate with traditional practitioners. Medical scientists, particularly pharmacologists, were urged to focus their research on validating the national materia medica. The directive also applied to the people who were exhorted by mass campaigns that were repeatedly reinforced to grow medicinal herbs. The result was a mass alignment of pharmaceutical personnel to study natural products of plant, animal and mineral origin [8, 9]. The news that leaked later indicated many achievements and great strides in improving the health standards of the country. The mission of our group was to learn about the progress, projects, and approaches the Chinese had made, especially in herbal pharmacology at both the basic and clinical levels.

We visited twenty-one institutions, both traditional Chinese and Western, in six major cities, that included hospitals, medical and pharmacy schools, research institutes, pharmacies, pharmaceutical firms and botanical drug gardens. Our perceptions were contingent on the place we visited and had a wide range that included skepticism, ambivalance, grudging acceptance and sheer admiration. A major annoyance at the time was the inseparability of medicine and politics which has now been greatly ameliorated. Our ignorance in the principles and language of ancient traditional medicine caused difficulties in translation. *Huo* or fire was not always a fever treatable by an antipyretic or febrifuge and measurable by a thermometer but on occasions a body heat reflecting an aberration in the five elements that affected a body essence or humor. A diurectic could be applied to decrease humidity; a cardiotonic to increase cardiac function by vaguely improving circulation. Problems surfaced from different cultural values and thinking habits. Western science has made its greatest advances by reducing variables while purposely manipulating one and keeping others fixed. It was difficult to accept, therefore, proof or evidence of efficacy of a recipe consisting of several products when the ingredients could be altered at any time based on the subject's physical condition or mental attitude. The traditional practitioners, on the other hand, seem quite convinced that the simultaneous application of several therapeutic modalities is neccesary and the validation comes from the test of time. Their faith resides in the glowing anecdotal testimonies from selected groups of patients who favor the healers with the beneficial and innocuous effects of their remedies. The summary and conclusions have been published and will be excerpted slightly modified [10–12]. The Chinese people consume considerable quantities of herbal remedies, many of which have been in use for centuries. Both laymen and scientists subscribe to the belief that these natural products have proved their efficacy and safety through years of consumer satisfaction. Medicines of plant, animal, and mineral origin are available both via prescription and "over the counter". The genesis of interest in herbal drugs lies in the perceived clinical benefits. The philosophic concepts of ancient Chinese medicine are closely intermeshed with such usage, but for the scientific-medical establishment, it is the empiric performance of these natural products that provides the basis for their use and for research. It soon became clear that even though many practical contributions could be versed with the theories of Chinese medicine, it was not always possible for us to make critical analysis of the information. This was due in part to our ignorance of the philosophic basis of Chinese traditional medicine. We were exposed to a great mass of information which appeared good and bad, but it was not possible to make critical judgements of the system by Western standards. In the traditional approach, whenever positive or negative findings were obtained, the data would be rationalized and incorporated into theory. In effect, there was no attempt to make observations or carry out experiments to test the theories. The theory of traditional Chinese medicine, being a rigid, closed system adhering strictly to dogma in terms of what was said and what was established, can neither be supported nor rejected by the experimental approach of Western science.

An example of the weakness in the traditional Chinese program was that little attempt was made to prove any of the many facets of the rationalizations. The possible efficacy of no treatment was, for instance, not considered; patients often do get well even though they are not treated. In tests for the efficacy of a drug, control studies to determine whether the remedy truly accelerates recovery or whether the patient is recovering unaided were not included. The holistic traditional Chinese approach, although highly commendable, seemed overly stressed. Although it is very important to treat the patient as a whole and Western medicine should emphasize this aspect more, the perspective can be distorted. Modern medicine clearly shows that many diseases can be associated primarily with the pathology of a particular organ or tissue and when the treatment is direct with specific drugs (or surgery), dramatic alleviation of the condition can occur. Prescription simplification is another facet that was not examined. In Western medicine, to avoid drug interactions the use of a single drug is preferred for treatment. Sometimes it is important to use drugs in combination because some substances administered alone may not be nearly as efficacious as when combined with others. In traditional Chinese medicine, however, nearly all the prescriptions contain several herbs, but if attempts were made to simplify the recipe the traditional practitioner would argue that any modification violates theory and, therefore, could alter the treatment outcome. Such concepts frustrate any attempts to establish drug efficacy on an objective basis.

The Western approach with crude drugs is to reduce the complexities by attempting to isolate and identify the active constituent. A single component assures uniformity in response, minimizes drug interaction and provides clues for the synthesis of superior surrogates. This approach combined with a suitable bioassay system is the main reason for the development of pharmacology as a modern scientific discipline. However, when no biologic activity could be demonstrated in the purified preparations, the traditional practitioner applied the same arguments as used against recipe simplification. Under the circumstances the traditional practitioner was in a no-lose situation, being able to accept credit when findings were affirmative and to resort to dogma when negative.

Despite this and the uncritical attempts of clinicians to validate the prescription remedies directly, the Western trained pharmaceutical chemists and pharmacologists in China were vigorously pursuing the isolation and characterization of active principles in plants. Considerable amounts of data were accumulated and the achievements are summarized in reference [10] and in a later report when a Chinese delegation reciprocated and visited the United States [11].

When the political leaders in China initiated the huge program to elevate traditional medicine, it was sheer pragmatism to place the traditional and the Western practitioners together because at the time there was a severe shortage of physicians in China. To implement the program, herbal doctors were placed alongside Western trained physicians in the hospitals and the latter group was required to learn some traditional medicine. However, the integration was not all that simple because the practitioners with their discrepant backgrounds tended to adhere to their own theories. To the traditional practitioners, even if their notions are difficult to understand in light of present day knowledge, cannot be improved upon or hamper scientific validation, their theories have not outlived their usefulness because new discoveries could be incorporated into their dogma. To the Western practitioners the validation of some herbal recipes and acupuncture were most positive experiences. The basic accomplishments were substantial and seemed to be well-grounded but this was not always the case with the clinical studies. Although interesting therapeutic claims were made for herbal medicines, and the biochemotaxonomic analysis sometimes supported these contentions, on the basis of the clinical evidence alone, it was not possible to come to firm conclusions about any specific traditional drug. The reasons for this are multiple and include the unpredictable course of most symptoms or diseases, the almost total absence of controlled trials, the cultural objection to the use of placebo controls, and the simultaneous administration of multiple forms of treatment, including Western drugs. A formidable barrier to identifying unequivocally effective elements from the field of herbal pharmacology is that there were so few clinical situations controlled enough to permit a positive statement. Herbal decoctions were widely used in conjunction with Western drugs, and often used in chronic diseases (such as degenerative neurological disorders or chronic angina or long-term recovery from stroke) where prognosis and critical evaluation are exceedingly difficult. A decoction of eight plants could contain literally hundreds of different chemicals. Finally, careful records and controls usually were not always kept. Morever, serious attempts to quantify treatment effects against knowledge of the course of the untreated disease or to evaluate herbal medicine with and without Western medicine were not made. Many Western scientists, with their background and bias, were troubled by traditional medicine, much of which represents a throwback to an earlier day in which the germ theory of disease and the etiology of many noninfectious diseases were unknown. Little of traditional medicine was subjected to scientific proof or even to semicritical scrutiny, and some patients may not have received the best treatment by Western standards. On the positive side, it must be stated that, on the whole, patients in China seem to do as well as those in the West at the hospitals we visited, and the present amalgam of Chinese and Western medicine may be as good as (or better than) any other system that might be devised for the Chinese population. Furthermore, the "marriage" of the two systems was moving ahead without obvious dislocation – e.g., the chiefs of service in the hospitals seemed to be trained in both. Nor did we really hear any criticism of Western medicine *per se* [10, 12].

From this integration there emerged many important and interesting findings, not only in treatment and practice but also with respect to the research facets concerned with a concerted approach to identify the active constituents of many natural products. Out of these efforts much botanical, chemical, pharmacological and clinical knowledge was gained, and there is now a vast literature in all these areas. Many works are appearing constantly in the current literature that are too numerous to cite; a few monographs indicate the intense activity in the field [13–24].

The successes called the attention of the West to the benefits of acupuncture and many herbal remedies. Perhaps the most significant impact felt by the scientific members of the delegation came from the challenge to basic assumptions long held by our own society. What we saw of acupuncture analgesia; Chinese orthopedic practices; their nonoperative approach to kidney stones, appendicitis, and perforated peptic ulcer; the geographical incidence of certain cancers; cataract surgery; burn treatment; their methods of dispensing drugs; and the respect for the opinions and experience of both patients and physicians was extremely provocative and suggested a need for Western scientists to reexamine some of their favorite dogmas.

4   The heritage of ancient traditional medicine

Despite the criticisms of the traditional theories, the beneficial consequences for mankind have been many and varied. It is irrefutable that a large number of useful preparations were discovered at the time the notions were in effect. No doubt the discovery of useful natural products in the beginning was empiric and serendipitous but the concepts formulated later from such findings were essentially a concept unique to Chinese civilization. The fruits from the *yin yang* and five elements doctrine include efficacious medicinal remedies still in use. Besides the therapeutic agents, the holistic prerequisites brought into focus the importance of calisthenics and massage that are so popular in modern health facilities. The theories facilitated the systematization and rationalization of a large mass of data on medicinal remedies, the development of proto-sciences that have become important basic and clinical disciplines related to pharmaceutics, and the compilation of invaluable compendia on *materia medica*, including the first pharmacoepia and the formulation of some principles in pharmacology that can be extrapolated for current application.

4.1   Medicinal remedies

The armamentarium numbers more than two thousand products of plant, animal and mineral origin that have been formulated into approximately eleven thousand recipes. However, a relatively recent manual contains 434 kinds of *materia medica* commonly used in clinical practice, including 382 plants, 36 animals and 16 minerals [21], although another comprehensive source lists the number of natural products in use today as probably less than 250, and less than 100 are popular [15].
The Chinese had considerable knowledge about endocrine function related to thyroid, diabetes and sex. For example, it was known in the fifth

century that solely drinking mountain water resulted in the development of goiters. Although the condition was not attributed to a lack of iodine, the treatment was seaweed or other plants high in iodine content [25]. Diabetes was diagnosed as a disease associated with polyuria and later with sweetness of the urine [26]. The urine was used also as a source for sex hormones. Approximately a millenium ago, crystalline gonadal principles could be obtained from urine by sublimation [27], a process used for processing mercury and its salts at least one thousand years earlier when the functional role of the male gonads was also recognized. General historic texts in Chinese history [28–32] reveal that during the Zhou dynasty (1030–221 B.C.) removal of the testes was a form of corporal punishment. Later on, intellectually talented men of humble birth were recruited as counselors to help govern, but they were deprived of their sexual capabilities by castration by their emperors to ensure that there would be no scandalous behavior with the ladies in court. Such imperial exploitation of eunuchs, whose services during their life helped to either build or destroy dynasties, prevailed for about two millenia from the Han (202 B.C.–220 A.D.) through the Qing (1644–1911) dynasty.

The best validated Chinese drug to the West is the chief active principle of *Mahuang* or *Ephedra sinensis*, isolated and identified as the alkaloid, ephedrine. The plant was described in the herbal literature more than two thousand years ago. Ephedrine is currently used to treat asthma, hypotension, colds, allergies, and as a central nervous stimulant. The wide application of the compound in the West is due primarily to Chen who, after extracting ephedrine from the plant he bought in a local herbal shop, made a thorough investigation of its pharmacologic profile. He and his associates noted that ephedrine could constrict blood vessels, relax bronchioles, dilate the pupils and stimulate the central nervous system [33]. It was a major break-through and stimulated much effort to improve on nature by the synthesis of novel sympathomimectic nervous system congeners; the new surrogates have been many including the alpha and beta blockers which have become most important for various cardiovascular disorders [34–36].

A few other early contributions include amalgam as filling for tooth decay, cannabis for anesthesia and analgesia, *Datura alba* or mandola blossoms containing scopolamine in combination with an anaesthetic to produce pain relief and amnesia, ergot for uterine conditions, and chaulmoogra oil for leprosy [6, 7, 21, 22]. Not all the natural products appear to have validity or a rational basis but were, nonetheless, incorporated into dogma. Blood might reasonably be used as replacement therapy in nose bleeding, post partum hemorrhage or from vomiting, but the basis for its application in birthmarks and warts is not clear. Even more questionable is the use of human hair for renal colic, abscesses, unexpelled placenta and stomach ache [37] and the theories frustrate any attempts to subject such applications to scientific test.

Ephedrine may be the most renown of the Chinese medications but it is by no means the most important which surprisingly is hardly recognized by the West. The greatest gift the Chinese contributed to preserving the health of all mankind, is the first immunologic procedure, smallpox inoculation. As the erudite historian Joseph Needham points out [38], this innovation was the beginning of immunology, the most beneficient department of modern medical science. He documents in considerable detail that smallpox inoculation was prevalent in China in the sixteenth century and traces its origin to as early as possibly 1000. Its derivation was based on Taoist concepts of *yang sheng* (nourishing life), literally, to preserve health by strengthening the natural healing power of the body. The notion, *i tu kung tu*, that is, use a toxin to combat the toxin, was applied to convey permanent immunity to smallpox by implantation of a pledget of the pustule contents or scab extract in the nose. To minimize the transmission of the disease by the inoculum, the preparation was taken from mild cases during the terminal recovery stage. Thus, the method of prophylaxis antedates Jenner's discovery of cowpox lymph in 1798 by about three hundred if not eight hundred years. Unfortunately, little attention was paid to letters before 1700 concerning smallpox inoculation from China to the Royal Society nor to those of the Jesuits living in China in the 18th century. Needham provides cogent plausible arguments how the Turks could have learned about the procedure from the Chinese via the Silk Road and passed it on to England. Certainly, more than two hundred years was time enough to communicate the information through such an important flourshing trade route as between China and Europe.

4.2   Development of pharmaceutical sciences and literature

The ends motivated the means and the proto-sciences that emerged were the offshoot of the Taoist notions to attain immortality. Such developments were extensively analyzed by Needham [27, 40, 41]. Besides the attempts to achieve longevity by exemplary ethical thoughts, moral behavior, calisthenic physical conditioning, etc., an elixir of immortality was intensively sought by the ancient rulers and the aristocracy who gave impetus by their rank and urgency. Thus, the priority was to promote and preserve health rather than to treat and cure illness. To prolong existence on earth, products of mineral, plant and animal origin were examined, and it is possible that the preparations not only might not have done the job but achieved just the opposite. In particular, salts of mercury, especially cinnabar were used as medicinals more than 2000 years ago, and any beneficial effects they elicited could have encouraged the use of higher doses or more chronic usage. The emperor Qin Shi Huang Ti, who united China in 221 B.C. and who was an ardent believer in the elixir of immortality, reigned only fourteen years. It would not be surprising that should ever his tomb in Xian become unearthed and his body found reasonably preserved, high levels of mercury might be found in his organs and tissues. It is no longer a revelation these days to find an intact two millenia old corpse since archeologists in China have unearthed quite a few from Han tombs only two hundred years less old than the ones of the Qin. Judging from the outer magnificient tombs of Emperor Qin with more than 7000 terra cotta soldiers guarding him, elaborate care must have been taken to preserve his body. Hence, such speculation that he may have been a victim of chronic poisoning is not beyond the realm of reality. In any event, if the body is there the mercury is not going away, and if mercury salts were used for embalming systemic levels should not be greatly altered. Perhaps I may live long enough to learn the answer.

Decoctions of animal (including human) parts, especially the gonads, were also tried to promote longevity. The belief in their efficacy remains today with many but no quantitative statistical data exist to substantiate the faith.

Nonetheless, in the process of seeking longer life something was learned about chemical substances of the body which may be considered in the realm of physiologic chemistry. In a similar vein, environmental ecology was appreciated by observations that certain insects were found to have active principles that were deadly to other insects and organisms [27,41]. The quest for immortality led to studies on gold which was also considered capable of prolonging life (aurifiction). The alchemical attempts to fabricate it from less noble elements (aurifaction) and the toxicity that could result gave need and importance to forensic toxicology [42], which interestingly was established not by physicians or pharmacists but by legalists concerned with judiciary matters involving homicides, suicides and accidental deaths. The over-riding interests to prolong life can be said to have led in part to proto-sciences that marked the beginnings of physiological chemistry, endocrinology, toxicology. Again, the reader can consult the many citations of Needham for a profound treatment of these topics [27,41,42]. Such concerns by the Chinese coupled to those for treating ills also resulted in the development of certain pharmaceutical sciences and their relationships [3, 22, 41, 42].

4.2.1   Pharmacognosy

The Chinese recognized early on that the active principles could be concentrated in specific plant and animal parts and the sources of these constituents might vary in potency and effectiveness. To ensure reliability of drug action they sought to obtain a standardized product. Hence a sketch of an herb, often elegant, was provided together with a detailed description of its source, part used, method of collection and storage as well as its pharmacologic properties. Similar care was applied to body fluids and organs of animal origin. The information was compiled into volumes on *materia medica* with the appellation *ben cao* or dispensatories that contemporary texts in pharmacognosy closely emulate. Such activities greatly stimulated interests in plants and led to many important early contributions in botanical science [48, 49].

4.2.2   Pharmacology

Some basic principles of drug action were enunciated by Zhang Zhongjing during the Late Han that may have reflected even earlier notions. His personal writings are lost but the contents were preserved by others who at the time had access to the originals. The most edifying extrapolator whose influence has endured is Tao Hongjing (451–526). Known foremost as a great alchemist, he was also equally qualified as physician, pharmacognocist, pharmacist and pharmacologist. Tao was not an idle philosopher but an active experimenter. He not only added to the repertory of remedies for health care but also enlarged Zhang's concepts that can be incorporated into modern principles concerned with drug action. Tao categorized medicinals according to potency and efficacy and took cognizance of the many factors that could alter their responses. He noted host, environmental and temporal facets that included age, sex, physical, mental and pathologic states, locale, climate, time of the day, season and circadian rhythm (chronobiology). His discourses on drug interactions use language that is easily translatable into such modern parlance as synergism, potentiation, agonism, antagonism and delivery systems. The major tenet of traditional treatment early on was the use of of several products in combination to achieve enhanced therapeutic effects. Thorough familiarity with the properties of each herb, organ part or mineral to be dispensed was required since the interactions between the components could be beneficial or adverse. Six types of mutual relationships were considered to exist in a highly complex and sophisticated manner that could be influenced by emotion or behavior. Literally, two or more drugs can "need, use, respect (or fear), dislike, kill or oppose each other". There are many traditional examples of such drug-drug interactions but it would be more meaningful to exemplify these relationships with agents selected from current pharmacologic textbooks of the West [34–36]:

xiang xu (need each other) additive or synergistic enhancement of pharmacologic action by two or more substances with similar properties, for example, certain oncolytics or antibacterials may be combined to reduce host toxicity while maintaining or increasing effectiveness against tumors or microorganisms.

xiang shi (use or reinforce each other) potentiation or synergism; enhancement of therapeutic action by substances with different properties, e.g. digitalis to increase cardiac contractility and diurectics to decrease the load on the heart; antitussives with expectorants to liquefy the mucus; opioid analgetics to decrease the dose of anesthetics.

xiang wei (mutual respect or restraint) inhibition or reduction of pharmacologic effects by two or more substances with properties in common; metals such as mercury and arsenic competing for sulfhydryl groups; partial agonists and agonists such as codeine reducing the potency of morphine.

xiang wu (mutual dislike), inhibition or reduction of an effect of one drug by another with an opposing action, e.g., physiologic or pharmacodynamic antagonism, that is, using a general central nervous system depressant such as a barbiturate (or diazepam) to antidote strychnine or metrazol convusions; may be exploited also to reduce an adverse effect of the principal drug, e.g. anticholinergics such as benzotropin to reduce the extrapyramidal effects of phenothiazine antipsychotics.

xiang sha (kill each other), the specific nullification of the effect of one compound by another agent by competitive antagonism such as between agonist and antagonist compounds, e.g. naloxone against morphine or calcium against magnesum.

xiang fan (oppose each other), incompatibility, not suitable for combination because severe adverse effects may result such as hyperpyrexia from the combined use of meperidine and monoamine oxidase inhibitors.

One of the components of a traditional prescription is the adjuvant, *yao yin zi*, that directs or leads the principal drug, *yin jing bao shi*, to the proper channel. In modern pharmacokinetic parlance this could be termed a drug delivery system for the site of action or receptor, e.g. the use of carbidopa in combination with levo-dopa to treat Parkinsonism, an affliction of the brain affecting motor function. Levo-dopa is the principal agent but its application alone is inefficient because it is destroyed in peripheral tissues. Carbidopa inhibits the enzyme that biotransforms levo-dopa peripherally thus allowing more of the active agent to gain access to the brain.

4.2.3   Pharmacy

Crude products had to be processed for ingestion and this necessitated the development of delivery systems to facilitate their administration. To augment drug potency, the techniques involved concentrating and reducing the bulk of the raw material by comminution, trituration and extraction.

Ingestability of the products was also improved by enhancing their appearance and palatability. Powders, pills and decoctions were formulated, and since these pharmaceutical preparations were documented 2000 years ago, the methodolgy must have been in existence well before this. In 1973, a Late Han tomb was excavated at Mawangtui near Changsha and found to contain parts of a formulary in varying states of preservation. The fragments were reconstituted into a volume *Wu Shih Er Ping Fang* [52], Prescriptions for Treatment of various ills. The recipes were derived from two hundred and twenty-four natural products and included directions for the preparation and dispensing of powders, pills, solutions in water, wine or vinegar for oral administration as well as ointments and paste for topical application [50]. Even earlier documentation for compounding is evidenced by a jade mortar and pestle stained with cinnabar unearthed in the tomb of a wife of a Shang dynasty ruler who died about 1200 B.C. [43, 44]. Bottle gourds, traditionally displayed at the front of shops as a sign for clinical practice or dispensing herbs, have been used in recipes as a diurectic to reduce edema and its shell as a container for drugs. Evidence that the bottle gourd was grown at least 6000 years ago was derived from the discovery of gourd seeds in excavations at Zhejiang province in 1973 [51].

4.2.4   Ben Cao (dispensatories and pharmacopeias)

The term *Ben Cao* is used generically for dispensatories and such application has been in evidence for describing materia medica since the Han dynasty. Although *Cao* refers to plants and the *Ben Caos* cover in the main drugs of vegetable origin, products derived from mineral and animal (humans also) sources are part of the subject matter. Hence it has become common to use the word "herbal" loosely to include all natural products.

The written record on pharmaceutics in China dates back approximately 3500 years to the Shang dynasty (ca. 1520 to 1030 B.C.). The Egyptians and Babylonians practiced a form of medicine that was probably older but the medical system in China is the oldest continuing one and its origin will almost surely date further back with archeologic excavations that are continuing. Inscriptions on animal bones and tortoise shells, found in Anyang at the site of the ancient capital city of the Late Shang, indicate that the civilization, as evidenced by the magnificient bronzes, was already quite advanced [43, 44]. The Chinese were cognizant of diseases and used wine, contained in ritual bronze vessels, extensively for religious and medical purposes. After the Shang, descriptions about treatment of certain ailments were recorded in the classical literature of the Zhou dynasty (1030 to 722 B.C.) when brush and lamp black were used for writing on silk, wood or bamboo slats [52]. Although legend claims that the compilation of the knowledge about pharmaceutical remedies derived from plants, animals and minerals began more than 5000 years ago, about 2500 seems more correct. The first events recorded in writing reflect to those handed down through generations by word of mouth about the contributions of great leaders whose existence cannot be demonstrated. Although a legendary hero could have been fabricated from thin air and the facts distorted over time by successive story-tellers, living proof for a problematic existence gains substance from noble deeds. It would seem that tales, communicated without resortment to the supernatural and subordinating anthropocentricity to acceptance of nature and the laws of the universe, could be true. Under such circumstances, although the person, the happening and the date can not be fixed, we can only surmise that the achievements of an illustrious figure made an impact that could not be ignored.

The first treatise devoted primarily to health and medical matters, *Huangdi Nei Jing* (Yellow Emperor's Classic on Internal Medicine) is ascribed to a legendary ruler Huangdi who supposedly lived 5000 years ago. However, the consensus of scholars is that the *Nei Jing*, even though it described some earlier history, could have been written only after the advent of brush writing, probably during the late Zhou dynasty (Warring States period, 480 to 221 B.C.) but perhaps even earlier (Spring Autumn, 722 to 480 B.C.) [53].

The first text on pharmaceutics, *Shen Nong Ben Cao Jing* (Canonical Text of the Divine Husbandman) is attributed also to another legendary ruler, Shen Nong, who preceded Huangdi. Based on archeologic evidence, however, the compendium is approximated to have been written more than 3000 years later. Hence, the use of Shen Nong's name in the title appears to be honorific rather than adjectival for ascribing authorship. Shen Nong was the second of three primordial sovereigns and is immortalized as the patron deity of agriculture, animal husbandry, pharmacy and medicine. He taught the people how to grow grain, till the land with a plough and assess the quality of spring water. He tasted hundreds of plants and learned what to avoid and accept for food. In the course of finding the esculent, he noted that some vegetation exhibited healing qualities and began a daily systematic search to evaluate products of plant, animal and mineral origin. He recorded and classified the pharmacologic properties of 365 substances.

Although no author's copy has been found, its existence is evidenced by citation in original prescriptions unearthed in Han tombs and its origin is approximated to be no earlier than 200 B.C. and no later than 200 A.D. The dates could be estimated from mention of the dispensatory in recipes found at burial sites of the Late Han (25 to 220 A.D.) but not Early Han (202 to 9 B.C.) even though many products and recipes of the two periods were found to be similar [54, 55]. Thus it would appear that the unknown author(s) of the Late Han were attempting to record the state ot the art before their time. Prior to these excavations, the most compelling evidence for the existence of *Ben Cao* was found in the revision by Tao Hong-jing (452 to 536) who based his information on articles long lost [27, 47].

In a span of approximately 1500 years between the Han and nineteenth century, the number of writings dealing exclusively with medical matters is quite extensive, exceeding more than 2600 [47]. During the Tang dynasty (618 to 906) a committee of twenty-two scholars and physicians appointed by the Emperor Kao Zung published a manual on the natural products of plant, animal and mineral origin, *Xin Xiu Ben Cao* (New Compilation on Materia Medica) in 659 A.D. The work was the first treatise on pharmaceutics to have official sanction and may be considered to be the first pharmacopeia [3, 27, 51].

The most celebrated compendium on materia medica, *Ben Cao Gang Mu* by Li Shih-Zhen, was published in 1596 during the Ming dynasty (1368 to 1644). The contents are contained in 52 volumes and nearly 11,000 prescriptions compounded from 1,892 substances described in detail with respect to appearance, properties, method of collection, preparation and use. The book took thirty years to write and is not only an encyclopedic dispensatory but a comprehensive work on natural history in botany, zoology, mineralogy that is worthy of comparison with the best scientific work of the Renaissance period in Western countries [57].

Li was a careful and competent investigator as well as a great physician. He personally studied the action of many drugs and discarded a lot of useless information and toxic preparations [57]. His monumental work remains the pandect for all subsequent texts on materia medica in China. Unfortunately, dogma prevailed increasingly after his death, and his results and conclusions became incorporated into metaphysical doctrines after the fall of the Ming dynasty. Indeed, during the ensuing Ching dynasty, traditional medicine not only ceased to advance but an erosion of its rational basis also occurred.

5   The validation of traditional medicines

Even though the Chinese theories on drug action have become dated, the frame in time has not been that long. Pharmacology did not emerge as a disciplinary entity in the West until the end of the nineteenth century, and only then did the textbooks begin to give attention to the factors that may alter drug action, which the Chinese had thought about and written about centuries earlier. However, rapid strides were made in the West during the twentieth century which truly was the Golden Age for the development of new pharmaceutical entities and mechanistic notions about drug action. Despite these major innovations, the Western approach to establishing the utility of an agent is by no means perfect and requires considerable expenditure of time, money and effort with no guarantee of success.

5.1   Deficiencies in the Western approach

It is not always a simple matter to establish drug efficacy. Even with the many methodologies available, many may not be applicable for validating the efficacy of traditional Chinese medicines. Moreover, the current screening programs by pharmaceutical companies to develop an agent superior to prototypic ones generally do not produce novel innovations. Some even deride such projects as "me tooism", but in fairness such an approach has yielded many useful agents better than their parent counterparts. However, there are also many medicaments being prescribed with only trivial advantages over their original models and these have reached the market place for economic rather than scientific reasons. With few exceptions, the truly novel discoveries have resulted from the serendipity of pharmacologists and clinicians rather than by design. The modern texts in pharmacology abound with accounts where luck and the prepared mind resulted in success [34–36, 39]. Most readers should be familiar with the classic examples mentioned below and should have no problem including a few others.
Antibiotics were developed because it was noted in contaminated culture media that bacterial growth was inhibited by the presence of a mold.

Antipsychotics arose from a project to find novel antihistamines to treat allergies but the peculiar sedative response elicited by certain congeners stimulated interest in their psychotropic properties. Diuretic drugs came from the initial attempt to design an agent to slow the excretion of penicillin which at the time of its inception was in short supply and expensive. Pethidine (meperidine), the first totally synthetic surrogate of morphine, resulted from a project to develop an antispasmodic agent but the pharmacologist tested it for analgetic properties when it elicited locomotor behavior in mice similar to morphine [62]. Subsequently other congeners of pethidine were developed to produce short-term anesthesia and to treat diarrhea. In such instances, trial and error played a more important role than mechanistic considerations.

The limitations of the Western method for validating a folkloric remedy can be further illuminated by taking the reader through the necessary experimental process for discovering a new product. Suppose that it becomes necessary to validate an ancient herbal remedy which has been used for centuries for treating pain. Conceivably, that plant may contain an active constituent capable of supplanting morphine in that it would possess superior analgetic potency and efficacy without addiction liability. In order for the chemist to extract, characterize and identify the active principle, a bioassay method must be available to measure its pharmacologic activity. Even though the herbal remedy may have been used for centuries and is believed to be effective and safe, it would not be feasible for medical, legal as well as ethical reasons to initiate the evaluation of the isolated principle on human subjects. Hence, prior to testing in the clinic, the putative analgesic would have to be assessed in the experimental laboratory. I should like to take the reader through the numerous processes required based on my own experiences in this area. A variety of experimental model systems are available for screening potential analgetic activity. Although a battery of tests on animals can easily be carried out, the screening tests provide useful data only for opioid-like substances and have poor predictive reliability for other types of anodynes such as the non-steroidal antiinflammatory agents.

To assess for opioid-like analgetic activity, the dog, cat, rabbit and guinea pig have been used but the animal of choice has been the mouse or rat. A noxious stimulus (thermal, chemical or electric shock) can be applied to the tail or foot and the rodent will respond by attempting to avoid the stimulus by flicking the tail or lifting the paw. The reaction time to the nociceptive stimulus can be recorded after which the test compound is injected into the animal. An "analgetic" response would be indicated by a prolongation in the reaction time by the tail or paw to the noxious stimulus. A dose-response curve can be plotted to provide a quantitative measure of the potency of the unknown substance when compared with a known standard such as morphine. It should be noted that the test provides only a measure of nociception and not analgesia because the antinociceptive response reflects a spinal reflex and/or supraspinal action. Since pain is a sensation and requires interpretation by the brain cortex, a true experimental test for analgesia could be performed only if the animal could say "ouch". No matter, the antinociceptive tests for morphine-like action provides data that correlates well with clinical findings. Indeed, *in vitro* assessments on an isolated strip of guinea pig longitudinal muscle (other species will not do) will provide data on rank potency in a series of opioid-like compounds that correlate surprisingly well with clinical findings. Even simple binding tests on homogenized brain tissue or cells in culture have predictive potential although it is necessary to differentiate between agonist and antagonist binding. However, even if a succession of experimental tests reveals the unknown plant constituent to be tenfold more potent than morphine, it is better not to be overly elated. Some current morphine congeners that have been synthesized are over a hundred-fold more potent than morphine but at therapeutic doses they produce no greater pain relief than that afforded by morphine. To date there have been many compounds discovered to be more potent than morphine but none have been demonstrated to be more efficacious, and that is not the end of the caveats.

If greater efficacy cannot be demonstrated, then to have any advantage over morphine, fewer undesirable side effects should at least be displayed by the test substance. In particular, the agent in question should exhibit low addiction liability, that is, it should not promote compulsive drug usage with ultimate detrimental effects on the user. Unfortunately, it would be even less ethical and practical to prove in the clinic lower addiction liability potential than greater analgetic efficacy. In this instance, the reader should not be burdened again with the experimental approach and recitation of the numerous model systems and tests that are available for providing the clues. Suffice it to say, all the tests are designed to compare the plant product with the prototypic compound, morphine [58–60]. The methodology involves assessments for opioid-like properties such as tolerance and physical dependence development as well as discriminatory tests on rodents and non-human primates to ascertain selective preference for a desired substance. However, decreased responsivity to an agent (tolerance) and enhanced rebound hypersensitivity upon discontinuance of an agent after frequent repeated exposure of the compound (physical dependence) do not always reflect a precise index of compulsive drug usage.

And although conditioned drug-seeking behavior provides a better indication, all the described tests are geared towards discovering a substance which displays lower drug-seeking behavior, less tolerance and less physical dependence than morphine. Thus, even though a product superior to morphine can be discovered by such an approach, since morphine is the prototype and the tests are designed to reflect its properties, the odds are against the discovery of a novel analgetic even if it is tailor-made. Such a view can easily be substantiated. After nearly five decades of a major program aimed toward developing a non-addicting analgetic under the initial sponsorship and coordination by an expert committee of the National Research Council acting in behalf of the prestigious National Academy of Sciences in the United States [61], only partial success was achieved. Several compounds have been marketed, but their advantages over morphine have been relatively minor and would be hardly missed if adequate supplies of morphine could be ensured.

Of course, those with expertise in opiate pharmacology can argue that morphine acts on at least four types of receptors, mu, kappa, delta and sigma; so the approach should be aimed to be more specific and since the mu receptor seems primarily involved with addiction liability, perhaps compounds selectively active on the other receptors should be made. This has been done with kappa agonists, and some potent analgetics with little addiction liability are commercially available. However, for reasons that are not entirely clear such substances have not gained wide popularity. In part, these agents at higher doses are usually dysphoric whereas in subjects with pain morphine generally produces a liking or euphoric effect. The undesirable psychotomimetic action of kappa agonists is thought to reflect a response on the sigma receptor [59]. Clearly, the reductionistic approach of the West cannot be applied to solve all ills; at times it can even be misleading. Success or failure can sometimes be attributed to being right for the wrong reason or wrong for the right reason.

To give a few examples, the analgetic pethidine was designed to be an antispasmodic and this was established by tests *in vitro* on excised tissue. As mentioned earlier, however, the compound was found by chance in mice to be a potential analgetic, and it did reach the market place as a highly useful anodyne [62,63]. Unfortunately, it was also asserted to be antispasmodic and non-addicting. Subsequent tests with pethidine on the biliary tract of human subjects, however, revealed that it not only did not relax smooth musculature but that it was actually spasmogenic. Moreover, it also turned out to be highly addictive, especially in physicians and nurses [63].

5.2   Computerized databasing of Chinese materia medica

Language barriers and the diffusion of vast amounts of data over centuries have greatly hindered the communication of information on Chinese medicinals to the West. With computerized data basing the access has been greatly facilitated. A unique Computerized Chinese Medicinal Database (CCMD) has been established at the Chinese University in Hong Kong to facilitate interchange and access to current activity in this area. The system provides on-line information on Chinese materia medica and includes botanical, chemical, pharmacological and clinical reports for instant retrieval and linking with Western biomedical databases [64].

Databasing is also being applied to facilitate the validation of traditional remedies [65]. The World Health Organization estimates that up to 80% of people in developing countries rely at some time on indigenous traditional medicine to meet their health care needs. Of the approximated 250,000 species of flowering plants on earth perhaps 20% have been used for treatment, and the therapeutic value of some 200–250 has been demonstrated scientifically to warrant their application in Western (allopathic) medicine. A combination of information indicating that a plant has been used in an indigenous health care system for centuries together with efficacy and toxicity data published by several laboratories yields a correlation that justifies further investigation. To validate additional useful products, the WHO has established a Collaborating Center for Traditional Medicine to draw on the vast published literature on the pharmacologic evaluation of plant extracts. A computerized data base NAPRALERT (NAtural PRroduct ALERT), housed at the University of Illinois, provides information on the world literature concerning the chemical constituents and pharmacology of plant, microbial and animal extracts, derived from about 700 scientific journals. The system can be used in a number of ways, ranging from simple retrieval of information to complex problem solving.

An important practical application of the database is analysis of data to determine the rational use of specific plants. One example was an analysis of plant extracts from 248 plants used in traditional medicine by "barefoot doctors " near Beijing to determine whether one or more components of certain prescriptions had a valid pharmacologic basis of action. The search included pharmacologic profile, ethnomedical claims and chemical constituents. If a prescription contained one or more drugs whose pharmacologic effects could be correlated with its traditional usage or if a principle was shown to elicit an appropriate pharmacologic response, the recipe was presumed to have a rational basis for application. Also, when the use of a plant by people geographically distant or with different cultural background was similar, the coincidence was considered unlikely to be due to chance. By such criteria, the analysis revealed that 45% of nearly 800 prescriptions had a valid rationale for their recommended use; lack of scientific data precluded substantiation for the use of the remainder [10, 12, 65].

5.3   The Japanese approach

The validation of a traditional Chinese prescription or formula is certainly more complex than that for assessing a pure constituent of plant or animal origin. In a given recipe, several natural products are combined to enhance therapeutic efficacy and/or to reduce undesirable side effects. When healing, the traditional practitioner is bound by ancient theory to alter the daily therapeutic regimen in accordance with the condition of the patient and under such circumstances a controlled study cannot be performed. However, Japanese herbal (*Kampo*) medicine, which has its roots in traditional Chinese medicine has provided some insight.

Diagnosis and treatment in *Kampo* medicine is alluded to as *Sho* and *Ko* but these two terms are not altogether synonymous with their Western counterparts. *Sho* circumscribes a profile of signs and symptoms without naming any actual disease, but once the syndrome is identified, treatment is initiated with a corresponding *Ko*. *Ko* consists of a decoction of fixed composition formulated from several natural products that is given after *Sho* is determined. Since *Sho* may vary from day to day, so then must *Ko*. Thus, as in traditional Chinese medicine, the absence of a stable steady-state for making assessments subjects *Kampo* medicine to criticism despite the fact that its empirically, in many instances, it may have withstood the test of time. To the proponents of the Western school who seek to isolate the active constituent of a natural product and evaluate it on a specific disease there is much skepticism about the merits of *Kampo* medicine. However, it is entirely conceivable, indeed to be expected, that the efficacy and toxicity of a drug can be altered by products with which it is combined. Hence, investigators in *Kampo* medicine have attempted to provide a rational pharmacologic basis for the claims of enhanced potency and lowered tendency for adverse effect of *Kampo* medicines. For example, by testing for antitussive activity in a concoction of several plants for treating asthma, Hosoya and associates found that the most active one was *Ephedra herba*. Although a decoction of this herb alone was potent pharmacologically, the complete prescription containing four products was longer-lasting. [66]. They also provided experimental data indicating that the anticonvulsant effects of a nine-herb decoction (TJ-960) could be assigned to one or two plants but potency was reduced when the other products were omitted from the recipe. Such controlled data provide clear validation of traditional theory concerning drug-drug interaction.

6   Regulatory problems for traditional remedies

There are regulatory agencies in some countries today that would like to require the purveyors of herbal remedies to provide scientific evidence on the efficacy of their products. In principle, it is difficult to argue against such a demand but the question is "What would be the scientific evidence"? Even with pure substances, as has been pointed out earlier, suitable model systems are not always available to provide the correct answer for certain diseases, and some might even give the wrong one. The cost in time and money today to market a new drug is considerable. It took on the average six to twelve years of basic and clinical investigation and an expenditure of $ 359 million [67] in order to get a new entity from the laboratory to the pharmacist's shelf in the United States in 1993. The pharmaceutical firm is required to establish both efficacy and safety and the approval process is extremely slow [68] but fortunately is improving [69]. A major problem is the extreme caution exercised by the regulatory agency that results in agonizing delays, the decision being weighted more towards demonstrating lack of toxicity and less towards loss of benefit.

One of the requirements by regulatory agencies for demonstrating drug efficacy is that double-blind methodology be applied, that is, the evaluation of the test compound must be compared with an inert substance (placebo) and the subject and investigator must remain ignorant of the nature of the medication. Thus, a positive finding leads to the conclusion that the test compound is better than the dummy. I have argued (to no avail) that the double-blind test for pain relief (and many other conditions) is difficult to defend both on medical and ethical grounds [70]. If a patient needs treatment, it is unethical to withhold medication by giving an inert substance. On the other hand, in evaluating a new medication, it is ethical to try to find out on a blind basis the lowest dose of the agent that will be effective without producing side effects. Thus, a dose-response evaluation could be performed double-blind on a test substance in comparison with a positive standard. Opponents to such an approach argue that such trials would be prohibitively expensive in time and money because the placebo response, especially in subjects with pain, may be as high as 30 percent. Should such factors be the decisive consideration, especially since the the costs can be recovered when the drug is marketed?

Apart from the economic facets, a high placebo response raises some semantic considerations. If the placebo produces an affirmative effect on a significant segment of the population, then it is better than nothing and is therefore a remedy. So when an herbal (or any test) substance turns out to be no better than a placebo, is it still not benefiting a lot of people? Unless natural remedies are demonstrated to be directly harmful, there seems to be little point in preventing their accessibility. Some might rightfully point out that their usage might delay critical life-saving intervention but unless this can be documented and the availability of modern drugs can be guaranteed for all people, especially the underprivileged, common sense dictates that the wisdom of the ages should allow nature to take its course.

The other side of the coin is that the traditional remedies used by the Chinese may display delayed long-term toxic effects [71, 72]. To counter it can be argued that the Chinese have time on their side. As early as two thousand years ago, natural products were grouped by their potency, and it would seem by now that any serious toxicity elicited by such substances after chronic usage should have surfaced. The possibility of latent undesirable effects emerging cannot be discounted and there have been recent reports on the toxicity of herbal remedies [71, 73, 74]. In some instances, the more serious adverse effects have been traced to proprietary remedies wherein a traditional recipe was adulterated with a potent drug developed in the West or a wrong plant product was substituted in a recipe [71, 72]. The marketing of such a preparation would appear tantamount to acknowledging lack of efficacy of the original product but this hardly justifies the act. Fortunately, these events have seldom been reported. Nonetheless, such happenings could be minimized by qualified organized traditional practitioners setting rules and standards for professional conduct and health care among themselves to protect the public.

Where there is lack of precise scientific data, anecdotal evidence cannot be easily dismissed. I recall vividly that when I was a graduate student more than fifty years ago, the U.S. Federal Trade Commission initiated a suit against Fong Wan, a highly popular herbalist in the San Francisco Bay area, for false advertising about the curative actions of herbal remedies. The government sought to establish by expert testimony that Chinese natural products did not have therapeutic value and in support of their case, brought in two eminent university pharmacologists, some prominent clinicians from two major medical centers, and several practicing physicians in the metropolitan area representing various specialties. Thus, town and gown served as friendly witnesses for the government.

The two pharmacologists testified in essence that people do get well especially from acute illnesses, that the efficacy of the herbal remedies was not unequivocally established and possibly therefore, many of the remedies may not have therapeutic value. However, when the defense displayed some plants for the two experts to identify and they could not, the defense queried "How can you opine a remedy is without value unless you know what it is?" The practicing physicians from academe and town also expressed skepticism of the healing feats of the recipes but the defense paraded a multitude of witnesses who gave personal testimony in vigorous support of Fong Wan. In virtual unison, they swore that they were cured by Fong, after having been treated without success by Western physicians. Finally, when Fong Wan took the stand he revealed that he had two sons, one a graduate and the other a student at distinguished U.S. medical schools, whom he treated with Chinese herbal tea when they were ill. Fong Wan was acquitted and afterwards advertised the proceedings verbatim in the city newspapers [75]. In twenty-two separate instances, governmental and professional regulatory agencies were unable to win their case against Fong Wan other than concessions to advertising claims. Of course, proponents for controlled clinical trials could emphatically point out, not to be proven legally wrong did not establish that Fong Wan's remedies are superior to those of the West. Winning battles in court hardly qualifies lawyers to replace pharmacologists for carrying out tests on drug efficacy and toxicity but the decisions point to the problems scientists, practitioners and regulators must face.

An open mind must be maintained with respect to the adequacy of experimental and clinical procedures for assessing traditional products. Systematic screening of compounds in the animal laboratory for efficacy and toxicity has been ongoing for over a century and applied in many instances with great success. Nonethless, as has been demonstrated, the methodology at times can be shown to have short-comings. In clinical assessments especially, the rigors of double-blind assessments tend to limit the sensitivity of the procedure. Hence, the inability to obtain affirmative data by the scientific approach does not necessarily mean negation. It is well-recognized that a failure might be due not only to inadequate sensitivity of the procedure but also to lack of suitable methodology or knowledge base to establish the fact. The validation of acupuncture is a case in point.

The procedure has long been viewed with skepticism by many Western-trained physicians despite its ancient history and wide application. Even though it has finally gained clinical respectability and sanction by governments and professional organizations, it was not until opiopeptins (brain peptides with opiate-like action, endorphins) were discovered in 1976 and acupuncture was shown to cause the release of these endogenous substances that the procedure gained scientific credence [76].

Among the armamentarium of natural products of the Chinese, tonics have long been popular and still are today, the most notable one being ginseng. Many principles have been isolated from ginseng and their pharmacologic actions studied [15, 22, 74]. Based on the findings, it is difficult to explain satisfactorily its putative beneficial effects, but has the correct methodology been applied? To demonstrate any merit to ginseng, perhaps the ancient concepts for longevity should be reconsidered. There has been insufficient focus on host factors that might be of benefit in prolonging life, and a longitudinal approach, difficult as it may be, should receive more attention. Perhaps the emphasis should be more towards identifying the appropriate physiologic systems primarily involved with maintaining health or promoting resistance to disease. Current knowledge concerning the role of suppressors and promoters in carcinogenesis has directed the focus towards finding promoter inhibitors or suppresser enhancers, and expectations are high. Until two decades ago the effects of drugs on the immune system had scarcely been studied. Only when it became necessary to suppress the immune system to facilitate organ transplantation were such compounds investigated. It may be necessary to remind the reader at this point that immunology had its roots in China when inoculation for smallpox was introduced in the sixteenth century [38], and now attempts are being made to provide an immunopharmacological and biochemical basis for Chinese herbal medicine [79]. In recent years the lay and semi-popular press have directed attention to anti-aging agents, and it has become difficult to extinguish in the minds of many that the antioxidant properties of vitamin C and E may prevent cancer and senescence by scavenging free radicals. More recently there have been two other putative rejuvenators that have received considerable attention. The sales of melatonin, the pineal gland hormone, which is easily available for sleep in health-food stores, has increased substantially in the wake of articles suggesting the agent is an antioxidant. For analogous reasons, DHEA, dehydroepiandrosterone, an androgenic hormone in the adrenal gland has stirred the public but economic considerations are not yet a factor because the compound is not easily available. In essence human nature has not changed over millenia and interest in ginseng will continue to prevail unless some striking adverse effect is found. Based on the long history of usage of the plant and current pharmacologic studies the possibility of discovering latent chronic toxicity seems rather remote. To my knowledge no remedy has been established to prolong longevity in humans, but the possibility does exist and if it is reasonably safe, why not?

7   Conclusions and perspectives

Some might assert that even though the Chinese system may have spawned some useful remedies, most have outlived their usefulness. However, even if these natural products become discarded, so also will the ones discovered in the West. To comprehend such suppositions, it is only necessary to consult any modern textbook in pharmacology or better yet a compendium on therapeutic agents that is published annually.

The 1995 edition of Physician's Desk Reference [76] lists nearly three thousand prescription drugs that are in current usage in the United States, and virtually all were introduced in the twentieth century. Indeed, roughly ninety percent of the innovations were made within the past five decades. These encompass new drug entities for the treatment of infectious diseases, allergies, cardiovascular complications, renal failure, mental states, and metabolic conditions. Medications among these groups include antibiotics, antihistamines, b-adrenergic blockers, calcium channel blockers, diuretics, antiepileptics, antipsychotics, steroid hormone congeners, etc., and each drug class may include as many as twenty or more related surrogates; some of the relatively recent innovations have already become obsolete. Thus, it should not be expected that the materia medica of the past can prevail forever.

These suppositions are to be anticipated and are inevitable in pharmacology. Although the discipline is defined as the study of the effects of chemical substances on living tissue, it cannot help but have a strong anthropocentric focus on drugs for diseases affecting humans. As the field broadens and the data base expands, a large body of the knowledge loses practical significance because the bulk of the information is concerned with details about the chemical and biologic properties of specific medications. Although the pharmacology of such agents retains scientific relevance, the interest in them wanes once they are replaced by surrogates with greater potency, fewer side effects and more profits. It should be apparent, therefore, that survival of a drug depends not only on its efficacy and lesser toxicity but also on economic factors associated with patentability, marketability as well as regulatory practices that can be biased by local attitudes and politics.

Despite the fact that new and better agents are being introduced at an unparalleled rate, there are still good reasons why the orthodoxy of the ancient healers can not be simply tossed aside. Even today, major improvements in therapy are more often the result of empiricism rather than reductionism, and well-established agents have often found new applications without regulatory approval. In most instances, the usage emanated not from design but from astute observation of their side effects. Familiar and surprising examples can be given. Aspirin has been available for headache and arthritic disorders for nearly a century but only recently has it been applied to thin the blood of patients with histories of stroke and myocardial infarct; now it seems only reasonable to exploit such action to prevent diabetic retinopathy. Articles now appear in the popular press on other investigational uses for aspirin, including to boost the immune system, to prevent toxemia of pregnancy and retard development of cataracts. Such applications are not established but are mentioned to point out the increasing attention being given to new uses for old drugs based on observations of their adverse as well as their beneficial effects. Carbamazepine was introduced in the 1960s for treatment of neuralgia but is now considered to be a primary drug for most types of epilepsy and is also used for treating certain psychotic conditions. Amantadine, marketed as an antiviral agent, was unexpectedly found to cause symptomatic improvement in parkinsonism, a motor nerve disease. Who would have imagined antibiotics being recommended as the agent of choice for the prevention and treatment of gastrointestinal ulcers [80]? Will the much aligned thalidomide that caused fetal malformations find application in tuberculosis [81] or AIDS [82] as it has in leprosy [83]?

Rapid studies are being made today with the basic receptor mechanisms involved in drug action, and this new knowledge will certainly facilitate the innovation of novel and better drugs. In particular, the biotechnical contributions on the genetic basis of diseases have been most rewarding even though progress in the main is applicable only in the treatment of some rare diseases. Nonetheless, such success portends undoubtedly that there will be significant advances made on ills that affect greater segments of the population. Hopefully, answers on the molecular basis of Alzheimer's disease, schizophrenia and cancer will be provided "soon" to facilitate the design of novel drugs by computer graphics technology. Such compounds are likely to be rigid proteinmimetic analogs of the native substances related to the aforementioned diseases. In such instances, the new technology of combinatory chemistry will enable the synthesis of new drug entities of known structure on an assembly line basis. By simultaneously creating compounds with shapes, charges and electrostatic characteristics, the odds of finding selectively active compounds with potential therapeutic activity are tremendously reduced. In addition, by merging combinatorial chemistry with silicon-pattering technics, intricate checkerboards of different nucleotide sequences anchored to a silicon chip can be produced to serve as detectors of aberrant genetic sequences [84]. This knowledge should facilitate the design of genetic sequences and facilitate the design of drugs for genetic diseases. However, "soon" is not yet precisely definable. In the meantime, traditional Chinese medicine with its herbal remedies is still widely prevalent and necessary because today's free enterprise system, however successful it may be, cannot assure immediate access to those who need immediate treatment.

References

1   K.C. Wong and L.T. Wu: History of Chinese Medicine. National Quarantine Service, Shanghai (1936).
2   M. Porkert with C. Ullman: Chinese Medicine, translated by M. Howson, William Morrow, New York (1988).
3   P.Y. Ho and F.P. Lipowski: Concepts of Chinese Science and Traditional Healing Arts. World Scientific, Singapore (1993).
4   P.U. Unschuld: Medicine in China, A History of Ideas. University of California, Berkeley (1985).
5   N. Sivin: Traditional Medicine in Contemporary China. University of Michigan, Center for Chinese Studies, Ann Arbor (1986).
6   F.F. Kao: Medicine in China: New Discoveries, New Concepts and New Frontiers. Amer. J of Chinese Med. 2, 171 (1974)
7   J.Y.P. Chen: Acupuncture and Pharmacology, in: J.R. Quinn (Ed.): Medicine and Public Health in the People's Republic of China, p. 63, U.S. Department of Health, Education and Welfare, DHEW Publication No. (NIH) 73–75. Washington, D.C. U.S. Government Printing Office (1973).
8   E.L. Way: Pharmacology, in: S.H. Gould (Ed.): Sciences in Communist China, American Association for the Advancement of Science, p. 363. Washington, D.C., publication no. 68 (1961).
9   E.L. Way: The Materia Medica Program in Communist China. Proc. West. Pharmacol. Soc. 4, 44 (1961).
10   Herbal Pharmacology in the People's Republic of China. A trip report of the American Herbal Pharmacology Delegation to the National Academy of Science, Washington, D.C. (1974).
11   J.J. Burns and P.J. Tsuchitani (Eds.): U.S.-China Pharmacology Symposium, Committee on Scholarly Communication with People's Republic of China. Washington, D.C. (1980).
12   L. Lasagna: Herbal pharmacology and medical therapy in the People's Republic of China. Annals of Internal Med. 83, 887 (1975).
13   C.P. Li: Highlights in Chinese Traditional Herbal Medicine. A trip report to J.R. Quinn, the International Cooperation and Geographic Studies Branch, Fogarty International Center, National Institutes of Health, Bethesda (1974).

14   H.M. Chang, H.W. Yeung, W.W. Tso and A. Koo: Advances in Chinese Medicinal Materials Research. World Scientific, Singapore (1985).

15   H.Y. Hsu, Y.P. Chen and M. Hong: The Chemical Constituents of Oriental Herbs. Oriental Healing Arts Institute, Long Beach (1982).

16   H.M. Chang and P.P. But: Pharmacology and Applications of Chinese Materia Medica. World Scientific, Singapore (1986).

17   B. Yu and K. Peng (Eds.): Colour Atlas of Chinese Traditional Drugs. Science Press, Beijing (1987).

18   T. Takemi, M. Hasegawa, A. Kumagai and Y.Otsuka (Eds.): Herbal Medicine, Past and Present. Tsumura Jutendo, Tokyo (1985).

19   A Barefoot Doctor's Manual. John E. Fogarty International Center, National Institutes of Health, Bethesda, DHEW Publication No. (NIH) 75–695.

20   E. Hosoya and Y. Yamamura (Eds.): Recent Advances in the Pharmacology of *Kampo* (Japanese Herbal) Medicines. International Congress Series *854*, Excerpta Medica, Amsterdam (1988).

21   M. Ou (Ed.): Chinese-English Manual of Common-Used in Traditional Chinese Medicine. Joint Publishing, Hong Kong (1989).

22   K.C. Huang: The Pharmacology of Chinese Herbs. CRC Press, Boca Raton (1993).

23   J. Ying, X. Mao, Q. Ma, Y. Zong and H. Wen, translated by Y. Xu: Icons of Medicinal Fungi from China. Science Press, Beijing (1987).

24   Z. Xie, Z. Zhao and Y. Huang: Medicinal Plants in China. Chinese Academy of Traditional Medicine and World Health Organization, Manila (1989).

25   S. Miyashita: An Historical Analysis of Chinese Drugs in the Treatment of Hormonal Diseases, Goitre, and Diabetes Mellitus. Am. J. Chin. Med. *8*, 17 (1980).

26   G.D. Lu and J. Needham: Records of Diseases in Ancient China. Am. J. of Chin. Med. *4*, 3 (1961).

27   J. Needham and G.D. Lu: Science and Civilisation in China. Chemistry and Chemical Technology, Vol. V Pt. 5. Cambridge University Press, Cambridge (1983).

28   L.C. Goodrich: A Short History of the Chinese People. Harper & Brothers, New York (1941).

29   R. Grousset: The Rise and Splendour of the Chinese Empire. University of California Press, Berkeley (1953).

30   C.P. Fitzgerald: The Horizon History of China. American Heritage, New York (1969).

31   W. Eberhard: A History of China. University of California Press, Berkeley (1977).

32   W.S. Morton: China, Its History and Culture. Lippincott and Crowell, New York (1980).

33   K.K. Chen: Half a century of ephedrine. Am. J. Chin. Med. *2*, 359 (1974).

34   B.G. Katzung (Ed.): Basic and Clinical Pharmacology. Appleton and Lange, Norwalk (1995).

35   T.M. Brody, J. Larner, K.P. Minneman and H.C. Neu: Human Pharmacology Molecular to Clinical. Mosby, St. Louis (1994).

36   A.G. Gilman, L.S. Goodman, T.W. Rall and F. Murad (Eds.): The Pharmacological Basis of Therapeutics. Macmillan, New York (1985).

37   W.C. Cooper and N. Sivin: Man as a Medicine, Pharmacological and Ritual Aspects of Traditional Therapy Using Drugs Derived From the Human Body, in S. Nakayama and N. Sivin (Eds.): Chinese Science. MIT Press, Cambridge, Massachusetts (1973).

38   J. Needham: China and the Origins of Immunology. L.S. Olschki Editore, Firenze (1987).

39   M. Silverman: Magic in a Bottle. Macmillan, New York (1941).

40   J. Needham and L. Wang: Science and Civilisation in China, History of Scientific Thought, Vol. II. Cambridge Press, Cambridge (1958).

41   J. Needham, P.Y. Ho, G.D. Lu and N. Sivin: Science and Civilisation in China, Spagyrical Discovery and Invention: Apparatus, Theories and Gifts, Vol. VPt. 4. Cambridge Press, Cambridge (1980).

42   G.D. Lu and J. Needham: A history of forsenic medicine in China. Med. Hist. *32*, 352 (1988).

43   H. Qian, H. Chen, and S. Ru: Out of China's Earth. Harry Abrams, New York and China Pictorial, Beijing (1981).

44   M. Sullivan: The Arts of China. University of California Press, Berkeley (1984).

45   F. Liu and Y.M. Liu: Chinese Medical Terminology. Commercial Press, Hong Kong (1980).

46   D. Bensky, A. Gamble, T. Kaptchuk and L.L. Bensky: Chinese Herbal Medicine. Eastland Press, Seattle (1986).

47   P.U. Unschuld: Medicine in China, A History of Pharmaceutics. University of California Press, Berkeley (1986).

48   J. Needham, G.D. Lu and H.T. Huang: Science and Civilisation in China, Biology and Biotechnology, Botany, Vol. VI Pt. 1. Cambridge Press, Cambridge (1983).

49   F. Bray: Science and Civilisation in China, Biology and Biotechnology, AgricultureVol. VI Pt. 2. Cambridge Press, Cambridge Press (1994).

50   *Wu Shih Er Ping Fang* (Prescriptions for 52 diseases). Wen Wu Publishers, Beijing (1979).

51   W.K. Fu: Traditional Chinese Medicine and Pharmacology. Foreign Language Press, Beijing (1985).

52   T.H. Tsien: Written on Bamboo and Silk, The Beginnings of Chinese Books and Inscriptions. Chicago University Press (1962).

53   I. Veith: *Huang Ti Nei Ching Su Wen.* The Yellow Emperor's Classic of Internal Medicine. University of California Press, Berkeley (1966).

54   A. Akahori: Chapters of *Huang-ti-nei-ching* derived from *yin-yang-shih-imo-chiuching.* Nihon Isshigaku Zasshi *25*, 288 (1979).

55   S. Miyashita: A historical analysis of Chinese formularies and prescriptions: three examples (dysentery and diarrhea, insanity, and the common cold). Nihon Isshigaku Zasshi *23*, 283 (1977).

56   G.D. Lu: China's Greatest Naturalist: A brief biography of Li Shih-Chen. Am. J. Chin. Med. *4*, 209 (1976).

57   E.L. Way (Ed.): New Concepts in Pain and its Clinical Management. F.A. Davis, Philadelphia (1967).

58   E.L. Way, H.H. Loh and F.S. Shen: Simultaneous quantitative assessment of morphine tolerance and physical dependence. J. Pharmacol. Exp. Ther. *167*, 1 (1969).

59   W.R. Martin (Ed.), in Handbook of Experimental Pharmacology, Vol.45/I, Drug Addiction I, Morphine, Sedative/Hypnotic and Alcohol Dependence. Springer Verlag, Berlin (1977).

60   J.V. Brady and S.E. Lucas (Eds.): Testing Drugs for Physical Dependence Potential and Abuse Liability. NIDA Research Monograph 52, DHHS no (ADM) *84*, 1332, Rockville (1984).

61   N.B. Eddy: The National Research Council Involvement in the Opiate Problem. National Academy of Sciences, Washington, D.C. (1973).

62   O. Eisleb and O. Schauman: Deutsche med. Wchnschr. *65*, 967 (1939).

63   J. Jaffe in A.G. Gilman, L.S. Goodman, T.W. Rall and F. Murad (Eds.): Opioid Anal-
      gesics and Antagonists (with W. Martin) and Drug Addiction and Drug Abuse, The
      Pharmacological Basis of Therapeutics. Macmillan, New York (1985).

64   W.S. Lee and H.M. Chang: Computerized Chinese Medicinal Database, in H.M.
      Chang, H.W. Yeung, W.W. Tso and A. Koo (Eds.): Advances in Chinese Medicinal
      Materials Research. World Scientific, Singapore (1985) pp. 9.

65   N.R. Farnsworth, C.W.W. Beecher and H.H. S. Wong: The NAPRALERT database:
      linking traditional and modern medicine. Essential Drug Monitor, *20*, 2 (1995).

66   E. Hosoya: Scientific Evaluation of *Kampo* Prescriptions Using Modern Technol-
      ogy, in Recent Advances in the Pharmacology of *Kampo* (Japanese Herbal Medi-
      cines), E. Hosoya and Y. Yamamura. Excerpta Medica, Amsterdam (1988).

67   D.E. Wierenga and J.F. Beary: The Drug Development and Approval Process, in New
      Medicines in Development for Cancer, Pharmaceutical Research Manufacturing
      Association, Washington, D.C. (1995).

68   B. Spilker: Multinational Drug Companies: Issues in Drug Discovery and Develop-
      ment. Raven, New York (1989).

69   K.I. Kaitin, M. Manocchia, M. Seibring and L. Lasagna: The new drugs approvals of
      1990, 1991 and 1992: trends in drug development. J. Clin. Pharmacol. *34*, 120 (1994).

70   E.L. Way: A Pharmacolgist's Concept of Narcotics, in C.S. Hill, Jr. and W.S. Fields:
      Advances in Pain Research Vol. II. Raven Press (1989).

71   T.Y.K. Chan, J.C.N. Chan, B. Tomlinson and J. Critchley: Chinese herbal medicines
      revisited: a Hong Kong perspective. Lancet *342*, 1532 (1993).

72   D.J. Atherton: Towards the safer use of traditional medicines. Brit. Med. J. *308*, 673
      (1994).

73   Y.T. Tai P.P.B. But, K. Young and C.P. Lau: Cardiotoxicity after accidental herb-
      induced aconite poisoning. Lancet *340*, 1254 (1992).

74   J. Cui, M. Garle, P. Eneroth and I. Bjorkhem: What do commercial ginseng prepar-
      ations contain? Lancet *344*, 134 (1994).

75   Federal Trade Comission: Official Report of the Proceedings. Docket No. 3964, San
      Francisco January 10, 1940.

76   Physician's Desk Reference 50th Edition, Medical Economics, Montvale (1996).

77   B. Pomeranz and D. Chiu: Naloxone blockade of acupuncture analgesia: endorphin
      implicated. Life Sci. *19*, 1757 (1976).

78   National Health and Nutrition Examinations Survey (NHANES D): Epidemiology
      5, 138 (1994),

79   E. Lien: Immunopharmacological and biochemical basis of Chinese herbal medi-
      cine. Prog. Drug Res. *46*, 263 (1995).

80   M.J. Blaser: The bacteria behind ulcers. Scient. Amer. *274*, 104 (1996).

81   J.M. Tramonta, U. Utaipat, A. Molloy, G. Kaplan et al.: Thalidomide treatment reduces
      tumor necrosis factor alpha production and enhances weight gain in patients with
      pulmonary tuberculosis. Molec. Med. *1*, 384 (1995).

82   S. Makonkawkeyoon, R.N.R. Limson-Probre, A.L. Moreira et al.: Thalidomide inhib-
      its the replication of human immunodeficiency virus type 1. Proc. Nat. Acad. Sci USA
      90, 5974 (1993).

83   C. Blaney: Second thoughts about thalidomide. NCCR Reporter, November/Decem-
      ber 1995.

84   J. Alpers: Drug discovery on the assembly line. Science *264*, 1339 (1994).

Progress in Drug Research, Vol. 47 (E. Jucker, Ed.)
© 1996 Birkhäuser Verlag, Basel (Switzerland)

Emerging drug targets in the molecular pathogenesis of asthma

By Jeanne Fürst Jucker and Gary P. Anderson

Asthma and Allergy Research, K-125.10.15 CIBA, 4002 Basel, Switzerland

1   Introduction

Although widely perceived as a disease that is little more than a trivial and transient nuisance of childhood, epidemiological statistics collected over the last decade clearly indicate that asthma is anything but unimportant. Across the developed world the incidence and prevalence of asthma have reached epidemic proportions. The reasons for this are unknown. Asthma is potentially a fatal disease afflicting as many as 5–9% of the population. Increasing evidence suggests that as well as causing episodic disease symptoms long-standing asthma is a serious risk factor for progression to irreversible debilitating fixed airway obstruction.

The magnitude of the asthma health problem has prompted intense research into the pathogenesis of this disease. Currently, asthma is viewed as an immunologically driven inflammatory disease of the airways associated with structural changes in mucosal and submucosal tissues that contribute to disturbed lung function (Fig. 1). Important advances have been made in recent years in designing better symptomatic and palliative therapy for asthma. This research has led to the development of novel leukotriene antagonists, phosphodiesterase inhibitors, long-acting bronchodilators, improved corticosteroids, neuropeptide antagonists, kinin and other mediator antagonists. These advances have been extensively reviewed (Nicholson, 1994) and will not be discussed here.

The purpose of this review is to outline the very recent advances in immunology and cell biology that suggest entirely new therapeutic approaches, not only to improve asthma symptoms, but also eventually to prevent and cure this disease. This review is structured in sections, each dealing with

---

Fig. 1.

Overview of key pathogenic mechanism in asthma

The figure shows the process of induction of T_H2 immunity and T cell driven cellular inflammation. During commitment allergen processed by antigen presenting cells (APC) is presented to CD4+ helper T cells. In the context of appropriate cytokine and cognate signals (e.g. from B7 family co-stimulation molecules) commitment to the T_H2 pattern of cytokine production occurs. During expansion, the T_H2 cells proliferate, drive B cell IgE production and release cytokines causing eosinophilia. In established disease mast cells may serve as an additional source of IL-4 driving commitment but macrophage-derived IL-12, TGF-β and IFN-γ may serve as important down-regulatory signals. During activation, in the inflamed mucosa antigen triggers IgE sensitized mast cells and other cells perpetuating inflammation, e.g. by promoting eosinophil activation leading to deposition of toxic major basic protein (MBP) in tissues. In established disease IL-1 probably acts to expand silent T_H2 committed „memory" T cells. In the long-term induction of tissue metalloproteases (MMPs), probably via receptor tyrosine kinase coupled growth factors (GF), promote proliferation of gland structures and the induction of epithelial differentiation/transdifferentiation causing an increased number of secretory cells. Microvascular proliferation also under GF/MMP influences is likely to occur and leads to plasma exudation.

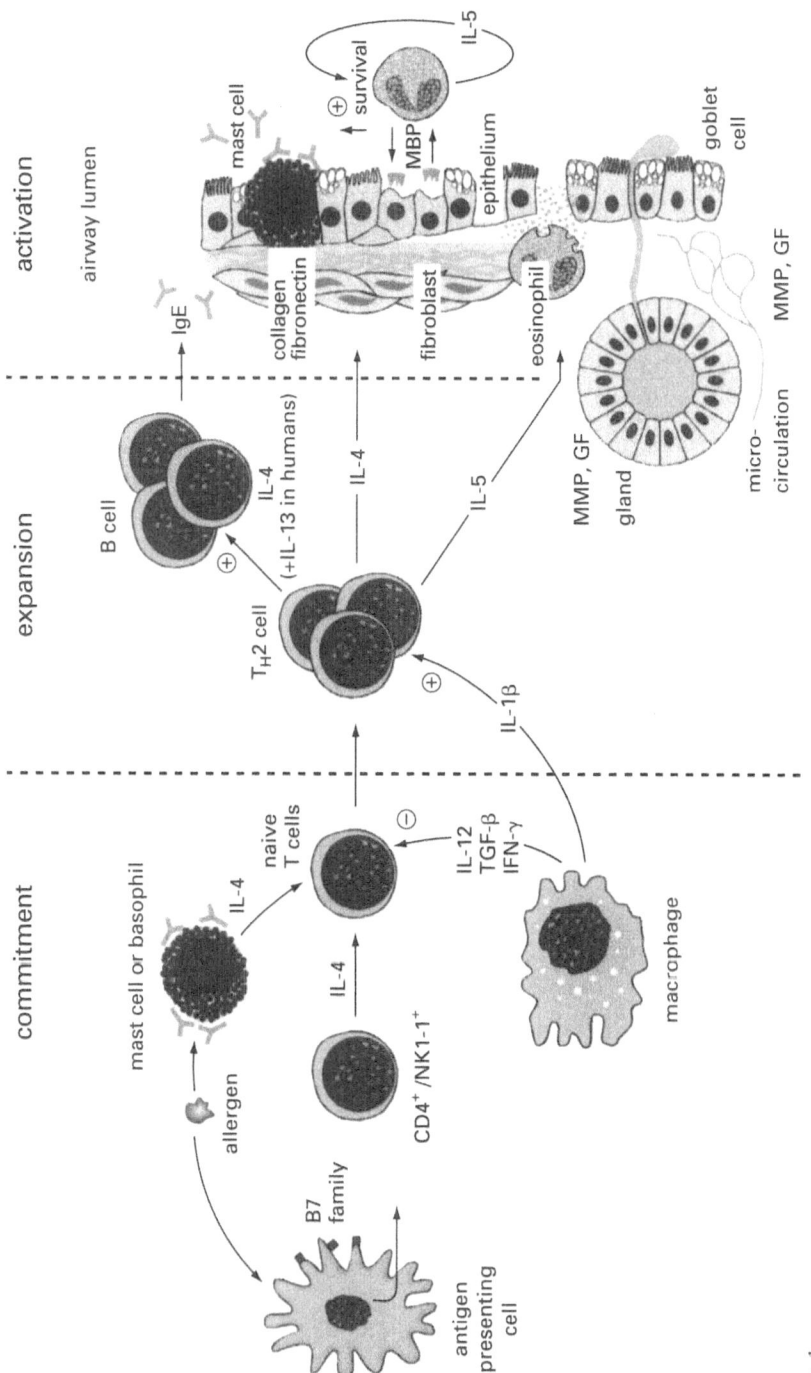

Fig. 1

important pathological processes believed to contribute to asthma. It outlines the principal molecular events likely to cause this pathology and it describes the pharmacological interventions that are, or will be in the near future, possible to alter these processes.

Many of the drugs mentioned here are experimental prototypes of new therapeutic classes. Although it is unlikely that any of the individual drugs described here will ever be used as therapeutic agents in humans, development of safe agents in each class will define the future of asthma therapy. In this review, the term drug is taken to include therapeutic use of recombinant proteins and agents based on synthetic or recombinant nucleotide technologies as well as more traditionally low molecular weight organic compounds.

2   Categories of asthma

The term „asthma" denotes a group of clinical presentations linked by the common features of episodic, reversible airflow limitation, bronchial hyperreactivity and eosinophilic inflammation of the conducting airways. Asthma has classically been divided into extrinsic and intrinsic asthma. Extrinsic asthma, defined as asthma in the presence of atopy, occurs as a response to inhaled allergens and it is most common in children. The presence of atopy is identified by elevated total and specific IgE and/or positive skin test reactions. Intrinsic asthma occurs most commonly in adults, may be of uncertain origin and skin reactivity is uncommon. This group includes the special subgroups of

- late onset asthma occurring in adults typically after the third decade of life, and
- asthma in response to industrial sensitizers.

Asthma is frequently subdivided into functional categories (Thurlbeck and Miller, 1988):

- Antigen-induced asthma: the most common form with known or suspected reactions to allergens.
- Occupational asthma: induced by sensitizing agents leading to an acquired hypersensitivity response that occurs only in a proportion of exposed subjects (i.e. animal handlers, bakers, workers with wood and vegetable dusts, metal salts, pharmaceutical agents, industrial chemicals).

- Environmental asthma: usually during episodes of massive air pollution.
- Drug-induced asthma: it occurs most commonly in patients with known asthma (i.e. induced by aspirin).
- Asthma produced by viral respiratory tract infections.
- Exercise-induced asthma in patients who already have the disease.
- Asthmatic bronchitis occurring in patients with chronic obstructive airway disease.

The clinical diversity of asthma must always be considered when considering the usefulness of new therapeutic intervention.

3   Overview of pathology and pathogenesis

The histopathologic findings of patients who have died in status asthmaticus are dramatic. Their airways are filled with thick tenacious adherent mucous plugs and the lungs are hyperinflated. The plugs contain strips of epithelium and many eosinophils. The extruded eosinophil granules can form needle-like crystals (Charcot-Leyden crystals). In some cases the mucous plugs form casts of the airways called Curschmann's spirals. Compact clusters of epithelial cells called Creola bodies can be seen in the sputum in some patients.
The epithelium loses the normal pseudostratified appearance and may if desquamated leave only the basal cells on the basement membrane. The epithelial cells are hyperplastic and squamous metaplasia may be present. Goblet cells, an important source of mucus, are also increased in number. The epithelial basement membrane is pseudothickened due to an increase of subbasement membrane collagen deposition and the smooth muscle is prominent because of muscle hyperplasia. The inflammatory cells, mainly eosinophils, are located in the lamina propria and edema and thickening of the bronchial walls are common. All these lesions vary in severity according to the state of the disease. Moreover, there are several additional lesions such as bronchiectasis in the upper lobes, probably due to the bronchial obstruction by mucous plugs as well as emphysema (Thurlbeck and Miller, 1988).
The etiology and the pathogenesis of bronchospasm and hypersecretion in bronchial asthma are complex. Bronchial muscle contraction and mucus secretion are, to some degree, under nervous control. Parasympathetic stimulation (vagus nerve) leads to bronchoconstriction and hypersecretion of mucus. The sympathetic stimulation through beta-adrenergic recep-

tors leads to vasodilatation and probably diminishes mucus secretion. There is a non-adrenergic (purinergic) inhibitory system that causes the relaxation of the airway smooth muscle. However, many mediators released from inflammatory cells such as histamine, bradykinin, leukotrienes, prostaglandins and thromboxanes cause bronchoconstriction and increase vascular permeability, and others serve as chemoattractants, e.g. for eosinophils, and directly cause mucus secretion.

In allergic asthma, the patient becomes sensitized. Although asthma can occur in the absence of IgE, IgE-mediated mechanisms play an important role in acute allergic asthma almost certainly by causing mast cell degranulation. The released mediators induce an immediate asthmatic response (Corrigan and Kay, 1992) but also induce the adhesion, diapedesis, directional migration and activation of eosinophils, possibly via synthesis/release of cytokines (Bradding et al., 1992).

3.1   Structural changes in the airways

Changes of the airway structure notably thickening of the airway walls lead to a progressive impairment of function which is increasingly recognized as a serious consequence of the disease that is poorly controlled by current therapies (Fig. 2).

3.1.1   Changes in the airway mucosa

Viscous, inspissated mucus, tenaciously blocking bronchi and bronchioles is an almost inevitable post-mortem finding in asthma deaths (Reid, 1987). Histopathological examinations of asthmatics who have died from causes other than asthma have also revealed extensive physical obstruction of the airways by mucus plugs. The term 'mucus plug' in this context is a misnomer: biochemical analysis of the constituent components of plug mate-

---

Fig. 2.
Growth factors in chronic airway disease and mechanism of mucus hyperproduction
The role of receptor tyrosine kinase (RTK) coupled growth factors in asthma is currently controversial but the established biology of many of these factors predicts that they will cause fibrosis matrix tissue remodelling, alter the nature of the epithelium, may lead to induction of proteolytic enzymes which could degrade the connections between the airway wall and lung parenchyma, promote the induction of glandular hypertrophy in the upper airways and may directly act on resident cells and tissues to promote inflammation.
Mucus, more correctly thought of as a plasma rich mucus containing exudate, is increased in asthma because the epithelium undergoes changes in its cellular composition leading to an increase area density of globlet cells and because mucus glands proliferate in the upper airways. The exact nature of the stimulus causing mucus release is unknown but it is likely that many inflammatory cells and mediators each contribute to hyperproducion of the mucus exudate.

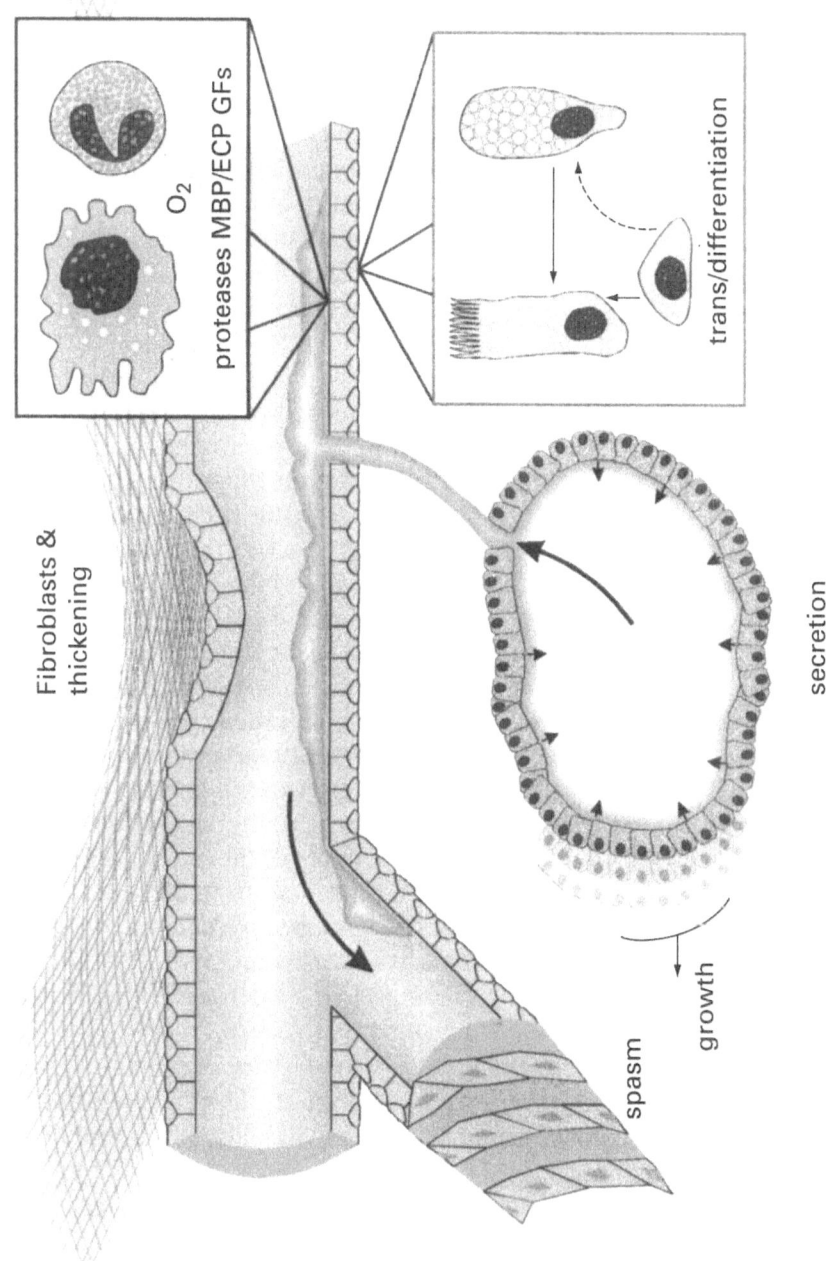

Fig. 2.

rial or expired mucus suggests that the asthmatic mucus plug is an admixture of mucus glycoproteins, an exudate rich in blood plasma proteins and cellular debris which together is the likely source of the minor eukaryotic DNA component. It is therefore important to realize that the hypersecreted material obstructing the airways in asthma is a mucus *exudate* formed by the interaction of increased mucus glycoprotein production and the leakage of plasma from inflamed microvessels of the airway submucosa (Brogan et al., 1975) (Fig. 2). Shimura et al. (1988) have demonstrated that the albumin content of human asthmatic mucus is more than 650% higher in fluid mucus secretions and more than 1700% higher in viscous mucoid sputum than that of saliva (saliva 0.03 ± 0.06; bronchorhea 0.2 ± 0.2; mucoid sputum 0.51 ± 0.21 mg/ml). This suggests that therapeutic strategies to control *mucus exudate* formation in asthma must consider both the altered nature of the asthmatic respiratory epithelium and alterations in the properties of plasma-leaking microvessels.

Three distinct problems must be considered in the therapy of mucus hypersecretion: (1) increases in the volume density of mucus gland structures, (2) increases in the surface density of mucus secreting cells in the airway epithelium, and (3) control of secretion from (1) and (2). Of these processes the epithelium and its regulation are the most likely to be of greatest importance in human asthma because bronchioles, the major site of mucus production and plugging, lack glands. It is, however, possible that some mucus in bronchioles is inspirated from mucus released glands in larger more central airways. The respiratory epithelium shows an increase in the density of mucus secreting goblet cells which is observed also in small bronchi and in the distal bronchioles (Dunhill et al., 1969; Cutz et al., 1978). In severe, fatal disease the extent of goblet cell hyperplasia can be striking: Aikawa et al. (1992) have observed up to 30-fold increases above control levels in airway goblet cell number particularly in bronchioles. Although the contribution of mucus gland secretion to airway obstruction remains an area of debate, there is clear evidence that mucus gland size and number are increased in asthma (Cutz, 1978; Aikawa et al., 1992; Houston et al., 1953; Dunhill et al., 1969). These pathological findings indicate that drugs which prevent mucus-secreting structures from proliferating, or drugs which suppress mucus release will be of considerable therapeutic value in asthma.

Chronic injury or irritation of the epithelium has been established for a long time as a cause of increased number of goblet cells in experimental animal models. However, almost nothing is currently known of the molecular mechanism(s) which underlay the increase in goblet cell number. The origin of goblet cells is disputed and the subject of continuing research.

Goblet cells may arise from basal cells, a cell type which may have a local stem cell function under baseline condition in the epithelium. However, in models of epithelial cell trauma goblet cells differentiate from type II cells or neighboring serous cell population. The capacity of proliferation of goblet cells to themselves has also been suggested but not unequivocally demonstrated. Conceptually, it is therefore important to distinguish between increases in mucus secreting cell number that follows injury resulting in stripping of epithelial cells from the basal cell stroma and chronic irritation which does not produce frank denudation of the epithelium since the patterns of tissue response and repair are likely to differ markedly. To date the possible role of EGF (Epithelial Growth Factor) has been established in the *in utero* generation of respiratory epithelium maturation. Evidence is lacking, but by inference from other models of repair and differentiation, two classes of signal, both of which represent drug targets, are relevant in epithelial mucus hypersecretion: growth factor interaction with receptor tyrosine kinase (RTK) coupled receptors and signals delivered to cells by the extracellular matrix and their neighbors.

Hyperplasia of the mucous glands probably occurs in response to large molecular weight growth factors and might be preceded by induction of gland cell metalloproteinase(MMP) secretion, a possible drug target (Fig. 3), causing digestion of the basement membrane. In the lower airways mucus is released by mucus cells and clara cells. An increase in the number of these cells has been observed and is the cause of hypersecretion in this area. The successful suppression of mucus hypersecretion is a highly desirable property of future drugs. Of therapies currently available only glucocorticosteroids exert a beneficial effect on hypersecretion due to their global effect on airway inflammation and reduction of microvascular leakage.

3.1.1.1 Mechanisms of mucus hyperproduction

Asthmatics normally die due to airway occlusion by mucus exudate. In living asthmatics hypersecretion is also a main factor of morbidity. The submucosal glands and the goblet cells are the major source of mucus glycoproteins in the lower airways (Fig. 2). The glands in the upper airways are at least partially under the control of the parasympathetic system, while goblet cells have no direct efferent innervation.

The endogenous stimuli leading to overproduction of mucus in asthma are obscure. Similarly, the endogenous mechanisms of the plasma leakage and plasma transudation, a critical pathological process leading to thickening of mucus, are poorly understood. Much more is known of the mechanisms and pharmacology of mucus release from both glands and goblet cells and plasma leak in model systems. The parasympathetic system

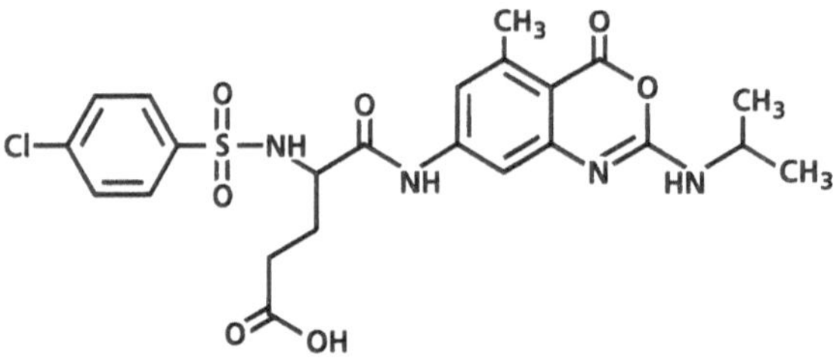

TEI-5624 (Tejin)

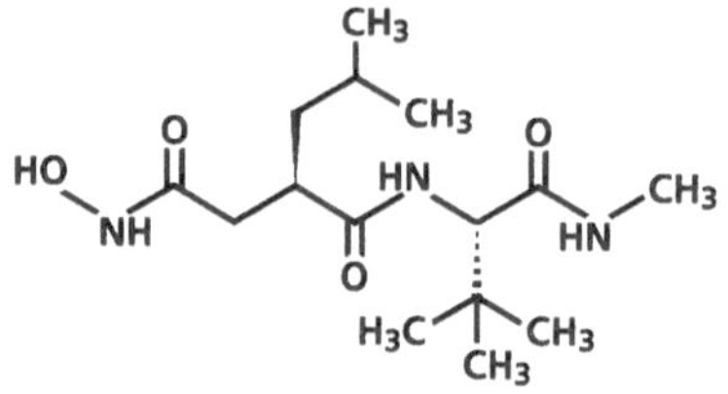

Ro-31-9790 (Roche)

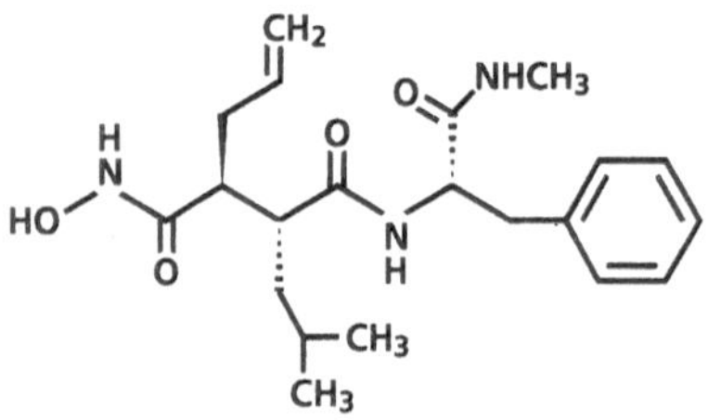

BB-1101 (British Biotech)

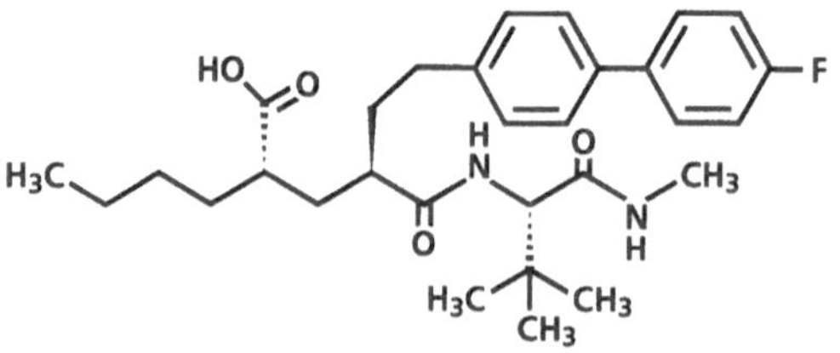

L-758354 (Merck)

Fig. 3.
Matrix degradation inhibitors

controls the secretion in the upper airways and stimulation of the vagi leads to prompt increasing secretion volume. Anticholinergics which are occasionally used in asthma as bronchodilators might therefore be expected to reduce mucus hyperproduction but this is not the case. A very large number of inflammatory mediators are also secretagogues and possibly have a role in mucus hyperproduction in established disease. The mediators include neuropeptide NK1 agonists, cysteinyl leukotrienes, histamine and bradykinin. Recent attention has focused on the capacity of proteases, notably neutrophil elastase, released from inflammatory cells to induce a very potent and efficacious mucus release from goblet cells. The precise mechanism of this release is unknown but it may represent a pathway of great importance in asthma exacerbation where inflammatory leukocytes flood into the inflamed mucosa. It is also of interest in this context that bacterial products, such as supernatants from *Pseudomonas auregenosa*, a very common pathogen in cystic fibrosis, cause mucus gene induction and are secretagogues for mucus. Neuropeptides such as tachykinins are thought to be key regulators of mucus release although to date no clinical evidence of the efficacy of pure neurokinin antagonists in mucus release in humans has been obtained.

3.1.2   Changes in the submucosa

3.1.2.1   Angiogenesis and vascular reactivity

The presence of exudated plasma in the airways suggest important contributions from disturbances in the airway microcirculation in chronic asthma. Blood vessels surround the bronchial walls with a dense plexus in the submucosa and peribronchial space, forming an interconnected capillary network that covers the tracheobronchial tree from the trachea to the terminal bronchioles. Due to this anatomical arrangement, an increase in bronchial blood volume leads to an decrease in the airway diameter and compromises therefore pulmonary mechanics (Gilbert and McFadden, 1992; McFadden and Gilbert, 1993; Gilbert et al., 1993).

In asthmatic patients, the thickening of the airway walls seems partially due to the dilatation of the submucosal vessels (Wilson, 1995) and the submucosal edema, but also to the smooth muscle hypertrophy and hyperplasia as well as the inflammatory cell infiltration. Airway wall thickening causes airway flow obstruction and hyperreactivity in asthma. Moreover, changes in blood flow may modulate the uptake, the release and distribution of inflammatory substances as well as the pharmacokinetics of administered substances. Vascular engorgement may contribute to airway obstruction, but can also increase airway reactivity. Rapid infusion of saline into normal asthmatic patients results in enhanced responsiveness to methacholine and frigid air. It can also develop airflow limitation. In addition, it has been shown, that patients with chronic pulmonary venous hypertension and prolonged bronchovascular congestion can have increased airway reactivity that is eliminated by methoxamine (potent vasoconstrictor without affecting the airway smooth muscle tone) and α-agonists (McFadden, 1993). Engorgement may be particularly important in exercise-induced asthma (McFadden, 1993) although this mechanism has been questioned.

Chronic inflammation is typically accompanied by angiogenesis in the inflamed tissue although the occurrence of true angiogenesis in human asthma is poorly documented. The study of Wilson et al. (1995) compared submucosal vascular volume in bronchial biopsy samples from mild asthmatics and normal controls. Vessel numbers were similar in both groups, but slightly increased in asthma. However, the vascular area was greater in asthmatics than in normal controls. Since angiogenesis requires degradation of basement membrane collagen it is possible that matrix metalloprotease inhibitor may emerge as unexpectedly useful new drugs (Fig. 3).

Gilbert and colleagues (1993) have shown that sudden elevations in intrathoracic vascular volume with warm saline produces airway obstruction that is quantitatively similar to that seen with hyperventilation in asthmatics suggesting vascular engorgement is important in airflow obstruction. This finding suggests that the two stimuli interact together so that a common mechanism may exist to produce the decrease in airflow. Hyperpnea and the magnitude of thermal differences are related and alterations in blood supply affect bronchial heat flux and influence obstruction (Gilbert et al., 1992).

3.1.2.2   Leak of plasma

Plasma extravasation is an important finding in asthmatics and leads to airway edema, but also to increased mucus viscosity, increased formation of mucus plugs and impaired mucocilliary transport. Mucosal exudation may reflect ongoing airway inflammation (Persson, 1993). Glucocorticoids can inhibit the leakage. The leakage occurs at the level of post-capillary venules and their permeability is increased by inflammatory factors and mediators (Kay et al., 1989; Persson, 1993). These mediators include histamine, bradykinin, cysteinylpeptide leukotrienes and platelet activating factor (PAF). In addition, stimulation of the vagus nerve by releasing sensory neuropeptides such as substance P, causes microvascular leakage in rodents (Kay et al., 1989). The airway mucosal surface seems to be the main destination of the plasma exudate. Mucosal exudation of plasma proteins can also occur without mucosal edema, or epithelial disruption or shedding. Indeed the epithelium may even be intact in patients dying from asthma (Persson, 1993).

3.1.2.3   Neuronal elements

The sensory innervation of the airways may be stimulated by cellular and plasma derived mediators, as well as by inhaled irritants, that may evoke cough, sneeze and tissue responses (hyperemia, secretion and mucociliary activity). It is not known if neurogenic inflammation (cell activation and plasma exudation) can occur in human airways (Persson, 1993).

The cholinergic, adrenergic and NANC (Non-adrenergic Non-cholinergic) mechanisms possibly involved in asthma have been reviewed by Barnes (1993).

There is a new evidence that neuronal control of the airways may be abnormal in asthmatic patients and that there is an imbalance between excitatory (muscarinic cholinergic, α-adrenergic and NANC-excitatory) and inhibitory β-adrenergic, NANC-inhibitory) components. Inflammatory mediators may have an effect of neurotransmission and neurotransmitters. Autonomic nerves regulate airway smooth muscle tone, secretions, blood flow, microvascular permeability and the migration and release of inflammatory cells.

The cholinergic nerves are the dominant bronchoconstrictor pathway in the airways and anticholinergic drugs are very effective bronchodilators in acute severe asthma but less useful in chronic asthma. There are several mechanisms contributing to cholinergic bronchoconstriction in asthma:

- an increase in vagal cardiac tone and an increase in sinus gap at night
- the stimulation of sensory receptors by inflammatory mediators, such as histamine, bradykinin, prostaglandins and cytokines, inducing reflex bronchoconstriction
- increased acetylcholine release in parasympathetic ganglia or from post-ganglionic nerve terminals (induced by inflammatory mediators)
- dysfunction of muscarinic autoreceptors (M_2) results in exaggerated cholinergic reflexes in asthma, as the normal feedback inhibition of acetylcholine release may be lost. Oxidants, eosinophil major basic protein and other products of the inflammatory response may possibly alter M2-receptors, which have the most high affinity to acetylcholine binding.

Adrenergic mechanisms involve sympathetic nerves, circulating catecholamines (noradrenaline, adrenaline and dopamine) and α- and β-adrenoceptors. Adrenergic nerves could influence cholinergic neurotransmission via α- and β-adrenoceptors. Beta-blockers cause bronchoconstriction in asthmatics but not in normal subjects. This suggests that adrenergic drive to the airways is important as a defense against bronchoconstriction. Moreover α-receptors may play an important role in regulating airway blood flow, that may influence airway responsiveness. There is some evidence that α-agonists may reduce airway narrowing in exercise-induced asthma.

VIP (vasoactive intestinal polypeptide) acts as a functional antagonist and is an inhibitor of release of acetylcholine. It is localized to cholinergic nerves in human airways and it is a potent bronchodilator in human airways *in vitro*. VIP could not be found in asthmatics, probably due to the enzymatic degradation i.e. by mast cell derived tryptase. As the neural bronchodilator response is not reduced by α-chymotrypsin (a reduction has been demonstrated in guinea pigs), it is most unlikely that VIP acts as a bronchodilator NANC transmitter in human airways.

In contrast, nitric oxide may modulate cholinergic contraction in human airways. Nitric oxide is rapidly degraded by superoxide anions released from inflammatory cells which contribute to the increased reflex bronchoconstriction in asthma.

Many neuropeptides have been identified in human airways. Unmyelinated sensory nerves (C-fibres) contain neuropeptides such as the tachykinins (substance P (sub P) and the Neurokinin A (NKA) as well as the calcitonin gene related peptide (CGRP). NKA is a potent human bronchial constrictor *in vitro* while sub P is a strong inducer of microvascular leakage and stimulates mucus secretion. No increase in the number and length of sub P immunoreactive fibres has been seen in asthmatic subjects (Jeffery, 1994). C-fibre endings can be stimulated by inflammatory mediators. The loss of surface epithelial cells enhances access of irritant and inflammatory mediators to the intraepithelial endings. In addition, epithelial damage due to viral infection or ozone increases the airway responsiveness. CGRP, localized with tachykinins in airway C-fibres, may contribute to the hyperemia of asthmatic airways.

3.1.2.4   Extracellular matrix (ECM) and resident cells
The lung function is disturbed by an irreversible airflow obstruction due to proliferative and fibrotic changes (Fig. 2). The thickening of the basement membrane is due to fibrosis, the deposition of types I, III and V interstitial collagen, that probably proceeds from the myofibroblast. In contrast, type IV collagen predominates in epithelium, blood vessels and smooth muscle cells. Phylogenetically the myofibroblast has a phenotype intermediate to both the tissue matrix fibroblast and the airway smooth muscle. Therefore drugs suppressing myofibroblast proliferation would also be of benefit in preventing airway smooth muscle proliferation, however this speculation is not proven.

The three principal components of the ECM are fibronectin, collagen and elastin forming complex molecules of varied structure due to alternate splicing of their genes. Cytokines, such as TGF-β (Transforming Growth Factor-β) are known to modulate the splicing of fibronectin genes (Borsi et al., 1990). It may also promote collagen deposition by increasing the rate of collagen synthesis and decreasing the rate of collagen turnover by decreasing the production of collagenase. In addition, leukocytes, such as eosinophils can be activated by adhesion to ECM components. On the other hand an intact ECM has an inhibitory effect on airway smooth muscle division. In contrast matrix degradation products are mitogens or co-mitogens.

3.1.2.5   Airway smooth muscle, increased airway wall thickness and bronchospasm
Structural changes in the airways occur in chronic asthma leading to alterations in their physical properties associated with disturbed lung func-

tion and in some cases progressive deterioration ending in fixed irreversible airflow obstruction. Changes in bronchi and especially in bronchioles may be particularly important because small airways are the major site of airway obstruction in human asthma (Hogg et al., 1968).

Two broad categories of growth factors, mitogens and co-mitogens are known to affect the mammalian cell cycle, and therefore the rate of cell proliferation (Fig. 4). Competence factors prepare the cell to enter the mitotic phase of the cell cycle but do not promote the cell division. In contrast, the progression factors act on cells prepared to enter the cell cycle releasing the mitotic event. It is unusual for a particular factor to act as both a competence and progression factor on mammalian cells and especially on smooth muscle. Competence factors of interest in asthma are endothelin, PDGF (Platelet Derived Growth Factor) and thromboxane A2. Progression factors include Epithelial Growth Factor (EGF), Transforming Growth Factor (TGF) and Insulin-like Growth Factor (IGF).

The molecular mechanisms of airway wall remodelling are very poorly understood although a body of *in vitro* evidence and some *in vivo* animal studies suggest that growth factors coupled to receptor tyrosine kinases may be important mediators of tissue structural and phenotype changes in chronic airway disease. Tissue phenotype changes and tissue remodelling are pathological processes which underlie the transition of the inflamed lung from mild, reversible to chronic disease. The known candidate growth factors of interest include FGFs (Fibroblast Growth Factor), EGF, VEGF isoforms (Vascular Endothelial Growth Factor), PDGF isoforms, and SCF (Stem Cell Factor). These factors signal via receptor tyrosine kinase (RTK) pathways which are important targets for new classes of inhibitors (Fig. 5).

The increased airway smooth muscle bulk is characterized by hyperplasia (increase in the total number of airway smooth muscle cells) or hypertrophy (increase of the cell size). This is one of the most important features contributing to the impaired lung function in asthma, because it could be responsible for the altered contractility. Morphometric analysis of airway tissue in fatal asthma has shown hyperplasia (Heard et al., 1973). However, the increase of airway smooth muscle mass seems to be a cumulative process with a slight increase in cell proliferation rate causing a slow accumulation of long-lived non-dividing cells. This suggests that therapy directed against proliferation of airway smooth muscle might be of benefit if administered early in disease.

In view of the likely central role of T cell mediated immunity in asthma it is of great interest that these cells stimulate a smooth muscle cycle and

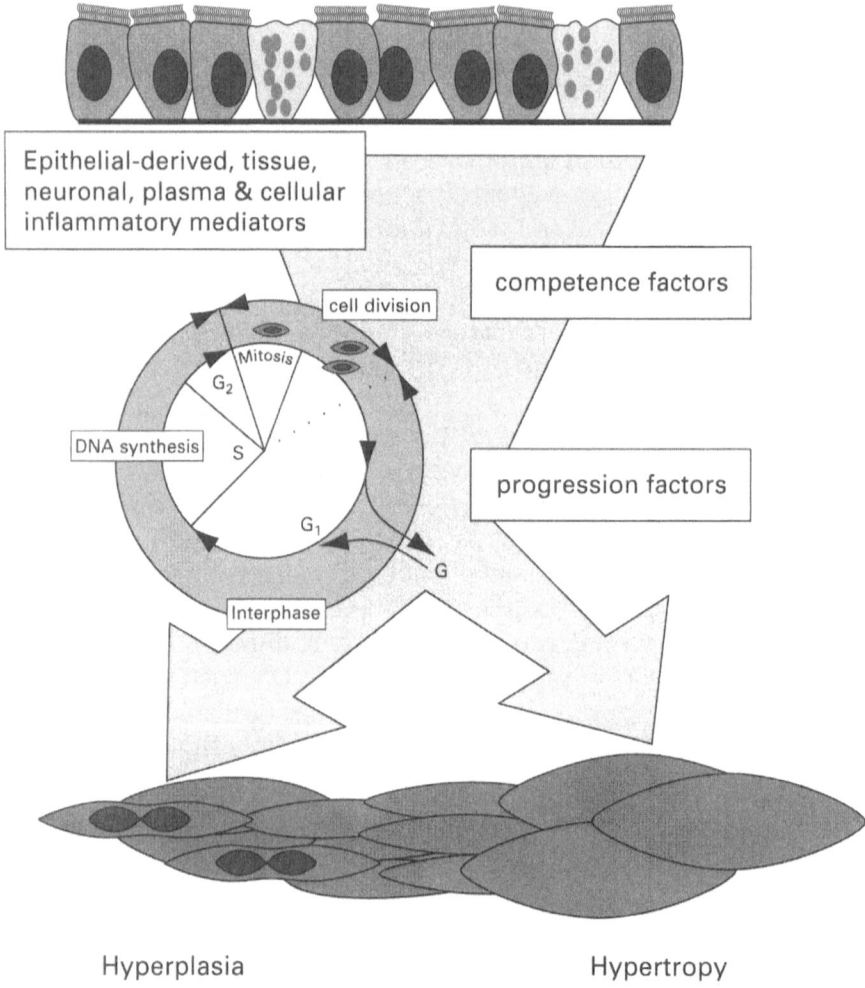

Fig. 4.
Overview of mechanisms leading to increase in airway smooth muscle mass in asthma (hyperplasia and hypertrophy).

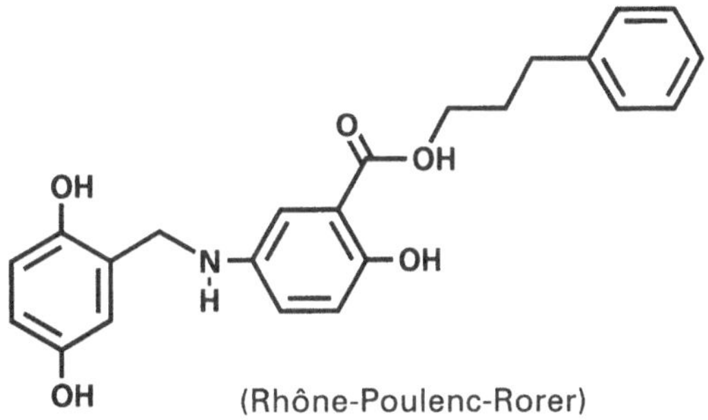

(Rhône-Poulenc-Rorer)

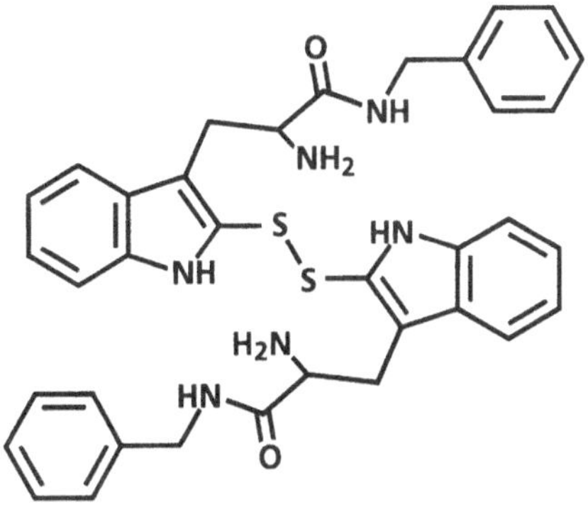

(Parke-Davis)

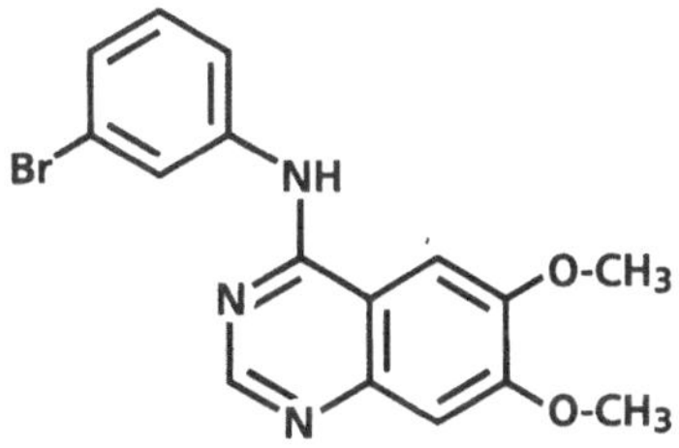

PD-153035
(Warner/Lambert/Parke-Davis)

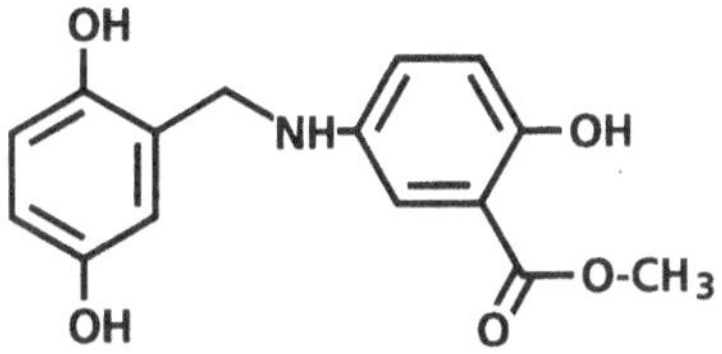

(Rhône-Poulenc-Rorer)

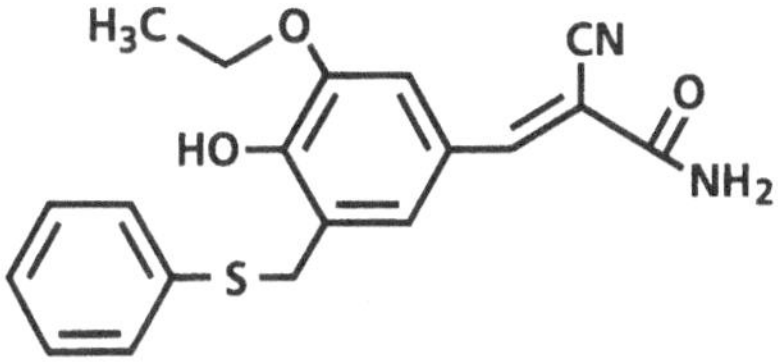

ST-638

Fig. 5.
RTK (receptor tyrosine kinase) inhibitors

have recently been identified as a source of growth factors (Blotnick et al., 1994; Lazaar et al., 1994) (Fig. 4).

Anti-inflammatory drugs may suppress smooth muscle increases indirectly but new direct inhibitors of airway smooth muscle growth have now been discovered (Fig. 6).

Episodic bronchospasm is one of the most important symptoms contributing to the morbidity of asthma. Several new classes of drugs such as kinase activators and PDE (phosphodiesterase isoenzyme) inhibitors may provide new classes of bronchodilators (Nicholson, 1994). However, much recent attention has focused on the biochemistry of smooth muscle contraction.

The contractile proteins actin and myosin, present in all smooth muscle, together with several other regulatory proteins such as tropomyosin, caldesmon, calponin and calmodulin are involved in the contractile mechanism. In addition, there are some other proteins that seem to form filaments to constitute the cytoskeleton of smooth muscle cells. Actin represents the major contractile protein in smooth muscle. It is 10 to 20 times more abundant than myosin. Actin filaments are composed of two linear proteins wrapped together in a helical configuration. Tropomyosin and caldesmon are placed along this helix. In contrast, myosin filaments are thick, arranged asymetrically in a hexameric structure. The myosin molecules are composed by a head section attached to a long spine or tail. The globular head possesses the binding sites for attachment to actin and the enzymatic sites (ATPase) that cleave ATP providing the necessary energy to fulfill the binding reaction. Inhibitors of MLCK have recently been discovered (Fig. 6).

There is a rapid cyclic attachment and detachment of cross-bridges between the globular heads of the myosin molecules and actin, responsible for the active force development in airway smooth muscle. The energy for this process derives from the breakdown of ATP by actin-activated myosin ATPase. The rate of force development is proportional to the rate of cross-bridge cycling. It is now accepted that phosphorylation of the light chains of myosin plays a crucial role in the initiation of the airway smooth muscle contraction. Many studies have shown that during contraction, the levels of light chain myosin phosphorylation is significantly increased and this kinase may represent a novel drug target. Moreover, the time courses of phosphorylation and dephosphorylation are related to the levels of free Ca^{2+} concentration in smooth muscle cells (Rodger, 1993).

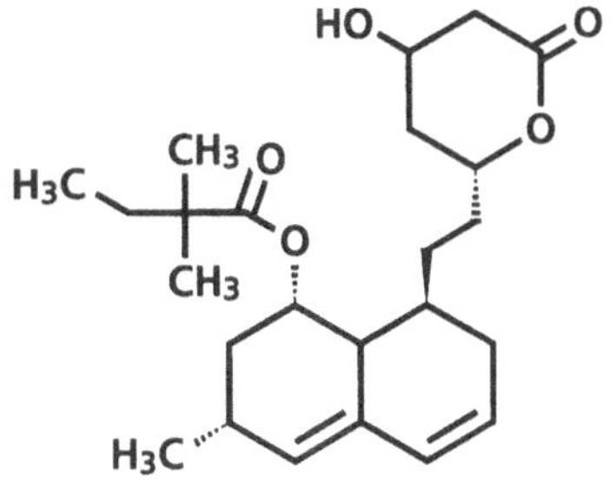

simvastatin (Merck) HMG-CoA reductase inhibitor

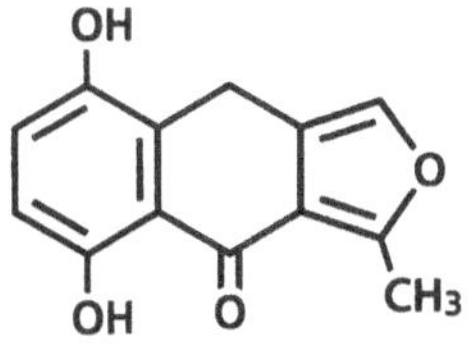

MS-444, from *Micromonospora* sp.
(Kyowa Hakko Kogyo)

Fig. 6.
Inhibitor of smooth muscle proliferation and myosin chain kinase inhibitor

3.2   Inflammatory cells

Inflammation is the response of vascularized tissue to injury and it serves to resolve and repair this effect (Kay et al., 1989). Histopathology, blood and BALF (bronchoalveolar lavage fluid) analysis confirmed the important role of the inflammatory cell response, especially that of eosinophils (Arm and Lee, 1992; DeMonchy et al., 1985; Frigas and Gleich, 1986), mast cells, macrophages and lymphocytes in the pathogenesis of bronchial asthma (Hill et al., 1991; Holgate et al., 1991; Iijima et al., 1987). Increased numbers of eosinophils, mast cells, neutrophils and lymphocytes as well as alveolar macrophages have also been found in the BALF and in biopsies of asthmatic patients (Arm et al., 1992; Berman et al., 1992; Djuka-novic et al., 1992; Hill et al., 1991; Mattoli et al., 1991). Mast cells as well as lymphocytes, eosinophils and many other migratory cells can release different mediators, enzymes and cytokines, which are important in the inflammatory processes (Persson, 1993).

It has been known for a long time that bronchial asthma is associated with eosinophilia in the blood and the lung. The intensity of blood eosinophilia correlates with the degree of the disease (Corrigan and Kay, 1992; Dur-ham et al., 1985; Frigas et al., 1986). It has been pointed out that asthma cannot be diagnosed in the absence of eosinophils (Saetta et al., 1989). Eosinophils degranulate at the bronchial wall and as a result induce tis-sue damage (Filley et al., 1982; Frew et al., 1990). Eosinophils may serve as a proinflammatory function, since they can release factors capable of eliciting tissue damage (Arm and Lee, 1992; Frigas et al., 1980; Kay, 1989). The released cytotoxic agents MBP (Major Basic Protein), ECP (Eosino-philic Cationic Protein), EDN (Eosinophil Derived Neuropeptide) and EPO (Eosinophil Peroxidase) destroy the mucociliary apparatus, after which bronchial secretions cannot be cleared. The release of leukotriene LTC4 and PAF contribute to the obstruction by causing bronchoconstric-tion and increased vascular permeability (Frigas and Gleich, 1986). More-over, eosinophils have the capacity to stimulate fibroblast growth *in vitro*, and may therefore be involved in the process of deposition of subepithe-lial collagen in asthmatic patients (Shock et al., 1991). Factors that may be responsible for stimulating eosinophilopoiesis are GM-CSF (Granu-locyte Macrophage Colony Stimulating Factor), IL-3 (Interleukin-3) and IL-5. IL-5 has been shown to promote the growth and differentiation of eosinophils in cell cultures while IL-3 and GM-CSF act as a terminal eosinophil-differentiation factor. Eosinophils can produce cytokines such as GM-CSF and IL-5, resulting in autocrine and paracrine modes of eosin-ophilic recruitment (Arm and Lee, 1992; Resnick and Weller, 1993).

Mast cells are an additional important cell type in T_H2 (T Helper-2) in-duced diseases like bronchial asthma. The released mediators induce an immediate asthmatic response (Corrigan et al., 1992) but also induce the adhesion, diapedesis, directional migration and activation of eosinophils. Mast cells are an alternative source of cytokines (Bradding et al., 1992; Galli et al., 1993; Gordon et al., 1990; Hansel et al., 1992) that amplify the vasoactive phase and attract inflammatory cells. Mast cells are certainly a key cell in the immediate response to allergens but their role in the chronic phase of the disease is less well established.

Alveolar macrophages and other macrophages located at the air-surface interface of the conducting airways in the lower respiratory tract may be important in chronic disease. Immunohistochemistry of bronchial biopsies has shown a significant increase in macrophages in the submucosa of asthmatics. These cells had phenotypic characteristics of peripheral blood monocytes, suggesting that they have migrated recently into the lung (Arm and Lee, 1992). Experiments in the rat have shown that macrophages can be activated by IgE-dependent mechanisms and that they possess a low affinity IgE receptor ($Fc_\varepsilon RII$). In atopic individuals the $Fc_\varepsilon RII$-positive lung macrophages and peripheral blood monocytes were increased in number. The treatment with corticosteroids reduced the number of cells, so that the expression of this receptor can be modulated by therapy. Moreover, molecules like IgE and cytokines are important regulators of mononuclear phagocyte $Fc_\varepsilon RII$ *in vivo*, capable of increasing the number of these cells. Activated macrophages can release factors like leukotrienes, prostaglandins, thromboxane, PAF and cytokines such as IL-5, GM-CSF, IFN-γ (Interferon-γ) and IL-3 that may contribute to the airway reactions. Macrophages manifest many different functional phenotypes, and therefore it is supposed that the airways of asthmatics contain macrophages which contribute to the disease and others that limit the extent of the inflammation and the pathophysiology (Kay et al., 1989).

In accordance with the expression of their surface receptor the majority of major T lymphocytes can be divided into two distinct phenotypes, CD4+ and CD8+ cells. CD4+ cells are activated by soluble foreign proteins such as allergens. These allergens are presented by major histocompatibility complex class II molecules (MHC class II restricted) as processed peptides on the cell surface by antigen-presenting cells. In contrast, CD8+ cells are activated by intracellular pathogens such as viruses. They are MHC class I restricted and have cytotoxic functions. Both cells can secrete cytokines. CD4+ T cells have been classified on the basis of their cytokine profile in T_H1 and T_H2 subsets.

T_H1 CD4+ T cells produce IFNγ, tumor necrosis factor beta (TNF-β) and IL-2 and are involved in delayed hypersensitivity responses. T_H2 cells produce IL-4, IL-5, IL-10 and IL-13. Both subsets produce IL-3 and GM-CSF (Mosmann and Coffman, 1989; Mosmann, 1991). IL-4 is essential in regulating T naïve cells to switch to the T_H2 phenotype. IL-5 is important in the terminal differentiation of eosinophils. Therefore the T_H2 panel of cytokines is essential in the pathogenesis of asthma and allergy.

Neutrophils seem to be important in the early phases of asthma. However, neutrophils count almost 50% of the total cell count in bronchial and in infectious exacerbations but their involvement in the chronic mechanisms of bronchial asthma is uncertain. After allergen and exercise challenge, a heat-stable-high-molecular-weight neutrophil chemotactic factor has been found in the peripheral circulation. This molecule is associated with increased expression of complement receptors (IgG Fc receptors) and enhanced cytotoxicity for complement-coated targets in asthmatic individuals (Arm et al., 1992). Neutrophils can cause tissue damage by releasing oxygen metabolites, proteases and cationic material. Neutrophils are also a potent source of mediators such as prostaglandins, thromboxanes, leukotriene B_4 and PAF which contribute to the airway responses or exacerbate the inflammatory response. In conclusion neutrophils probably participate in the functional alterations of asthma (Kay et al., 1989).

The recruitment of leukocytes to an inflammatory focus is enhanced by the expression of adhesion molecules. VCAM-1 (Vascular Cell Adhesion Molecule-1) is a surface glycoprotein found on endothelial cells. It is known that VCAM-1 selectively recruits eosinophils to the airways in asthma (Arm et al., 1992). The mechanism of binding is based on complementary adhesion molecules expressed on leukocytes. The counterligand for VCAM-1 is termed VLA-4 (integrin 4) and eosinophils possess this counter-receptor (Albeda, 1993). In addition, IL-4 stimulates eosinophil and basophil adhesion, by inducing endothelial cells to produce VCAM-1, which binds to eosinophil and basophil VLA-4. Therefore, *in vivo* local release of IL-4 in allergic diseases or after experimental allergen challenge, may partly explain the increase of eosinophils and basophils in these situations (Albeda, 1993; Briscoe et al., 1992; Schleimer et al., 1992). Much research has been focused on discovering low molecular weight adhesion molecule inhibitors (Fig. 7).

4   Humoral and cellular immunity

In this section important advances in the understanding of T lymphocyte (T cell) mediated immunity of the respiratory mucosa are discussed, which have not only led to a better understanding of normal host defense mechanisms in the lung but which have also provided important insights into how aberrations of these processes may result in disease. Specialized subsets of T-cells, identified by the distinctive patterns of the soluble factors (cytokines) that they produce, have been demonstrated in both animal models and human disease to be central regulators of immune and inflammatory responses in the lung.

T_H1 and T_H2 cells are generally believed to arise from a common precursor phenotype termed T_H0 during a process termed commitment which is closely cross-regulated by soluble and physical immunological signals

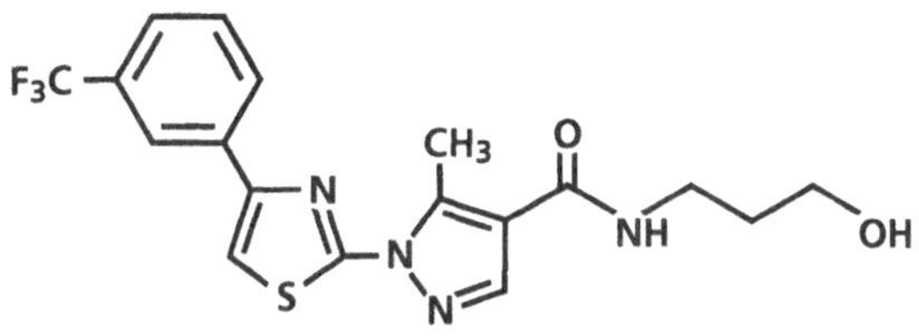

RWJ-50271 (R.W. Johnson)

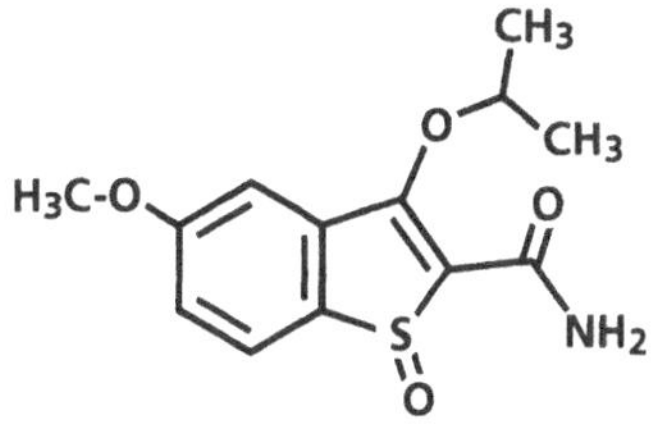

(Warner-Lambert/Parke-Davis

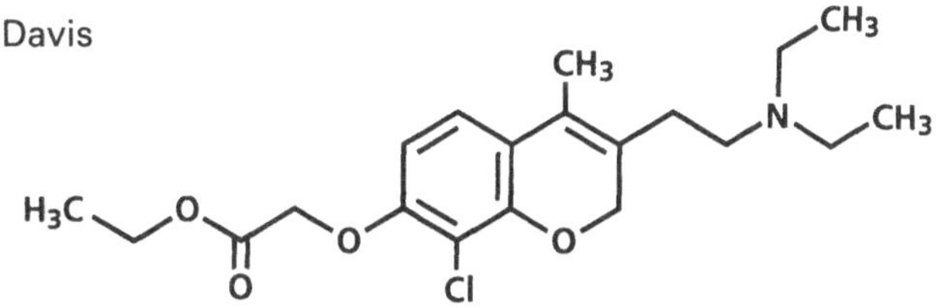

(cloricromene)

Fig. 7.
Cell adhesion inhibitors

(Fig. 1 and 8). The mechanism of commitment and cross regulation, which are more complex than outlined here, provide excellent opportunities to therapeutically manipulate the T_H1/T_H2 balance in disease. It should, however, be clearly understood that the concept of highly polarized T_H1/T_H2 responses is based on studies of long-term mouse T cell clones after intense stimulation. T cells producing mixed patterns of cytokines have been identified in *in vitro* culture studies and *in vivo* studies (Bucy et al., 1994; 1995). Especially in human disease, it is more reasonable to consider a bias towards T_H2 response reflected in the *net cytokine production of T cell populations* and never to exclude the existence of more subtle, intermediate patterns of cytokines in some T cells. Understanding how and why the immune response becomes biased towards a T_H2 response has not only provided important clues to finding advanced therapies (Anderson and Coyle, 1994) but may also challenge our current views of disease progression and management.

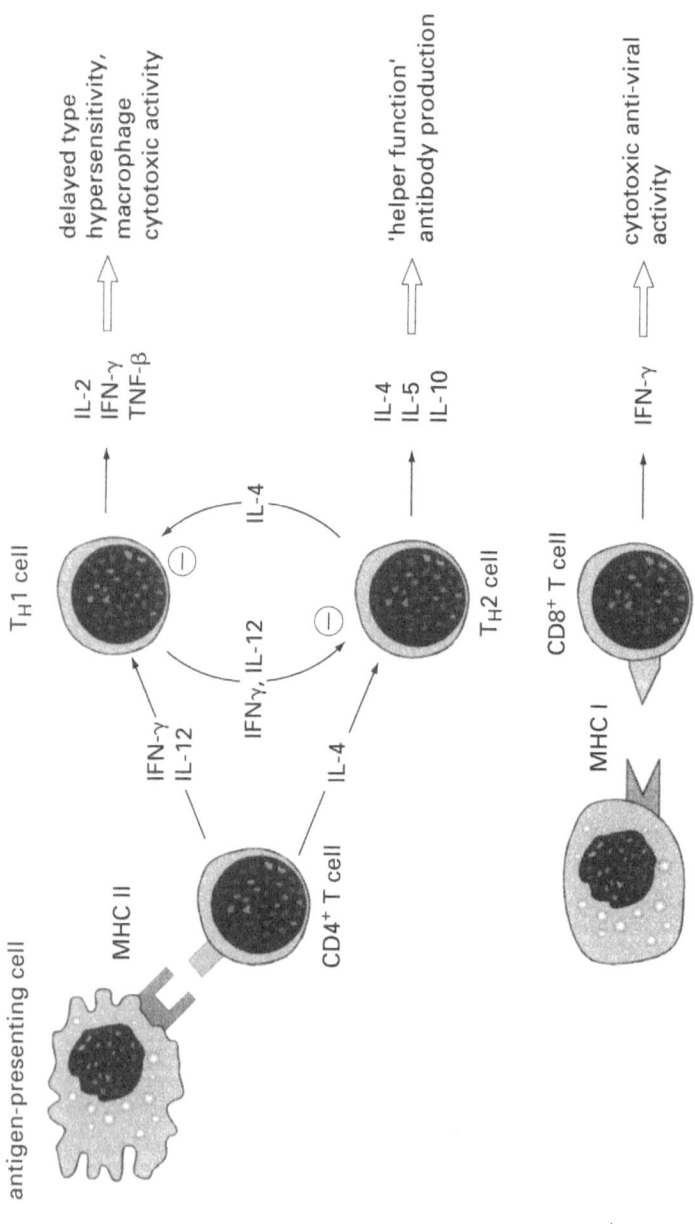

Fig. 8.
Regulatory mechanisms influencing cytokine producing cellular phenotypes in asthma. The diagram shows important cross regulatory pathways between T_H1 and T_H2 cells.

4.1   Is airway inflammation in asthma due to aberrant T cell mucosal immunity?

Inflammation of the airways occurs, to variable degrees, at all levels of the airways in asthma. The co-existence of eosinophilic inflammation with elevated IgE titers in allergic asthma has led to the widely held (but still not rigorously proven) belief that the inflammatory response in asthma is governed by the release of cytokines from T cells. This belief is strongly supported by a large number of experimental and clinical findings. Eosino-philia is strictly IL-5 and T cell dependent (Lopez et al., 1988; Baston and Beeson, 1974; Sanderson et al., 1986; Yamaguchi et al., 1991). Eosinophils are important sources of lipid mediators, especially cysteinyl leukotrienes, cytotoxic highly-charged degranulation products, and some growth factors such as transforming growth factors (TGF isoforms). IL-4 and IL-13 have central roles triggering B cells expressing surface IgM and IgD to undergo rearrangement of their genomic DNA, via a process termed „class switching" resulting in IgE production. When cross-linked by antigen IgE bound to specific high (Fce IR) and low (Fce IIR) affinity receptors triggers degranulation of metachromatic (mast cells, basophils and so-called Non-B/Non-T or NBNT cells) and other cells to release diverse pro-inflammatory mediators (Coffman et al., 1986; Snapper and Paul, 1987; Pene et al., 1988). The predominant, but not exclusive, source of these cytokines is the CD4+ T cell. In turn, elevated IgE and mucosal inflam-mation are thought to contribute directly to antigen-mediated bronchos-pasm, disturbances of normal lung function including exacerbations of bronchial hyperreactivity, wide spontaneous variation in airway caliber and perhaps as a consequence of persisting inflammation, mucous hyper-secretion (Busse and Reed, 1988; Mc Fadden and Gilbert, 1992).

4.2   Surface markers and cytokine patterns define important subtypes of T cells

The majority of mature T cells in the peripheral circulation or tissues express the surface markers CD4+ or CD8+ on their cell membranes. These markers are functional molecules and define fundamental biological dif-ferences in cell function. CD4+ bearing cells mainly recognize foreign anti-genic protein after it has been digested and presented in the context of major histocompatibility class two molecules (MHC class II restricted pre-sentation) by specialized antigen presenting cells such as the lung den-dritic cell. A major function of CD4+ T cells is to provide help in the form of soluble cytokines which induce B cells to produce antibodies and regulate the antibody isotype class (IgG, IgA, IgE etc.). In contrast CD8+ cells recognize somatic (self) antigens or intracellular pathogen antigens, notably viral antigens, which are presented by MHC class I molecules, and typically kill infected cells by direct cytolysis (Zingernagel and Doherty, 1977; Lukacher et al., 1984; Morrison et al., 1986).

As described before, the CD4+ subset has been subdivided into two further functional phenotypes termed T_H1 and T_H2. To date no surface marker which unequivocally identifies these subsets has been identified: instead they are defined by the characteristic panels of cytokines they secrete which in turn mediate their contrasting biological functions. The relevance of T_H2 derived IL-4 and IL-5 to asthma and allergy is immediately obvious. The presence of T_H2 cells, or a T_H2 pattern of cytokines has now been extensively documented in human allergy and asthma. T cells from the peripheral blood characteristically produce IL-2 and IFNγ when restimulated *ex vivo* but clones (clones are expanded populations of T cells derived from one original cell) derived from atopic patients produce elevated IL-4 and IL-5 but lower levels of IFNγ (Romagnani, 1992; Yssel et al., 1992). More importantly, *in situ* hybridization studies and immunohistochemistry studies have demonstrated respectively the presence of T_H2 pattern mRNA and protein in biopsies from human asthmatic airways (Hamid et al., 1991; Kay et al., 1991) and these cytokines are also present in elevated concentrations in bronchoalveolar lavage fluid aspirated from the airways of asthmatics after allergen challenge (Robinson et al., 1992). Perhaps even more important are the advances in the molecular genetics of asthma. Segregation analyses which link a region proximal to the T_H2 cytokine gene cluster (IL-4, IL-13, IL-5, IL-3, GM-CSF) mapped at human chromosome 5q31-33 to association with high serum IgE titer, bronchial hyperresponsiveness and asthma (Marsh et al., 1994; Meyers et al., 1994).

The T_H1 and T_H2 subsets are generally believed to arise from a common non-specialized precursor with a less restricted cytokine profile termed T_H0. This process, termed "commitment" is itself regulated to a large degree by the pattern of soluble cytokine signals a T_H0 cell encounters during antigen presentation (reviewed by Seder and Paul, 1994). IL-4 has a central role in the induction of the T_H2 subset whereas IFNγ promotes T_H1 responses (Mosmann, 1991a; Powie and Coffman, 1993; Romagnani, 1992). These regulatory pathways have been clearly demonstrated in *in vitro* studies of T cell commitment and unequivocally proven to be of *in vivo* relevance in animal models using neutralizing antibodies to block the action of given cytokines and more recently, using the highly sophisticated technique of homologous recombination gene targeting which allows the actual cytokine gene to be inactivated by deletion in living animals (Kopf et al.,

1993; Coyle et al., 1995). Furthermore, the T_H1 and T_H2 subsets negatively crossregulate each other (Mosmann, 1991): T_H2-derived IL-10 and IL-4 inhibit T Helper cells whereas T_H1-derived IFNγ suppresses T_H2 responses. IL-12 and IFNγ, both perhaps derived from macrophages indirectly suppress T_H2 response by promoting IFNγ production and increasing the frequency of IFNγ secreting T cells respectively. The mechanisms which regulate the commitment of T_H0 cells to the T_H1 or T_H2 phenotype has been extensively investigated using *in vitro* techniques. IL-4 is a critical factor promoting T_H2 responses (Finkelman et al., 1990; Demeure et al., 1994). However, T_H1 differentiation to the same stimuli can be induced by IFNα (Brinkmann et al., 1993; Demeure et al., 1994), IFNγ (Demeure et al., 1994), or IL-12 (Hsieh et al., 1993; Seder et al., 1994). IL-10 favors the development of T_H2 responses indirectly by suppressing IFNγ production. This suggests that the soluble cytokine signal(s) present at the time of T_H0 commitment is possibly more important than the type of inhaled allergen as a determinant of the nature of the airway mucosal immune response. IFNα, IFNγ, and IL-12 represent potential therapeutic paradigms for re-directing T_H2 commitment and suppressing T_H2 function. In contrast, neutralization of IL-4, IL-13, IL-10 or IL-5 are approaches that would suppress the effects of established T_H2 cells in human asthma.

Very recent studies have revealed a fascinating biochemical basis for crossregulation. IL-4 has been shown to induce a state of physical unresponsiveness to IL-12 in CD4+ T cells. This effect terminates the potential cross regulatory effects which would otherwise counteract an established T_H2 immune response (Szabo et al., 1995). Conversely, T_H1 cells appear to prevent autosuppression by down regulating surface expression of their own IFNγ receptor beta-chain, a structural component of the receptor complex essential for IFNγ signaling (Pernis et al., 1995). These findings have important clinical relevance because they suggest that T_H2 responses may be more readily influenced at the outset of disease but may be refractory to selective suppression in long-standing chronic asthma.

4.3   IL-10 and IL-12 in the regulation of T_H cell phenotype

IL-4 is not the sole cytokine capable of dampening T_H1 immune responses. IL-10 plays a major role in suppressing immune and inflammatory responses. IL-10 is produced by various cell types, including CD4+ and CD8+ T cells, B cells, and macrophages/monocytes (De Waal Malefyt et al., 1992). The inhibitory effect of IL-10 on the secretion of proinflammatory cytokines, and the enhancing effect on the production of IL-1 receptor antagonist (IL-1RA), which itself is an anti-inflammatory agent, suggests a role of IL-10 as a natural dampener of immune proliferative and inflammatory responses (De Waal Malefyt et al., 1992). In the context of allergy/asthma it may be important that IL-10 inhibits the production of IFNγ by T cells via an effect on the antigen-presenting cells and thereby favoring T_H2 responses (Powrie and Coffman, 1993). IL-10 inhibits several T_H1 effector functions, notably the induction of cytokine production (IL-1, TNFα, IL-6) by IFNγ (De Waal Malefyt et al., 1991; Fiorentino et al., 1991), and inhibits the production of reactive nitrogen oxides by macrophages and monocytes. The inhibitory effects of IL-4 and IL-10 seem to be complementary, since both cytokines synergize with TGFβ to inhibit macrophage cytotoxicity (Oswald et al., 1992), and a combination of IL-4 and IL-10 inhibits DTH (delayed-type hypersensitivity) responses more efficiently than either cytokine alone (Powrie and Coffman, 1993). Pretolani et al. (1993) have elegantly demonstrated that exogenous IL-10 can suppress T_H2-mediated allergen-induced eosinophilia in mice. In these studies a marked reduction in bronchoalveolar lavage fluid TNFα was observed suggesting a possible down regulation of airway macrophage activation. IL-12 has received a great deal of recent interest because of its possible role in regulating T_H2 immunity. Important *in vivo* experiments using infection of mice with *Leishmania major* (where disease outcome is governed by the capacity of mice to mount a protective T_H1 response) or the nematode *Nippostrongylus brasiliensis*, a natural stimulus of intense T_H2 immune reponses, have demonstrated that exogenously administered IL-12 can dampen T_H2 immunity. *In vivo* studies showed that neutralization of IFNγ in *Leishmania major* resistant mice favored an inappropriate T_H2 response (Heinzel et al., 1992). Conversely, neutralization of IL-4 in susceptible mice favored generation of IFN γ-producing T_H1 cells and allowed mice to heal (Sadick et al., 1989). Prophylactic immunization (vaccination) of susceptible mice with *Leishmania* antigens alone induced a T_H2 response but the addition of IL-12 to the same antigen mix induced protective T_H1 cells (Afonso et al., 1994). The data clearly show that the induction of either T_H1- or T_H2-like cells is genetically linked, but also demonstrate that the genetic predisposition to mount a T_H2 response can be overcome by supplying cytokines that favor T_H1 responses. A genetic basis of a predominately T_H1 or T_H2 response has been confirmed in the recent studies of Hsieh et al. (1995) who demonstrated that genetic background rather than antigen presenting cell types is the most important determinant of T_H phenotype commitment *in vitro*. Further evidence of an important modulatory role of IL-12 in disease models has been found in studies of *Schistosoma mansoni* whose eggs normally induce a T_H2-mediated immune response in mice. In these studies IL-12 was found to suppress production of mRNA for the cytokines IL-2, IL-4 and IL-13 via induction of IFNγ (Shu et al., 1994). Very little data is presently available on IL-12 effects in human tissues although it is noteworthy that IL-12 has been shown to redirect human T_H2 cytokine response to recall antigen towards a T_H1 type pattern (Shu et al., 1994).

Analysis of the stage in T_H2 commitment at which IL-12 is most effective suggests that the usefulness of IL-12 in realigning disease may be limited to the earliest stages of disease. T_H2 cells very rapidly lose the capacity to be downregulated by IL-12 due to an acquired failure to phosphorylate the intracellular signal transducing molecules Jak2, Stat3 and Stat4 (Szabo et al., 1995). The adjuvant effect of IL-12 suggests the possibility of co-administering this cytokine together with native or recombinant epitopes of major aero-allergens to realign immune response early in childhood. However, in view of the recently revealed severe toxicity of IL-12 in human cancer trials, it is uncertain whether this avenue can be pursued in children who would be the most likely candidates to receive such a therapy. Perhaps even more importantly, IL-12 has been discovered to severely exacerbate viral infections, the major cause of severe asthma exacerbations, in some animal models due to incapacitation of CD8+ T cell mediated anti-viral defenses (Orange et al., 1995). It should also be noted that studies to date with IL-10 and IL-12 have concentrated on their capacity to induce non-lung *macrophage* cytokine production or modulate macrophage antigen presentation. Since the alveolar macrophage (and to a lesser extent the airway interstitial macrophage) is an extremely inefficient antigen presenting cell, direct extrapolation of these results to human asthma would seem injudicious at the present time. Comparable studies of the effects of IL-10 and IL-12 on pulmonary dendritic cell function will be invaluable in understanding the role of these cytokine in modulating lung mucosal immunity.

4.4   Co-stimulation molecules and the induction of T_H2 immunity: B7-1, B7-2, CD28 and CTLA-4

The balance of evidence is overwhelmingly in favor of soluble factors, and particularly IL-4, as the most important signals that the naive CD4+ cell encounters during primary stimulation leading to commitment to the T_H2 phenotype. However, when T cells, via their T cells receptor complex proteins, first recognize processed antigen peptides bound to MHC molecules they may also encounter a number of differentially expressed surface markers on the antigen presenting cell which convey additional information to the T cell. This phenomenon is called co-stimulation and is a central regulatory process in immune recognition and activation. Co-stimulation of T cells can be provided by two members of the B7 protein family termed B7-1 (CD80) and B7-2 (CD86) which are variably expressed on antigen presenting cells. B7 members bind to the surface molecules CTLA-4 (cytotoxic T-lymphocyte associated molecule-4) and CD28 (Linsley et al., 1990; 1991; 1992).

Several major lines of evidence suggest that B7 molecules may be important in the early induction of T_H2 responses. In an *in vivo* model of autoimmune encephalitis, where T_H1 cells are formed in pathogenic numbers and mediate nerve damage, administration of antibodies against B7-1 leads to increased numbers of IL-4 secreting T_H2 cells and to the reduction in disease severity. Similar differential induction of T_H1 or T_H2 responses was observed *in vitro* (Kuchroo et al., 1995). In separate studies Freedman et al. (1995) showed that B7-2 caused human naive T cells to express IL-4 whereas memory T cells produced IL-4 in response to both B7-1 and B7-2. The molecular basis of this finding is difficult to explain with current knowledge since both B7-1 and B7-2 can bind to the same molecules, suggesting the likelihood of either differential time courses of expression and/or divergent signaling mechanisms (which, when clarified, may offer yet another approach to regulating T_H2 immunity). The prospect of selectively manipulating co-stimulation for asthma therapy is suggested by the observation that CD28 stimulation can lead to an *in vitro* T_H2 response in the absence of exogenous IL-4 (King et al., 1995). These data suggest that early B7-2 co-stimulation could slightly bias immune response in favor of early IL-4 production favoring development of T_H2 immune responses.

It seems unlikely however that B7 molecules dominate T_H1 or T_H2 commitment. CD28 triggering causes IL-2 production which is consumed by T cells during subsequent proliferation. IL-2, at least *in vitro*, is the second soluble signal need by T_H0 cells to commit to the T_H2 phenotype (Le Gros et al., 1990; Seder and Paul, 1994). Activation of CTLA-4 has generated great interest in transplantation research because a chimeric form of this molecule fused to human immunoglobulin G (CTLA-4-Ig) which has been used to provide an incomplete activation signal to T cells and thereby producing complete anergy of T cell responses *in vivo* preventing allograft rejection. However, in view of the role of CD28+ in early IL-2 production and the immunosuppressive action of CTLA-4 engagement blocking co-stimulation experiments may reflect broad spectrum immunosuppression rather than a selective T_H2 suppression more desirable in asthma therapy. Not all findings with B7-2 support a role in T_H2 induction. Lanier et al. (1995) found that B7-2 stimulation of human T cells lead to similar T_H1 and T_H2 cytokine levels. Moreover if co-stimulation were to be essential

for expression of T_H2 immunity diverse antigen presenting cells populations would be expected to differ in their ability to contribute to T_H2 commitment due to innate differences in their expression levels of co-stimu-
latory molecules. Although some antigen presenting cell populations may
more efficiently stimulate T_H2 cell proliferation than others there is evidence from studies using transgenic mice expressing defined antigen-spe-
cific T cell receptors at high frequencies that antigen presenting cell type,
and by inference co-stimulation, is *not* the central determinant of T_H2 commitment (Seder et al., 1992). Furthermore, Hsieh et al. (1995) have demonstrated in normal Balb/c and B10.D2 mouse strains that antigen presenting cell type appears relatively unimportant in regulating T_H2 commitment. An apparent explanation for these seemingly contradictory findings
is that the signal transduction mechanisms activated in T_H cells which
induce proliferation are almost certainly distinct from those required to
induce T_H2 commitment. Bluestone (1995) has suggested an alternative
"avidity model" where T_H1 or T_H2 immune responses are determined by
the interaction of the intensity of co-stimulation and the degree of T cell
receptor complex ligand density/affinity. This area is currently the subject of intense research.

4.5   Cytokine suppression of primary T_H2 commitment and
         secondary T_H2 immune responses to allergen are not
         identical

A clear distinction must be made between the role of cytokines in the
earliest molecular events causing T_H2 commitment and the maintenance
of responsiveness (memory/effector function) after the T_H2 phenotype
is established. We have demonstrated in a mouse model of T_H2-mediated
lung eosinophilic inflammation that the timing of anti-IL-4 antibody administration is critical. Neutralizing monoclonal antibodies administered
in doses preventing B cell IgE switch were without benefit in the aller-
gen-challenged mouse, where administered immediately prior to allergen
challenge (Coyle et al., 1995). This suggests that IL-4 is not as important
for eosinophil recruitment as supposed from the results of *in vitro* experiments (Moser et al., 1994). However, pronounced inhibition of pulmonary eosinophil influx was observed when monoclonal antibodies were
administered prior to secondary immunization suggesting an important
role for IL-4 in expanding or maintaining the T_H2 population induced on
primary allergen exposure (Coyle et al., 1995). This raises two issues of
therapeutic relevance. Firstly, drugs which affect IL-4 are more likely to
be of value given early in the natural history of asthma before or at the

time when patients begin to acquire specific sensitivity to aeroallergens. Secondly, drugs affecting IL-4 may not be effective in reversing or suppressing established T_H2 immunological "memory" to specific allergens. Indeed the balance of evidence currently available suggests that allergic hypersensitivity persists in humans in an IL-4 independent manner. Recently, a second cytokine, IL-13 which is closely related to IL-4, has been characterized. There is emerging evidence that IL-13 may be more important than IL-4 in the maintenance of allergic responses after initial IL-4 dependent commitment has occurred (Zurakawski et al., 1993; 1994). The IgE response has provided a useful alternative to eosinophilic inflammation to study T_H2 immune regulation. CD4+ T cells present antigen bound to MHC class II surface molecules to naive B cells and provide co-stimulation cognate (e.g. T cell CD40+ ligand binding to B cell CD40+ receptor) and soluble signals (e.g. cytokines) which activate B cells. Second soluble cytokine signals supporting cell proliferation and which have a profound effect on the *isotype* of antibody that is subsequently produced by B plasma cells (isotype switch). Studies in IL-4 knockout mice have formally demonstrated that *in vivo* IgE production is almost entirely dependent on a IL-4 co-signal at the time of antigen presentation (Kopf et al., 1993). However, once B cells isotype switch has occurred IL-4 seems less important in maintaining IgE production. Brinkmann et al. (1995) have demonstrated that naive CD4+ T cells (defined as those lacking the marker CD45RO) stimulated via CD3+ can be induced to secrete IL-5 and IFNγ and to help B cells make IgE in an IL-13 dependent manner whereas antigen experienced CD45RO+ "memory" CD4+ T cells use both IL-4 and IL-13 to support IL-4 and IL-5 production and B cell IgE switch.

4.6   IL-1 inhibitors may prevent reactivation of antigen experienced "memory" CD4+ T_H2 cells in chronic asthma

Although the differences in regulation of primary compared to secondary T_H2 response might seem to reduce therapeutic options in chronic disease, more detailed examination of established T_H2 immunity has revealed alternative potential therapeutic strategies. IL-1, a cytokine class with a very diverse biology, is an excellent example. IL-1α and IL-1 β are produced rapidly by mononuclear/macrophage lineages in response to insult but are also very widely expressed in other cell types. The proliferation of T_H2, but not T_H1 cells which do not express the functionally coupled type 1 IL-1 receptor, is promoted by IL-1 (Weaver et al., 1988; Solari et al., 1990). A subset of antigen-experienced or "memory" (recently activated) CD4+ cells is particularly sensitive to IL-1 induced proliferation. Indeed there is evi-

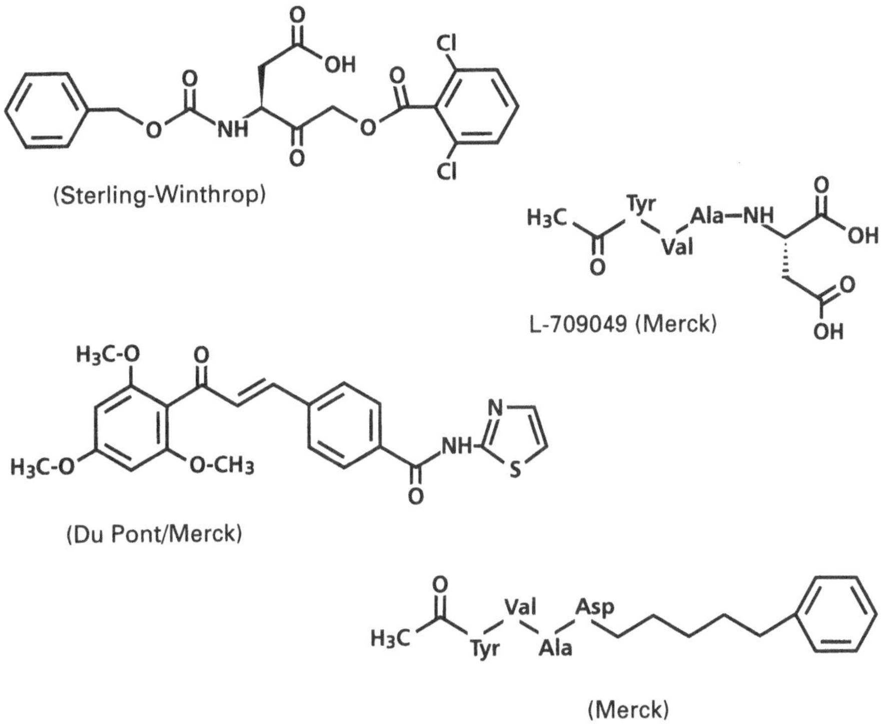

Fig. 9.
IL-1 synthesis inhibitors

dence that T_H2 cells produce IL-1 as an autocrine growth factor (Zubiaga et al., 1991) and that IL-1 favors the *in vitro* development of T_H2 cells (Manetti et al., 1994) acting via IL-4 upregulated type 1 receptors (Koch et al., 1992). A therapeutic potential was suggested by experiments where the naturally occurring human IL-1 receptor antagonist was produced in pure recombinant form (rhIL-1RA) and when administered *in vivo* was found to substantially reduce the intensity of inhaled allergen provoked eosinophilic airway inflammation and hyperreactivity in guinea pigs (Watson et al., 1993). In view of the selective action of IL-1 on post-committed T_H2 cell drugs targeted at IL-1 may be used preferentially in established rather than early disease. The situation in allergic asthma may, however, be somewhat more complex than predicted by animal models since IL-4 has recently been discovered to upregulate the synthesis and release of the soluble IL-1 type II receptor which serves as a decoy for IL-1 reducing its biological effects (Colotta et al., 1993). The intense research into inhibition of IL-1 has led to the discovery of several novel agents (Fig. 9).

4.7   Suppression of IL-5: clinical benefit in established T$_H$2 disease *in vivo*?

IL-5 supports the terminal differentiation of lineage committed progenitors into mature eosinophils *in vitro*, and to date it is the only cytokine known to exert this effect (Sanderson et al., 1986). IL-5 is critical for the manifestation of eosinophilia and eosinophilia is CD4+ T cell dependent (Baston and Beeson, 1976). In humans, IL-5 has been located by immunohistochemistry and identified in lung lavages and blood suggesting that IL-5 is a major determinant of eosinophilic inflammation consequent to allergen challenge in asthmatics (Walker et al., 1991; Ohishi et al., 1993). Similarly antibodies against IL-5 have been used to suppress eosinophilic inflammation in a number of animal models of allergen-induced airway inflammation (Chand et al., 1992; Nakajima et al., 1992; Van Oosterhout et al., 1993). Importantly, suppression of eosinophilia has been associated with a reduction in disturbed lung function in some but not all of these studies. With the exception of high toxic isothiazolones which covalently bind to the IL-5 receptor alpha chain, safe pharmacological inhibitors of IL-5 production or action have not yet been discovered although a number of unique monoclonal antibodies and IL-5 mutants have been constructed (Devos et al., 1995). Animal experiments with neutralizing antibodies suggest such drugs would be useful in asthma. In pre-sensitized mice or guinea pigs, allergen challenge leads to an eosinophilic inflammation of the airways which is profoundly suppressed by neutralizing antibodies against IL-5 (Chand et al., 1992). Similarly soluble recombinant IL-5 receptors reduce eosinophilia. However, as predicted by *in vitro* studies anti-IL-5 has no effect on IgE production.

4.8   IL-4 and IL-13 signal transduction: can specific inhibition be achieved?

To date several IL-4 blocking antibodies have been produced which are useful in understanding the *in vivo* biology of IL-4, but selective inhibitors of IL-4 and IL-13 have not been discovered. Given the complexity of the IL-4/IL-13 receptor complexes, which involve interaction with the IL-2 receptor common gamma chain, it is possible that classical receptor antagonists may never be found. However, molecular dissection of the means by which IL-4 and IL-13 achieve their signal transduction is already suggesting alternative strategies to selectively inhibit the effects of these cytokines (Fig. 10). Unlike IL-13, IL-5 and GM-CSF, IL-4 induces a pattern of phosphorylation of numerous intracellular substrates that is unlike

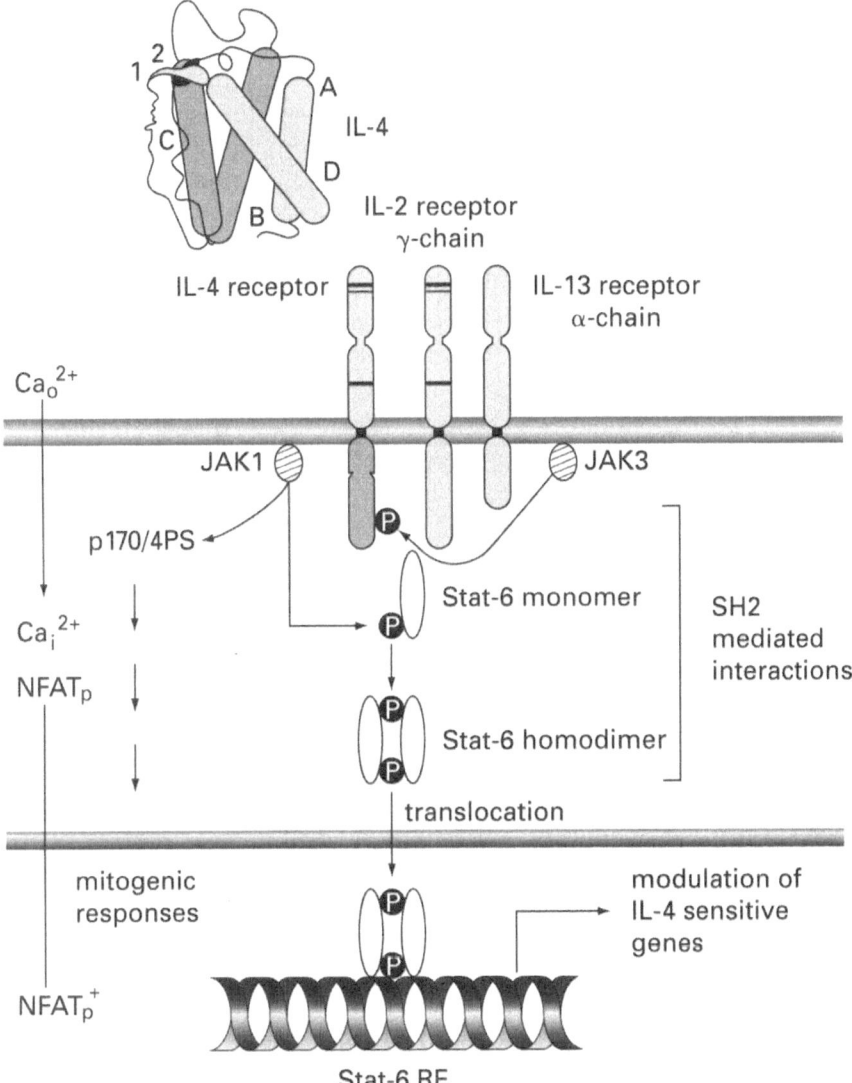

Fig. 10.
IL-4 (and IL-13) as a drug target
IL-4 signals via a receptor complex comprising the IL-4 alpha receptor chain the common gamma chain of the IL-2 receptor. Occupancy of the complex facilitates phosphorylation of the alpha chain by JAK3. Alternative signals transduced via the p170/PS4 pathway are concurrently produced. The transcription factor STAT-6 interacts with the phosphorylated alpha chain SH2 domain allowing its phosphorylation by JAK1 which allows the monomer to form a STAT-6 homodimer. This homodimer regulates IL-4 sensitive genes by binding to the STAT-6 regulatory element (STAT-6 RE). IL-13 is currently believed to use an analogous signalling pathway. The most promising drug targets are SH2 blockers and STAT-6 RE blockers. NFAT$_p$ regulation of IL-4 sensitive genes has also recently been demonstrated.

related hematopoietins (Keegan et al., 1994). These substrates are typically phosphorylated on tyrosine residues by receptor tyrosine kinase (RTK) enzymes. Phosphorylation in turn facilitates the physical interaction between signal transduction molecules by increasing their binding affinity. Unlike some cytokines and many growth factors, the IL-4 receptor complex lacks intrinsic RTK activity, and phosphorylation of diverse substrates is achieved via intermediate adapter molecules. Tyrosine phosphorylation is possible after IL-4 activates its receptor complex because Janus Kinase RTK family members Jak 1, Jak 3 and/or Fes RTKs are rapidly activated by the occupied IL-4 receptor (Witthuhn et al., 1994). Since these molecules have intrinsic RTK activity a cascade of phosphorylation ensues resulting in tyrosine phosphorylation of the IL-4 receptor itself, a 170 KD molecule termed 4PS, the insulin-related substrate molecule (IRS-1). The phosphotyrosine residues that are formed allow binding to intermediates bearing c-src homology domains (SH2-domains), notably the signal transduction coupled intermediates the 85 KD regulatory subunit of PI-3 kinase (activating the PKC signaling), Syp (SHPTP-2, a phosphatase down regulating phosphorylation) and Grb-2 (Growth factor receptor binding protein 2), an adapter protein bearing SH-2 domains that mediates activation of guanine nucleotide exchange on ras). In this way the IL-4 receptor can rapidly entrain a series of important signal transduction pathways and mediate mitogenic response. It is also certain that IL-4 receptor occupancy leads to the phosphorylation and interaction of specific transcription factors or patterns of transcription factors which translocate to the cell nucleus where they regulate the transcription of IL-4 inducible or suppressible genes by binding to recognition sequences. Notable amongst these molecules is the very recently discovered IL-4 STAT (signal transduction and activation molecule) also termed STAT-6 (Hou et al., 1994).

Although the signal transduction molecules mentioned above are often viewed as "generic and non-specific" several levels of selective coding allow highly directed interactions to occur. STAT-molecules for example can bind to at least ten recognition sequences (GAS-sequences) but the specificity of their binding is strongly influenced by the *pairing* of diverse STATS to form heterodimers. SH-2 (and related SH-3) domains also appear as a simple class of interaction sites yet the subtle difference which occurs in the structure of individual SH2 sites and their environs suggest that selective SH-2 antagonists are feasible (Fig. 11). Indeed prototype inhibitors have already been identified (Burke et al., 1995; Morelock et al., 1995). While selective IL-4 / IL-13 inhibitors based on signal transduction are not yet available the success in identifying selective PDGF

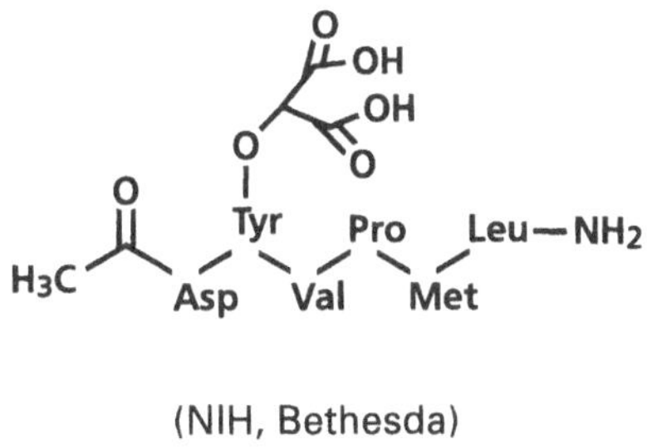

(NIH, Bethesda)

Fig. 11.
Src homology 2 (SH2) domain inhibitor

(platelet derived growth factor) (Buchdunger et al., 1995) and EGF (epidermal growth factor), RTK inhibitors (Fry et al., 1994) have already demonstrated the promise of this avenue of research.

5   Molecular genetics

Recently, considerable advances have been made in unravelling the genetic
basis of allergy and asthma (Marsh et al., 1994; Shirakawa et al., 1994).
Genetically, asthma belongs to a group of complex diseases, so termed
because their pattern of inheritance and expression is regulated by multiple genetic elements and does not follow the simple rules of Mendelian
genetics, characteristic of single gene diseases. For this reason identification of candidate genes has been extremely elusive and requires highly
complex analytical techniques. The problem of genetic analysis is made
more complex by the lack of an internationally agreed upon asthma phenotype and because of the changes which can occur over time in the severity of disease which may obscure inheritance patterns. Nevertheless, per-
sistence in analyzing traits associated with asthma such as bronchial hyperresponsiveness and, in the case of allergic disease, elevated serum IgE have
led to the identification of markers proximal to candidate genes. The methods which have been employed to date use generic DNA markers, usually highly poylmorphic regions which are easy to track and localize to

defined regions of chromosomal DNA. Linkage analysis of the trait to the marker is made in computerized segregation studies where the outcome is a series of probability values that the marker may co-segregate with the candidate gene. Several groups have reported linkages in atopic disease and very recently in asthma which are narrowing the gap between marker and gene. The most usual strategy being pursued in most laboratories is to further narrow the distance between marker and gene by using more markers in a candidate region. This will lead to efforts to positionally clone candidate genes. It is of great interest that of the linkages identified to date several are proximal to the IL-4/IL-13 gene cluster on chromosome 5q31-3 believed to be important in the expression of $T_{H}2$ immunity. Several groups have already advanced the concept that genetic variation in the IL-4 gene promoter (or perhaps a transcription factor regulating IL-4) may be central to the induction of asthma. This suggestion has not been confirmed to date. This 5q31 region also contains the genes for the beta-2 adrencoceptor, where clear polymorphic variants have been identifed in asthma (Green et al., 1995) and the glucocorticoid receptor as well as the genes for several growth factors of their receptors. One concept that is also emerging from the scant genetic information already at hand is that asthma may actually comprise a related group of disorders, manifesting similar lung pathology but different pathogenic defects. If this proves to be the case the dream of a single therapy for asthma will evaporate. However, if asthma is a group of diseases the availability of genetic analysis will allow highly specific diagnosis and, as our understanding increases, specific curative and preventative therapy will be designed.

6   Conclusion

As outlined in this brief review the better understanding of the role of growth factors, protease biology and molecular mechanisms of $T_{H}2$ mediated immunity which has been gained over the last several years has revealed clues about the fundamental regulatory defects linked to the clinical expression of asthma. More broadly the genetic regulation of $T_{H}2$ immunity is likely to be discovered in coming years as the fundamental predisposing factor in disease induction. This, together with other insights, will offer the possibility of definitive early prediction of disease onset, and if medicinal pharmacology succeeds in developing safe agents to realign mucosal defenses, the possibility of realizing the long-awaited goal of preventive and perhaps even curative therapy for asthma.

Acknowledgment

We would like to thank our colleagues Dr S. Alkan, Dr C.P. Bertrand, Dr M.A. Bray, Dr A. Coyle, Dr F. Erard, Dr Ch. Heusser, Dr M. Kopf, Dr G. LeGros, Prof. Th. Staehelin, Mr S. Tsuyuki and Mrs S. Tsuyuki, for the invaluable assistance and support in many of the basic studies which are drawn upon in this paper.

References

Afonso, L.C., T.M. Scharton, L.Q. Vieira, M. Wysocka, G. Trinchieri and P. Scott. (1994): The adjuvant effect of interleukin 12 in a vaccine against *Leishmania major*. Science *263*, 235.

Aikawa, T., Shimura, S., Sasaki, H., Ebina, M. and Takishima, T. (1992): Marked goblet cell hyperplasia with mucus accumulation in the airways of patients who died of severe acute asthma attack. Chest *101*, 916–921.

Albeda S.M. (1991): Endothelial and epithelial cell adhesion molecules. Amer. J. Respir. Cell Molec. Biol. *4*, 195–203.

Albeda S.M. (1993): The role of cell adhesion molecules in asthma. N. Drugs in Allergy, Asthma *43*, 141–150.

Anderson, G.P. and Coyle, A.J. (1994): TH-2 and TH2-like cells in allergy and asthma: pharmacological perspectives. Trend Pharmacol. Sci. *15*, 324–332.

Arm J.P. and Lee T.K. (1992): The Pathobiology of Bronchial Asthma. Adv. Immunol. *51*, 323–382.

Barnes P.J. (1993): Neural mechanisms in asthma. In: Holgate S.T., Austen K.F., Lichtenstein L.M. and Kay A.B. (eds.): Asthma: physiology, immunopharmacology, and treatment. Academic Press, London 1993, 259–273.

Baston, A. and P.B. Beeson (1970): Mechaism of eosinophilia. II. Role of the lymphocyte. J.Exp.Med. *131*, 1288.

Bentley A.M., Maestrelli P., Saetta M., Fabbri L.M., Robinson D.S., Bradley D.L., Jeffery P.K., Durham S.R. and Kay A.B. (1992): Activated T-lymphocytes and eosinophils in the bronchial muscosa in isocyanate-induced asthma. J. Allerg. Clin. Immunol. *89*, 821–829.

Berman J.S. and Weller P.F. (1992): Airway eosinophils and lymphocytes in asthma. Amer. Rev. Resp. Dis. *145*, 1246–1248.

Blotnick S., G.E. Peoples, M.R. Freeman, T.J. Eberlein and M. Klagsbrun (1994): T lymphocytes synthesize and export heparin-binding epidermal growth factor-like growth factor and basic fibroblast growth factor, mitogens for vascular cells and fibroblasts: differential production and release by CD4$^+$ and CD8$^+$ T cells. Proc. Natl. Acad. Sci. USA *91*, 2890.

Bluestone J.A. (1995): New perspectives of CD28-B7-mediated T cell costimulation. Immunity *2*, 555–9.

Borsi L., Castellani P., Risso A.M., Leprini A., Zardi L. (1990): Transforming growth factor beta regulates the splicing patern of fibronectin messenger mRNA precursors. FEBS Lett. *261*, 175–178.

Bradding, P., I.H. Feather, P. Howarth, S.R. Muller, J.A. Roberts, K. Britten, T. Hunt, Y.

Okayama, C. Heusser, G. Bullock, M.K. Church and S.T. Holgate (1992): Interleu-kin 4 is localized to and released by human mast cells. J. Exp. Med. *176*,1381–1386.

Bradding P., Feather I.H., Howarth P.H., Mueller R., Roberts J.A., Britten K., Bews J.P.A., Hunt T.C., Okayama Y., Heusser C.H., Bullock G.R., Church M.K. and Holgate S.T. (1992): Interleukin 4 is localized to and released by human mast cells. J. Exp. Med. *176*, 1381–1386.

Brinkmann, V., T. Geiger, S. Alkan and C. Heusser (1993): IFN α increases the frequency of IFN γ-producing human CD4-positive T cells. J. Exp. Med. *178*, 1655.

Brinkmann V. and Kristofic C. (1995): TCR-stimulated naive human CD4+ 45RO-T cells develop into effector cells that secrete IL-13, IL-5, and IFN-gamma, but no IL-4, and help efficient IgE production by B cells. J. Immunol. *157*, 3078–3087.

Briscoe D.M., Cotran R.S. and Pober J.S. (1992): Effects of tumor necrosis factor, lipopol-ysaccharide, and IL-4 on the expression of vascular cell adhesion molecule-1 *in vivo*. J. Immunol. *149*, 2954–2960.

Brogan, T.D., Ryley H.C., Neale, L. and Yassa, J. (1975): Soluable proteins of bronchopul-monary secretions from pateients with cystic fibrosis, asthma and bronchititis. Tho-rax *30*, 72–79.

Bucy, R.P., Karr, L., Huang, G.Q., Li, J., Carter, D., Honjo K., Lemons, J.A., Murphy, K.M. and Weaver, C.T.(1995): Single cell analysis of cytokine gene coexpression during CD4+ T-cell phenotype development. Proc. Natl. Acad. Sci. (USA) *92*, 7565–7569.

Bucy, R.P., Panoskaltsis-Mortari, A., Huang, G.Q., Li, J., Karr, L., Ross, M., Russell, J.H., Murphy, K.M.,Weaver, C.T. (1994): Heterogeneity of single cell cytokine gene expres-sion in clonal T cell populations. J Exp Med 180, 1251–1262.

Busse, W.W. and Gaddy, J.N. (1991): The role of leukotriene antagonists and inhibitors in the treatment of airway disease. American Review of Respiratory Diseases 143, S103–S107.

Busse, W.W., and C.E. Reed. (1988): Asthma: definition and pathogenesis. In: Allergy, prin-ciples and practice, 3rd ed., Middleton, E., Jr., C.E. Reed, E.F.Ellis, N.F. Adkinson, Jr. and J.W. Yunginger (eds.). C.V.Mosby, St.Louis. 969–998.

Cardell, B.S. and Pearson, R.S.B. (1959): Death in asthmatics. Thorax *14*,341–352.

Chand, N., J.E. Harrison, S. Rooney, J.Pilar, R. Jakubicki, K. Nolan, W. Diamantis and R.D. Sofia. (1992): Anti-IL-5 monoclonal anyibody inhibits allergic late phase bronchial eosinophilia in guinea pigs: a therapeutic approach. Europ. J. Pharmacol. *211*, 121–123.

Coffman, R.L., J. Ohara, M.W. Bond, J. Carty, A. Zlotnik and W.E. Paul. (1986): B cell stim-ulatory factor-1 enhances the IgE response of lipopolisaccharide-activated B cells. J. Immunol. *151*, 5053.

Coffman, R.L., B.W.P. Seymour, D.A. Lebman, D.D. Hiraki, J.A. Christiansen, B. Shrader, H.M. Cherwinski, H.F.J. Savelkoul, F.D. Finkelman, M.W. Bond and T.R. Mosmann. (1988): The role of helper T cell products in mouse B cell differentiation and iso-type regulation. Immunol. Rev. *102*, 5.

Colotta, F., F.R.M. Muzio, R. Bertini, N. Polentarutti, M. Sironi, J. G. Giri, S.K.Dower, J.E. Sims and A Mantovani (1993): Interleukin-1 type II receptor: a decoy target for IL-1 that is regulated by IL-4. Science *261*,472–475.

Corrigan C.J., Kay A.B. (1992): Role of T-lymphocytes and lymphokines. Brit. Med. Bull. *48*, 72–84.

Coyle, A.J. , G. Le Gros, C. Bertrand, S. Tsuyuki, C.H. Heusser, M. Kopf and G.P. Ander-son (1995): IL-4 is required for the induction of lung Th2 mucosal immunity. Am. J. Respir. Cell Mol. Biol. *13*, 54–59.

Cutz, E., Levison, H. and Cooper, D.M. (1978): Ultrastructure of airways in chilrdren with asthma. Histopathology 2, 407–421.

Demeure, C.E., C.Y. Wu, U. Shu, P.V. Schneider, C. Heusser, H. Yssel and G. Delespesse (1994): *In vitro* maturation of human neonatal CD4 T lymphocytes. II Cytokines present at priming modulate the development of lymphokine production. J. Immunol. *152*, 4775.

DeMonchy J.G.R., Kauffman H.F., Venge P., Koëter G.H., Jansen H.M., Sluiter H.J. and deVries K. (1985): Bronchoalveolar eosinophilia during allergen-induced late asthmatic reactions. Amer. Rev. Resp. Dis. *131*, 373–376.

Devos R., Plaetinck G., Cornelis S., Guisez Y., Van der Heyden J. and Tavernier J. (1995): Interleukin-5 and its receptor: a drug target for eosinophilia associated with chronic allergic disease. J. Leukoc. Biol. *57*, 813–9.

De Waal Malefyt, R., H. Yssel, M.G. Roncarolo, H. Spits and J.E. de Vries (1992): Interleukin-10. Curr. Opin. Immunol. *4*, 314.

Djukanovic R., Lai C.K.W., Wilson J.W., Britten K.M., Wilson S.J., Roche W.R., Howarth P.H. and Holgate S.T. (1992): Bronchial mucosal manifestations of atopy: a comparison of markers of inflammation between atopic asthmatics, atopic nonasthmatics and healthy controls. Eur. Resp. J. *5*, 538–544.

Dunhill, M.D. (1960): The pathology of asthma with special reference to changes in the bronchial mucosa. J. Clin. Pathol. *13*,27–33.

Dunhill, M.D., Massarella, G.R. and Anderson, J.A. (1969): A comparison of the quantitative anatomy of the bronchi in normal subjects, in staus asthmaticus, in chronic bronchitis and in emphysema. Thorax *24*,176–179.

Filley, W.V., Holley, K.E., Kephart, B.M. and Gleich, G.J. (1982): Indentification by immunofluorescence of eosinophil granule major basic protein in lung tissues of patients with bronchial asthma. Lancet *2*,11–15.

Finkelman, F.D., J. Holmes, I.M. Katona, J.F. Urban, M.P. Beckmann, L.S. Park, K.A. Schooley, R.L. Coffman, T.R. Mosmann and W.E. Paul (1990): Lymphokine control of *in vivo* immunoglobulin isotype selection. Annu. Rev. Immunol. *8*, 303.

Fiorentino, D.F., A. Zlotnik, T.R. Mosmann, M. Howard and A. O'Garra (1991): IL–10 inhibits cytokine production by activated macrophages. J. Immunol. *147*, 3815.

Freedman A.S., Freeman G.J., Rhynhart K. and Nadler L.M. (1991): Selective induction of B7/BB-1 on interferon-gamma stimulated monocytes a potential mechanism for amplification of T cell activation through the CD28 pathway. Cell Immunol. *137*, 429–37.

Frew A.J. and Kay A.B. (1990): Eosinophils and T-lymphocytes in late-phase allergic reactions. J. Allerg. Clin. Immunol. *85*, 533–539.

Frigas, E., D.A. Loegering and G.J. Gleich (1980): Cytotoxic effects of guinea pig major basic protein on tracheal epithelium. Lab. Invest. *42*,35.

Frigas E. and Gleich G.J. (1986): The eosinophil and the pathophysiology of asthma. J. Allerg. Clin. Immunol. *77*, 527–537.

Galli S.J., Gordon J.R. and Wershil B.K. (1993): Mast cell cytokines in allergy and inflammation. N. Drugs in Allergy, Asthma *43*, 209–220.

Gilbert I.A. and McFadden E.R. (1992): Airway cooling and rewarming. The second reaction sequence in exercise-induced asthma. J. Clin. Invest. *90* (3), 699–704.

Gilbert I.A., Winslow C.J., Lenner K.A., Nelson J.A. and McFadden E.R. (1993): Vascular volume expansion and thermally induced asthma. Eur. Respir. J. *6*(2), 189–197.

Gordon J.R., Burd P.R. and Galli S.J. (1990): Mast cells as a source of multifunctional cytokines. Immunol. Today *11*, 458–464.

Green S.A., Turki J,. Bejarano P., Hall I.P. and Liggett S.B. (1995): Influence of beta 2-adrenergic receptor genotypes on signal transduction in human airway smooth muscle cells. Am. J. Respir. Cell Mol. Biol. Jul. *13*(1), 25–33.

Griffiths M.H., Hansel T.T., Blaser K. and Walker C. (1992): The role of T lymphocytes in the pathogenesis of asthma. Schweiz. med. Wschr. *122*, 294–297.

Hamid, Q., M. Azzawi, S. Ying, R. Moqbel, A.J. Wardlaw, Corrigan, B. Bradley, S.R. Durham, J.V. Collins, P.K. Jeffery, D.J. Quint and A.B. Kay (1991): Expression of mRNA for interleukin-5 in mucosal bronchial biopsies from asthma. J. Clin. Invest. *87*, 1541.

Heard B.E., Houssain S. (1973): Hyperplasia of bronchial smooth muscle in asthma. J. Pathol. *71*, 319–331.

Heinzel. F.P., M.D. Sadick, S.S. Mutha and R.M. Locksley (1991): Production of interferon γ, interleukin 2, interleukin 4, and interleukin 10 by CD[4+] lymphocytes *in vivo* during healing and progressive murine leishmaniasis. Proc. Natl. Acad. Sci. *88*, 7011.

Hill M.R. and Kamada A.K. (1991): Pathogenesis of asthma: therapeutic implications. Ann. Pharmacotherapy, DICP *25*, 993–1001.

Hogg, J.C., Macklem, P.T. and Thurlbeck, W.M. (1968): Site and nature of airway obstruction in chronc lung disease. N. Eng. J. Med. *278*, 355–1360.

Holgate S.T., Roche W.R. and Church M.K. (1991): The role of the eosinophil in asthma. Amer. Rev. Resp. Dis. *143*, S66–S70.

Houston J.C., De Navasquez, S. and Thoimce, J.R. (1953): A clinical and pathological study of fatal cases of status asthmaticus. Thorax *8*, 207–213.

Hsieh, C.S., S.E. Macatonia, C.S. Tripp, S.F. Wolf, A. O'Garra and K.M. Murphy. (1993): Development of T_H1 CD4+ T cells through IL-12 produced by Listeria-induced macrophages. Science *260*, 547.

Hsieh C.S., Macatonia S.E., O'Garra A. and Murphy K.M. (1995): T cell genetic background determines default T helper phenotype. J. Exp. Med. *181* (1), 713–721.

Iijima H., Ishii M., Yamauchi K., Chao C.L., Kimura K., Shimura S., Shindoh Y., Inove H., Mue S. and Takishima T. (1987): Bronchoalveolar lavage and histologic characterization of late asthmatic response in guinea pigs. Amer. Rev. Resp. Dis. *136*, 922–929.

Jeffery P.K. (1994): Innervation of the airway mucosa: structure, function and changes in airway disease. In: Goldie Roy (ed.): Immunopharma-cology of epithelial barriers. Academic Press, London, San Diego 85–118.

Jeffrey P. (1991): Morphology of the bronchial wall in asthma and in chronic obstructive pulmonoary disease. Am. Rev. Respir. Dis. *143*, 1152–1158.

Kay, A.B., S. Ying, V. Varney, M. Gaga, S.R. Durham, R. Moqbel, A.J. Wardlaw and Q. Hamid (1991): Messenger RNA expression of the cytokine gene cluster, interleukin (IL)-3, IL-4, IL-5 and GM-CSF in allergen-induced late phase reactions in atopic subjects. J. Exp. Med. *173*, 775.

Kay A.B., Henson P.M., Hunninghake G.W., Irvin C., Lichtenstein L.M. and Nadel J.A. (1989): Cellular Mechanisms In: Holgate S.T. (ed.): The role of inflammatory processes in airway hyperresponsiveness. Blackwell Scientific Publications, Oxford, London, Edinburgh, Boston, Melbourne 151–178.

Keegan, A.D., K. Nelms, L.-M. Wang, J.H. Pierce and W.E. Paul. (1994): Interleukin 4 receptor: signaling mechanisms. Immunol. Today *15*, 423.

King C.L., Stupi R.J., Craighead N. and June C.H.. Thyphronitis G. (1995): CD28 activation promotes Th2 subset differentiation by human CD4+ cells. Eur. J. Immunol. *25*, 587–95.

Koch, K.C., K. Ye, B.D. Clark and C.A. Dinarello (1992): Interleukin (IL) 4 up-regulates gene and surface IL1 receptor type 1 in murine T helper type 2 cells. Europ. J. Immunol. 22, 153–157.

Kopf, M., G. Le Gros, M. Bachmann, M.C. Lamers, H. Bluethmann and G. Köhler (1993): Disruption of the murine IL-4 gene blocks Th2 cytokine responses. Nature 362, 245.

Kuchroo V.K., Das M.P., Brown J.A., Ranger A.M., Zamvil S.S., Sobel R.A., Weiner H.L., Nabavi N. and Glimcher L.H. (1995): B7-1 and B7-2 costimulatory molecules activate differentially the Th1/Th2 developmental pathways: application to autoimmune disease therapy. Cell 80, 707–18.

Lanier L.L., O'Fallon S., Somoza C., Phillips J.H., Linsley P.S., Okumura K., Ito D. and Azuma M. (1995): CD80 (B7) and CD86 (B70) provide similar costimulatory signals for T cell proliferation, cytokine production, and generation of CTL. J. Immunol. 154, 97–105.

Lazaar, A., S.M. Albelda, J.M. Pilewski, B. Brennan, E. Puré and R.A. Panettieri, Jr. (1994): T lymphocytes adhere to airway smooth muscle cells via integrins and CD44 and induce smooth muscle cell DNA synthesis. J. Exp. Med. 180, 807.

Le Gros, G., S.Z. Ben Sasson, R. Seder, F.D. Finkelman and W.E. Paul. (1990): Generation of IL-4-producing cells in vivo and in vitro: IL-2 and IL-4 are required for the in vitro generation of IL-4 producing cells. J. Exp. Med. 172, 921.

Lopez, A.L., C.J. Sanderson, J.R. Gamble, H.D. Campbell, I.G. Young and M.A. Vardas (1988): Recombinant human interleukin 5 is a selective activator of human eosinophil function. J. Exp. Med. 167, 219.

Lukacher, A.E., V.L. Braciale and T.J. Braciale (1984): In vivo effector function of influenza-virus specific cytotoxic T lymphocyte clones is highly specific. J. Exp. Med. 160, 814.

Manetti, R., P. Parronchi, M.G. Giudizi, M.P. Pichinni, E. Maggi, G. Trinchieri and S. Romagnani (1993): Natural killer cell stimulatory factor (interleukin 12) induces T helper type 1 (TH1)-specific immune responses and inhibits the development of IL-4-producing Th cells. J. Exp. Med. 177, 1199.

Mosmann, T.R. (1991): Cytokine secretion patterns and cross-regulation of T cell subsets. Immunol. Res. 10, 183.

Marsh, D.G., J.D. Neely, D.R. Breazeale, B. Ghosh, L.R. Freidhoff, E. Ehrlich-Kautzki, C. Schou, G. Krishnaswami and T.H. Beaty (1994): Linkage analysis of IL-4 and other chromosome 5q31.1 markers and total serum immunoglobulin E concentrations. Science 264, 1152.

Mattoli S., Mattoso V.L., Soloperto M., Allegra L. and Fasoli A. (1991): Cellular and biochemical characteristics of bronchoalveolar lavage fluid in symptomatic nonallergic asthma. J. Allerg. Clin. Immunol. 87, 794–802.

McFadden E.R. and Gilbert I.A. (1993): Vascular responses and thermally induced asthma. In: Holgate S.T., Austen K.F., Lichtenstein L.M. and Kay A.B. (eds.): Asthma: physiology, immunopharmacology, and treatment. Academic Press, London 1993, 337–343.

Morison, L.A., A.E. Lukacher, V.L. Braciale, D.P. Fan and T.J. Braciale (1986): Differences in antigen presentation to MHC class I and class II restricted influenza virus specific CTL clones. J. Exp. Med. 163, 903.

Moser, R., J. Fehr and P.L. Bruijnzeel (1992): IL-4 controls the selective endothelium driven transmigration of esoinophils from allergic individuals. J. Immunol. 149, 1432.

Mosmann, T.R. (1991): Cytokines: is there biological meaning? Curr. Opin. Immunol. 3, 511.

Mosmann, T.R. (1991): Cytokine secretion patterns and cross-regulation of T cell subsets. Immunol. Res. 10, 183.

Nakajima, H., A. Nakao, Y. Watanabe, S. Yoshida, I. Iwamoto (1994): IFNα inhibits antigen-induced eosinophil and CD4+ T cel recruitment into tissue. J. Immunol. *153*, 1264.

Nicholson, C.D. (1994): Inhbitors of cyclic nucleatide phosphodiesterase isoenzymes-thier potential utitlity in the therapy of asthma. Pulmonary Pharamcology *7*, 1–18.

Ohishi, T., K. Kita, D. Weiller, S. Sur, W.J. Calhoun, W.W. Busse, J.S. Anrams and G.J. Gleich (1993): IL-5 is the predominate eosinophil-active cytokine in the allergen-induced pulmonary late phase reaction. Am. Rev. Respir. Dis. *147*, 901.

Orange J.S., Wang B., Terhorst C. and Biron C.A. (1995): Requirement for natural killer cell-produced interferon gamma in defense against murine cytomegalovirus infection and enhancement of this defense pathway by interleukin 12 administration. J. Exp. Med. Oct. 1, *182*, 1045–56.

Oswald I.P., Wynn T.A., Sher A. and James S.L. (1992): Interleukin 10 inhibits macrophage microbicidal activity by blocking the endogenous production of tumor necrosis factor alpha required as a costimulatory factor for interferon gamma-induced activation. Proc. Natl. Acad. Sci. (USA) *89*, 8676–80.

Pene, J., F. Rousset, F. Briere, I. Chretien, J.Y. Bonnefoy, H. Spits, T. Yokota, N. Arai, K. Arai, J. Banchereau and J.E. De Vries (1988): IgE production by normal human lymphocytes is induced by interleukin 4 and suppressed by interferons gamma and alpha and by prostaglandin E2. Proc. Natl. Acad. Sci. (USA) *85*, 6880.

Pernis A., Gupta S., Gollob K.J., Garfein E., Coffman R.L., Schindler C. and Rothman P. (1995): Lack of interferon gamma receptor beta chain and the prevention of interferon gamma signaling in T_H1 cells. Science *269* (5221), 245–247.

Persson C.G.A. (1993): Airway mucosal exudation of plasma as a measure of subepithelial inflammation. In: K. Fan Chung and P.J. Barnes (eds.): Pharmacology of the respiratory tract. Marcel Dekker Inc. New York, Basel, Hong Kong 1993, 483–499.

Powrie, F., and R.S. Coffman (1993): Cytokine regulation of T-cell function: potential for therapeutic intervention. Immunol. Today 14, 270.

Reid L.M. (1987): The presence or absence of bronchial mucus in fatal asthma. J. Allergy Clin. Immunology. *80*, 415–416.

Resnick M.B., Weller P.F. (1993): Mechanims of eosinophil recruitment. Amer. J. Respir. Cell Molec. Biol. *8*, 349–355.

Robinson, D.S., W. Hamid, S. Ying, A. Tsicopoulos, J. Barkans, A.M. Bentley, C. Corrigan, S.R. Durham and A.B. Kay (1992): Predominant Th2-like broncho-alveolar T-lymphocyte population in atopic asthma. New Engl. J. Med. *326*, 298.

Rodger I.W. (1993): Airway smooth muscle: signal transduction and contractile mechanisms. In: Holgate S.T., Austen K.F., Lichtenstein L.M. and Kay A.B. (eds.): Asthma: physiology, immunopharmacology, and treatment. Academic Press, London 1993, 243–257.

Romagnani S. (1992): Induction of TH1 and TH2 responses: A key role for natural immune response? Immunol Today *13*, 529.

Sadick, M.D., F.P. Heinzel, B.J. Holaday, R.T. Pu, R.S. Dawkins and R.M. Locksley (1989): Cure of murine leishmaniasis with anti-IL-4 monoclonal antibody. J. Exp. Med. *169*, 115.

Saetta M., Fabbri L.M., Danieli D., Picotti G. and Allegra L. (1989): Pathology of bronchial asthma and animal models of asthma. Eur. Resp. J. *6*, 477s–482s.

Sanderson, C.J., O'Garra, A., Warren, D.J, Klaus and G.G.B. (1986): Eosinophil differentiation factor also has B cell growth factor activity. Proposed name interleukin-4. Proc. Nat. Acad. Sci. (USA) *83*, 437.

Schindler C., Kashleva H., Pernis A., Pine R. and Rothman P. (1994): STF-IL-4: a novel IL-4-induced signal transducing factor. EMBO J. *13*, 1350–6.

Schleimer R.P., Sterbinsky S.A., Kaiser J., Bickel C.A., Klunk D.A., Tomioka K., Newman W., Luscinskas F.W., Gimbrone M.A., McIntyre B.W. and Bochner B.S. (1992): IL-4 induces adherence of human eosinophils and basophils but not neutrophils to endothelium. J. Immunol. *148*, 1086–1092.

Seder, R.A., W.E. Paul, S.Z. Bensasson, G.S. LeGros, A. Kageyobotka, F.D. Finkelman, J.H. Pierce and M. Plaut. (1991). Production of interleukin-4 and other cytokines following stimulation of mast cell lines and in vivo mast cells/basophils. Int. Arch. Allergy Appl. Immunol. *94*, 137.

Seder R.A., Paul W.E. (1994): Acquisition of lymphokine-producing phenotype by CD4+ T cells. Annu. Rev. Immunol. *12*, 635–73.

Shimura, S., Sasaki, T., Sasaki, H., Takishima, T.and Umeya, K. (1988): Chemical properties of bronchorhea sputum in bronchial asthma. Chest *94*, 1211–1215.

Shirakawa, T., A. Li, M. Dubowitz, J.W. Dekker, A.E. Shaw, J.A.Faux, C. Ra, W.O.C.M. Cookson, and J.M. Hopkin (1994): Association between atopy and variants of the β subunit of the high-affinity immunoglobulin E receptor. Nature Genetics *7*, 125.

Shock A., Rabe K.F., Dent G., Chambers R.C., Gray A.J., Chung K.F., Barnes P.J. and Laurent G.J. (1991): Eosinophils adhere to and stimulate replication of lung fibroblasts *in vitro*. Clin. Exp. Immunol. *86*, 185–190.

Shu U., Demeure C.E., Byun D.G., Podlaski F., Stern A.S. and Delespesse G. (1994): Interleukin 12 exerts a differential effect on the maturation of neonatal and adult human CD45R0-CD4 T cells. J. Clin. Invest. *94*, 1352–1358.

Snapper, C.M. and W.E. Paul (1987): Interferon gamma and B cell stimulatory factor-1 reciprocally regulate Ig isotype production. Science *251*, 949.

Solari, R., N. Smithers, K. Page, E. Bolton and B.R. Champion (1990): Interleukin 1 responsiveness and receptor expression by murine Th1 and Th2 clones. Cytokines *2*, 129–141.

Street N.E., Schumacher J.H., Fong T.A.T., Bass H., Fiorentino D.F., Leverah J.A. and Mosmann T.R. (1990): Heterogeneity of mouse Helper T cells: evidence from Bulk cultures and limiting dilution cloning for precursors of TH1 and TH2 cells. J. Immunol. *144*, 1629–1639.

Szabo S.J., Jacobson N.G., Dighe A.S., Gubler U. and Murphy K,M. (1995): Developmental commitment to the Th2 lineage by extinction of IL-12 signaling. Immunity *2*, 665–75.

Thurlbeck W.M. and Miller R.R. Asthma. In: Rubin E. and Farber J.L. (eds.): Pathology. J.B. Lippincott Co., Philadelphia 1988, 587–590.

Van Oosterhout A.J., Ladenius A.R., Savelkoul H.F., Van Ark I., Delsman K.C. and Nijkamp F.P. (1993): Effect of anti-IL-5 and IL-5 on airway hyperreactivity and eosinophils in guinea pigs. Am. Rev. Respir. Dis. *147*, 548–52.

Walker, C., J.C. Virchow, P.L.B. Bruijnzeel and K. Blaser (1991): T cell subsets and their soluble products regulate eosinophilia in allergic and non allergic asthma. J. Immunol. *146*, 1829.

Watson, M.L., D. Smith, A.D. Bourne, R.C. Thompson and J. Westwick (1993): Cytokines contribute to airway dysfunction in antigen challenged guinea-pigs: inhibition of airway hyperreactivity, pulmonary eosinophil accumulation, and tumor necrosis factor generation by pretreatment with an interleukin-1 receptor antagonist. Am. J. Respir. Cell Mol. Biol. *8*, 365.

Weaver, C.T., C.M. Hawrylowicz and E.R. Unanue (1988): T helper cell subsets requires the expression of distinct costimulatory signals by antigen presenting cells. Proc. Natl. Acad. Sci. (USA) *85*, 8181–8185.

Wilson J.W., Li X. and Walters E.H. (1995): The increased submucosal vascular volume in asthmatic airways. Am. J. Respir. Critic Care Med. *151*, A 390.

Witthuhn B.A., Silvennoinen O., Miura O., Lai K.S., Cwik C., Liu E.T. and Ihle J.N. (1994): Involvement of the Jak-3 Janus kinase in signalling by interleukins 2 and 4 in lymphoid and myeloid cells. Nature *370*, 153–157.

Xu J., Levitt R.C., Panhuysen C.I., Postma D.S., Taylor E.W., Amelung P.J., Holroyd K.J., Bleecker E.R. and Meyers D.A. (1995): Evidence for two unlinked loci regulating total serum IgE levels. Am. J. Hum. Genet. *57*, 425–30.

Yamaguchi, Y., T. Suda, S. Ohta, K. Tominaga, Y. Miura and T. Kasahara (1991): Analysis of the survival of mature human eosinophils: interleukin 5 prevents apoptosis in mature eosinophils. Blood *78*, 2542.

Yamaguchi, Y., T. Suda, S. Ohta, K. Tominaga, Y.Miura and T. Kasahara (1991): Analysis of the survival of mature human eosinophils: interleukin 5 prevents apoptosis in mature eosinophils. Blood *78*, 2542.

Yssel, H., K.E. Johnson, P.V. Schneider, J. Wideman, A. Terr, R. Kastelein and J.E. De Vries (1992): T cell activation-inducing epitopes of the house dust mite allergen Der p I. Proliferation and lymphokine production patterns of Der p I-specific CD4+ T cell clones. J. Immunol. *148*, 738.

Yssel, H., K.E. Johnson, P.V. Schneider, J. Wideman, A. Terr, R. Kastelein and J.E. De Vries (1992): T cell activation-inducing epitopes of the house dust mite allergen Der p I. Proliferation and lymphokine production patterns of Der p I-specific CD4+ T cell clones. J. Immunol. *148*, 738.

Zingernagel, R.M. and P.C. Doherty (1977): Major transplantation antigens, viruses and specificity of surveillance T cells. Contemp. Top. Immunol. *7*, 179.

Zuany Amorim C., Haile S., Leduc D., Dumarey C., Huerre M., Vargaftig B.B. and Pretolani M. (1995): Interleukin-10 inhibits antigen-induced cellular recruitment into the airways of sensitized mice. J. Clin. Invest. *95*, 2644–2651.

Zubiaga, A.M., E. Munoz, B.T. Huber (1991): Production of IL-1α by activated Th type 2 cells. Its role as an autocrine growth factor. J. Immunol. *146*, 3849–3856.

Zurawski, S.M., F. Vega, B. Huyghe and G. Zurawski (1993): Receptors for interleukin 13 and interleukin 4 are complex and share a novel componenet that functions in signal transduction. EMBO J. *12*, 2663–2670.

Zurawski, G. and J.E. De Vries (1994): Interleukin 13, an interleukin 4-like cytokine that acts on monocytes and B cells, but not on T cells. Immunol. Today *15*, 19.

Progress in Drug Research, Vol. 47 (E. Jucker, Ed.)
© 1996 Birkhäuser Verlag, Basel (Switzerland)

Therapeutic applications of cytokines for immunostimulation and immunosuppression: An update

By Gaetano Cardi[1], Thomas L. Ciardelli[2] and Marc S. Ernstoff[3]

[1]Instituto Nationale per la Ricerca sul Cancro, Genova, Italy; [2]Dartmouth Medical School, Hanover, NH 03755, USA and Research Service, Veterans Administrations Hospital, White River Junction, VT 05009, USA; [3]Dartmouth Medical School and Norris Cotton Cancer Center, Hanover, NH 03755, USA

1   Introduction

As we indicated in an early review on this subject [1], the clinical use of proteins as drugs is not a new practice. What is new is the ability to produce almost limitless quantities of many clinically relevant proteins, and our depth of understanding of the mechanisms underlying their physiologic function. Unfortunately, neither of these aspects guarantees a successful transition from the laboratory to a meaningful clinical application. Despite being endogenous mediators of cell function, systemic administration of cytokines resulting in supraphysiologic levels often leads to toxicity [2]. Nevertheless, as predicted in our previous discussion, activity over the past four years in the field of clinical applications of cytokines and interleukins has been of sufficient volume to preclude a comprehensive overview in a single chapter. For some cytokines, such as the interferons and IL-2, a clinical role has been established and much of the recent work has focused on refining dosages, routes of administration, and schedules as well as investigations of combining these agents together or with other drugs with the goal of improving efficacy. In other cases, for example TNF and IL-1, despite being among the first cytokines to be characterized, clearly defined successful therapeutic applications remain elusive. For more recently identified cytokines such as IL-12 and IL-15, clinical trials remain in the earliest stages.

The range of therapeutic applications of cytokines has also expanded during the past four years. Trials in the area of infectious diseases and septic shock have been carried out but the major emphasis remains in the field of cancer and related therapies. This review will serve as an update to our previous discussion [1] and will focus on the specific use of cytokines for direct immunomodulatory therapy in humans during the past four years. These cytokines are listed along with their important characteristicis in Table 1. We will include the use of cytokines in combination with cancer vaccines and gene therapy but not for hematopoietic reconstruction. The latter field, although highly successful, contributes indirectly to immunostimulation and has been extensively reviewed [3–7]. We will present an overview of each clinically relevant cytokine, primarily, in terms of recent findings regarding both mechanistic and therapeutic data and provide more detailed background where appropriate.

Table 1.
Immunostimulatory cytokines

Cytokine	Function	Receptor	Source	Application
Interleukins				
IL-1(α and β) MW 17.5 kDa	Stimulates inflammation by inducing TNF, IL-6 and IL-8. Possesses hematopoietic and induces the CSFs. Stimulates hepatic acute phase proteins and can initiate shock syndrome.	Two receptors have been identified (I & II) with only I being functional. A third accessory protein may be required. Receptors present on a variety of cell types and tissues.	Produced by monocytes macrophages, fibroblasts and endothelial cells.	Cancer therapy, hematological reconstitution.
IL-1 receptor antagonist (IL-1Ra)	Unknown, may limit severity of mild inflammation.	IL-1Ra binds to both classes of IL-1R but with greater affinity to class I.	Similar to IL-1.	Sepsis, graft vs. host disease, possible reduction of IL-2 toxicity.
IL-2[a] (TCGF) MW 15.5 kDa	T-cell, B-cell and NK cell proliferation, lymphocyte differentiation, NK cell activation. IL-2 induces secondary release of cytokines such as TNF, GM-CSF and INFγ.	Receptors[b] are present on activated T-cells, B-cells, NK cells and at low levels on several other tissues. Three cell surface proteins (IL-2Rα,β & γ) combine to form sites of varying affinities.	Produced primarily by activated T$_H$1 CD4+ helper T-cells (some CD8+ cells may produce IL-2).	Cancer therapy, HIV and vaccine adjuvant.

Table 1. (continued)
Immunostimulatory cytokines

Cytokine	Function	Receptor	Source	Application
IL-4[a] (BSF-1) (BCGF-1) MW 25 kDa	Stimulates the growth of activated B cells. Some T-cell growth activity, promotes antibody isotype switching, induces MHC class II expression.	Receptors[b] present on a variety of lymphoid cell types. Shares IL-2Rγ.	Produced primarily by activated CD4+ T-cells.	Potential use in cancer therapy.
IL-6[a] (BSF-2, INF-ß2) MW 26 kDa	Co-factor for the growth and maturation of early progenitor cells, induces B-cell differentiation, induces acute phase proteins in the liver, some stimulation of activated T-cells.	Receptors[b] present on a variety of cell types. Two subunits cooperate to form the high affinity binding site, one subunit may be shared with other cytokine receptors.	Produced by a variety of cell types including T-cells, monocytes, fibroblasts and endothelial cells.	Potential use in cancer therapy.
IL-10 (CSIF) MW 18 kDa (functional form is a homodimer, structurally similar to INFγ)	Inhibits the production of IL-1, IL-2, IL-3, IL-6, IL-8, GM-CSF, TNF and INFγ. Stimulates production of IL-1Ra and down-regulates class II MHC. Suppresses T-cell proliferation.	Receptor is structurally related to the INFγ R (may share subunits) and is expressed primarily on hematopoietic cells.	Produced by activated T-cells, B-cells, monocytes and keratinocytes.	Sepsis (immunosuppression)

Cytokine	Function	Receptor	Source	Application
IL-12[a,b] (CLMF, NKSF) MW 75 kDa (Disulfide linked heterodimer having 40 and 35 kDa subunits. One subunit shares homology with the hematopoietic receptor family.)	Stimulates proliferation of T_H1 subpopulations. Increased cellular response.	Low affinity receptor[b] is found on activated T-cells and NK cells and has homology to gp130 of the IL-6 receptor.	Macrophages Monocytes Dendritic cells	Cancer therapy, HIV and vaccine adjuvant
IL-15[a] MW 15 kDa	Stimulates lymphocyte proliferation and NK cell activation with a profile similar to IL-2. Anabolic effects on skeletal muscle.	Shares the IL-2Rβ&γ subunits but has a unique α-subunit. IL-15Rα receptors are expressed on most tissues (highly expressed in the liver, heart and skeletal muscle).	IL-15 is produced by most tissues including skeletal muscle but not by activated lymphocytes.	Potential use in cancer therapy.
Interferons				
Interferon-α (leukocyte interferon) MW 17-23 kDa	Anti-viral and anti-proliferative activity due, in part, to inhibition of RNA synthesis and induction of RNA degradation, stimulates NK-cells	Receptors on a variety of cells and tissues. Interferons α and β share the same receptors.	More than 20 subtypes, produced by leukocytes.	Viral diseases, cancer therapy.
Interferon-β (fibroblast interferon) MW 20 kDa	Similar to interferon-α	Similar to interferon-α	Single protein product produced by fibroblasts and endothelial cells.	Cancer therapy, multiple sclerosis.

Table 1. (continued)
Immunostimulatory cytokines

Cytokine	Function	Receptor	Source	Application
Interferon-γ (immune interferon) MW 20 kDa	Similar to interferon-α, induces cytokine production, enhances expression of a variety of receptors including Fc receptors, induces MHC class II expression.	Receptors on a variety of cells, single protein distinct from the α and β receptor.	Single protein product produced primarily by activated CD4+ T-cells and NK cells.	Inherited and acquired granulocytic diseases (chronic granulomatous disease), cancer therapy.
Tumor Necrosis Factors				
TNFs α and β (Cachectin, α, Lymphotoxin, β) MW 50–75 kDa (as trimer)	Pleotropic activities toward a variety of tissues, including cytotoxicity toward tumor cells, induction of secretion of cytokines and other factors, induction of acute phase proteins.	Two structurally related receptors (55 kDa and 75kDa) have been identified on a variety of tissues	Produced primarily by monocytes, macrophages and T-cells.	Potential use in cancer therapy.

a Share similar core α-helical molecular tertiary structure.
b Belong to the hematopoietic receptor family based on structural homology.

Alternative nomenclature: BCGFs, B-cell growth factors; BSFs, B-cell stimulatory factors; CLMF, cytotoxic lymphocyte inhibitory factor; CSIF, cytokine synthesis inhibitory factor; INF-β2, interferon β2; NKSF, NK cell stimulatory factor;TCGFs, T-cell growth factors.

2   Interleukin-1 related proteins

Interleukin-1 possesses a number of characteristics that remain unique among proteins classified as interleukins or cytokines. Its three dimensional structure is unlike any of the other cytokines [8]. IL-1 is mostly produced by activated macrophages and has no secretory signal peptide and thus often remains largely cell associated. The class of IL-1 receptors identified thus far exhibit wide tissue distribution and seem to be triggered at exceptionally low receptor occupancy [9]. A structurally similar endogenous inhibitor of IL-1 has been identified (IL-1Ra). *In vivo*, IL-1 has a short half-life yet it induces a wide spectrum of biological effects and it is critically involved in inflammation. These characteristics describe a molecule whose activities are tailored to a very localized response. It is not surprising then that systemic administration of IL-1 is associated with profound toxicity resembling septic shock, even at very low doses [10].

The therapeutic potential as well as the biological properties of IL-1 have been extensively discussed [1, 11–14]. The systemic administration of IL-1 results in multiple toxicities that include fever, headache, anorexia, somnolescence, gastrointestinal disturbances and most notably hypotension that limits the acceptable dose to 300 ng/kg [14]. Clinical trials of IL-1 and related cytokines have continued, however, and recent clinical experiences are worth noting.

Although IL-1 can induce a great variety of biological responses, it has little direct immunostimulatory activity. Combined with the observation that IL-1 may induce growth, either directly or indirectly, of some malignant cell types [11], it would seem an unlikely candidate for the treatment of cancer. In one trial of the treatment renal cell carcinoma, albeit at low dose levels, no evidence of favorable responses were noted [15]. In contrast, in a recent trial for the treatment of a variety of solid tumors, where escalating doses of IL-1β were administered by brief IV infusion in combination with a fixed dose of IL-2 (given by continuous infusion over 4 days), beneficial results were reported [16]. At the lower IL-1 doses (5–50 ng/kg/d), CD4/CD8 cell ratios were significantly greater than for patients receiving IL-2 alone, while at higher doses (100–200 ng/kg/d), white blood cell counts were higher in the IL-1 treated group. Notably, toxicity was less than expected at the higher IL-1 doses and may reflect a protective effect of the combined therapy. Although a 27% response rate was reported, it was not possible to assess the influence of any additional immunostimulatory activity due to IL-1. It is likely, however, that the hematopoietic effects observed at the higher doses were beneficial. Similar hematopoietic activity has been reported in trials supplementing IL-1 therapy to the treatment of advanced malignancies [17, 18] and after autologous transplantation [19]. Significant toxicities were encountered in these trials as well, and it remains to be demonstrated that IL-1 is superior to other hematopoietic cytokines for the acceleration of hematological reconstitution.

Since IL-1 is intimately involved in the inflammatory response, due in part to its ability to induce other cytokines such as Tumor Necrosis Factor (TNF), IL-6, IL-8 and the colony stimulating factors (CSFs), some attention has been given to blocking IL-1 activity by therapeutic intervention (see [13, 14, 20, 21]). The inhibition of IL-1 activity could prove useful in immunosuppressive therapies as well as in the treatment of septic shock. Agents that have been considered for IL-1 receptor blockade include anti-receptor antibodies [22] and soluble IL-1 receptors [23]. Although these proteins are beyond the scope of this discussion, one agent that has been investigated as an IL-1 inhibitor is worthy of mention. The discovery of a naturally occurring, structurally related IL-1 receptor antagonist was a unique finding in cytokine biology [24, 25] and provided an opportunity to block IL-1 activity with an endogenous molecule. This molecule apparently has a greater affinity for IL-1R type I than for type II. Since it is only the IL-1RI that signals, the rationale for the use IL-1Ra as a therapeutic IL-1 inhibitor was clear. Initial studies of the pharmacokinetics and toxicity of IL-1Ra indicated rapid elimination (terminal half-life = 108 min after IV infusion) and few side effects [26]. There is one report, however, of possible IL-1 like agonist activity on human decidual cells [27]. Clinical experience with IL-1Ra has been limited and the results have been mixed. In a phase I/II trial for the treatment of steroid resistant graft-versus-host disease, doses up to 3,200 mg/d were administered by continuous IV infusion over seven days without complications and improvement was noted in 63% of the patients [28]. In contrast, in a much larger phase III for the treatment of sepsis syndrome, IL-1Ra provided no increase in survival time [29, 30].

Perhaps it is not surprising that initial clinical results employing IL-1Ra should be less than encouraging. To effectively block IL-1 receptor activation, virtually all of the receptors must be occupied throughout the inflammatory response. If the data concerning IL-1 dose-response relationships and receptor affinities are to be believed, triggering of only a few receptors per cell is sufficient to elicit a response; hence, the requirement for full blockade requiring large and prolonged dosages of any IL-1 antagonist (the recent report of the existence of an IL-1R accessory protein that boosts affinity about five-fold [31] does not greatly alter this requirement).

In conclusion, clinical experience with the use of IL-1 and IL-IRa for immunomodulation has been limited and the results have not been overly encouraging. This is due, in part to the extreme toxicity of IL-1 and its unique receptor-signaling properties. If IL-1 is to play an important clinical role, it will likely be due to its hematopoietic activity in hematological reconstitution.

3   Interleukin-2

Interleukin-2, one of the first cytokines to be characterized [32], continues to be the focus of both vigorous scientific study and greatly expanded clinical investigation. Over the past four years, significant progress has been achieved in understanding the nature of the heterotrimeric IL-2 receptor [33, 34] and the signal transduction mechanisms employed by this and related cytokine receptor complexes [35–38]. Although these pathways are very complex and much remains to be learned, the mechanisms underlying the pleiotropic and sometimes overlapping biologic activities of cytokines can now be understood in the context of receptor subunit sharing and convergent signaling pathways [39].

Progress on the clinical front, however, has been much slower. A large number of trials of the use of IL-2 in cancer therapy have now been carried out. These include a variety of dosing strategies, alone, in combination with cellular therapies and with other cytokines. Although most trials have focused on improving the early results obtained for the treatment of renal cell carcinoma and melanoma, IL-2 therapy has now been attempted for a number of other malignancies. The results of these expanded clinical trials have been summarized in several recent reviews [40–48]. Previously, we have presented the background and rationale for the early clinical trials of IL-2 [1]. In this discussion, we will attempt to update and highlight the pharmacological aspects of the most recent studies.

The first clinical use of IL-2 for cancer therapy was in conjunction with adoptive cellular therapy in which IL-2 mediated *ex vivo* expansion of the patient's own lymphocytes resulted in the generation of a subset of lymphokine-activated killer (LAK) cells. These cells, when re-infused with IL-2 into the patient, displayed potentiated antitumor activity [49]. Ten years of clinical investigation have failed to improve upon these initial findings and, in fact, have demonstrated that the initial interpretations may have been overly optimistic. It is now clear that LAK cells are a subset of natural killer (NK) cells activated by IL-2 to express increased non-

specific cytotoxicity [50]. The majority of these cells express the intermediate affinity ($\beta\gamma$) receptors [51, 52] and thus require a 100-fold greater
cytokine concentration for activation than is required for initiating proliferative responses on antigen-activated T-lymphocytes bearing high affinity receptors.

This "high-dose" regimen employed in these early studies was associated
with severe toxicity (see below). Although it has now been convincingly
demonstrated that *ex vivo* adoptive cellular therapy is no more effective
than high-dose IL-2 alone [53–56], the elimination of the difficult and
expensive *ex vivo* cell culture and re-infusion has had only a minor impact
on toxicity. The results of a recent phase III trial comparing IL-2 alone or
with LAK cells at lower doses for the treatment of advanced renal cell
carcinoma confirmed the lack of improvement in response rate for the
LAK cell treated group [57]. This study concluded that the weighted
response rate for IL-2 treatment (over a wide dose range) of over 1200
renal cell carcinoma patients was 16% and was independent of LAK cell
administration.

A second approach employing re-infusion of host immune cells activated
ex vivo by IL-2 uses lymphocytes isolated directly from the tumor itself.
Termed tumor infiltrating lymphocytes (TILs), it was assumed that these
cells, once expanded and activated, would home-in to tumor sites upon
re-infusion [58]. Unlike LAK cells, TILs seem to be heterogeneous in cell
type with greater proportions of non-cytolytic CD4+ cells [59]. Initial trials
of adoptive cellular therapy with TILs, either with or without IL-2 administration, have generated mixed results with low response rates and significant toxicity. One recent study employing both IL-2 and interferon-α
for TIL priming in patients with renal cell carcinoma, however, achieved
responses of greater than 30% without an apparent advantage to *ex vivo*
CD8+ cell enrichment prior to re-infusion [60]. This suggests that TIL therapy holds promise and is, therefore, currently the focus of several studies
employing combinations of cytokines as well as genetic manipulation. At
present, this approach remains costly and unpredictable and it is still difficult to predict what future role combined cytokine and adoptive cellular therapy will have in cancer treatment.

Considerable effort has been invested in studying the dose and route of
IL-2 administration with the goal of reduction in toxicity without loss of
efficacy. The initial studies employing IL-2 therapy, either with or without cellular re-infusion, encountered a range of significant and often life-
threatening toxicities [49]. The most serious manifestation of IL-2 toxicity has been vascular leak syndrome or increased vascular permeability.
This phenomena leads to a variety of problems including pulmonary ede-

ma, peripheral edema, hypotension and renal toxicity. Other toxicities observed in patients receiving high-dose IL-2 include flu-like symptoms (nausea, vomiting, chills, diarrhea), neural dysfunction, hepatic toxicity and sepsis. Although most of the toxicities are controllable and reversible upon cessation of treatment, they have precluded the continuation of high-dose IL-2 therapy in a significant number of patients. Consequently, the addition of drugs such as pentoxifylline and ciprofloxacin [61], methyl-l-arginine or aminoguanidine [42] to IL-2 protocols targeted specifically at reducing some of the toxicities is under evaluation. For pentoxifylline, a preliminary report suggests that it is of no benefit in alleviating IL-2 toxicity and may even exacerbate side effects [62].

Since most NK cells and activated T-cells have IL-2 receptors with greatly different affinities [52] and studies suggest that the majority of toxicities result from IL-2 initiated release of secondary mediators from NK cells [63], several trials have attempted to reduce the dose below that required to activate NK cells. The results of many of these trails are difficult to interpret since the definition of "low-dose" varies considerably and several routes of administration have been employed. A direct comparison of high- versus low-dose therapy suggests similar response rates [64] and in several trials using continuous infusion protocols of doses ranging from 3–18 $\times 10^6$ IU/m^2, response rates for renal cell carcinoma of $\approx 20\%$ were noted [41, 65]. Although milder, toxicities remained significant in these studies. In trials in which the doses were lowered even further, toxicity was less severe but efficacy was also reduced [66]. Subcutaneous administration of low-dose IL-2 has also lead to response rates comparable to continuous infusion with fewer side effects and may be the route of choice for many patients [67, 68].

In addition to systemic routes, local administration of IL-2 has also been attempted in an effort to confine the location close to the tumor site and reduce toxicity [69]. The pharmacokinetics of intraventricular, intralymphatic, intravesicular, intraperitoneal, intrapleural and inhalational administration of IL-2 have been reviewed [70]. In most instances, although doses were in the low range, these routes resulted in longer local half-lives and lower toxicity. In some instances, sufficient responses were noted to encourage continued investigation.

Other approaches to potentiating IL-2 therapy are being considered and include administration via liposomes [71], polyethylene glycol conjugated (PEG) IL-2 [72] and co-administration with anti-IL-2 antibodies [73]. It is possible that one or more of these methods will result in a marginal improvement of IL-2 efficacy or reduction in toxicity. It is unlikely, however, that the general issues of low and unpredictable response rates associated with IL-2 cancer therapy will be addressed by modifying routes of administration or formulations by themselves.

One potential avenue to improved clinical responses that has also been extensively investigated is the combination of IL-2 with other therapies. The combination of either low-dose or high-dose IL-2 with other cytokines has been attempted in several trials (see [40–42]). Although most of these trials have focused on the interferons (α, β and γ), combinations of IL-2 with IL-4 [74], IL-1 [16] and TNF [75] have also been attempted. Many of these trials have resulted in significant response rates in the treatment of melanoma and renal cell carcinoma, however, none of the combined protocols have demonstrated a clear advantage over single agent therapy. Combination therapy requires choice of dose and route of administration for each agent as well as timing. Since, for IL-2 and other cytokines, these variables have not been optimized in single agent therapy, effective combination protocols are difficult to define. It is possible that improved response rates will be achieved once these factors have been optimized and other cytokines have been investigated.

Approaches that combine IL-2 with chemotherapeutic agents have also been attempted. Many chemotherapeutic agents including cisplatin, carmustine, tamoxifen, doxorubicin, dacarbazine, vinblastine, 5-fluorouracil and cyclophosphamide have been used in combination with IL-2 or with IL-2 and other cytokines [41, 42, 45, 76]. One feature complicating this approach is the potential damage to the immune system by the chemotherapeutic agent employed [77]. Perhaps this is a factor contributing to the observation that in the majority of these trials, favorable responses do not appear to exceed those of single agent treatment. In the case of advanced melanoma, however, a combination of IL-2 and interferon-α with chemotherapy may prove to be synergistic [78].

One criticism of systemic cytokine therapy is that although physiologic levels at the local sites of an immune response may reach or exceed therapeutic levels, the systemic level of cytokines remain far below those attained during therapy and are often undetectable [79]. Hence, systemic toxicity is encountered during therapy. Genetic approaches have now opened the possibility of achieving high local concentrations of cytokines in the context of tumor antigen. By transducing tumor cells with vectors designed to allow the expression of cytokines, the old concepts of active immunotherapy and cancer vaccines have been revitalized [40, 79]. The introduction of the IL-2 gene into tumor cells was one of the first successful attempts in this direction [80] and clinical trials employing IL-2 transduced tumor cells are in progress [81-83]. It is not certain, however, whether IL-2 will prove to be the best choice for tumor vaccine-gene therapy since there is some indication in animal models that the degree of immunization achieved using IL-2 secreting tumor cells is very dose dependent. Too high a level of IL-2 secretion may impair cytotoxic T-cell production [84].

Finally, as mentioned in our previous review [1], the treatment of infectious disease might be the application in which IL-2 makes the greatest impact. Although several infectious diseases continue to pose significant health problems, worldwide, due to the emergence of new resistant strains, HIV infection remains at center stage. From the beginning, the use of IL-2 for the treatment of HIV has presented a dilemma. The potential of this drug to inhibit or reverse the inexorable decline in CD4+ cells in HIV patients has always been weighed against the danger of activating new viral replication as a result of increased proliferation. Limited trials of low-dose IL-2 therapy in conjunction with antiviral drugs have attempted to shed some light on this problem. In a recent study employing IL-2 plus at least one approved antiviral agent, the cytokine was administered by continuous infusion [6–18×10^6 IU/d) for 5 days every 8 weeks during 7 to 25 months [85]. In more than half of the 10 patients that began the trial with CD4+ cell counts greater than 200/ml, increases in CD4+ cells exceeding 50% were achieved. In those patients with less than 200/ml CD4+ cell counts, little improvement was noted. Typical IL-2 related toxicities were encountered in the majority of patients as well as an increase in viral activation, particularly in the population with less that 200 CD4 cells/ml. The conclusion from this study was that IL-2 therapy could improve the immune status of HIV patients whose CD4+ cell counts were greater than 200/ml, where increased viral activation was, at worst, transient. In another trial employing daily subcutaneous low-dose IL-2 combined with antiviral therapy in patients suffering from HIV-associated malignancies, improved immunologic parameters were observed even in some patients with CD4+ cell counts < 200/ml without a significant increase in viral burden [86]. The consensus from most of the other preliminary trials support these studies [87,88]. In general, IL-2 can improve the immune status of patients suffering from HIV infection, particularly in patients whose CD4+ counts remain relatively high, since the danger of increased viral activation appears less likely in this group. It should be noted, however, that there is no evidence that IL-2 helps to reduce or inhibit the progression of the disease as measured by viral burden. The major benefit to improved immune status is likely to be greater resistance to opportunistic infections and improved quality of life. Thus, for HIV infection, IL-2 may yet play an important role in combination therapy with antiviral drugs or in vaccine protocols as they develop.

In conclusion, IL-2 continues to be an important drug in an expanded spectrum of clinical applications. Despite considerable effort, progress over the past 5 years in IL-2 tumor therapy has remained disappointing. Approaches such as gene therapy combined with tumor vaccines are now being examined and may prove to be the most efficacious. The use of IL-2 for the treatment of infectious disease remains a promising area of investigation.

4   Interleukin-4

IL-4 was originally called BSF1 or BCGF1 on the basis of its ability to induce B cell proliferation in culture when co-stimulated with antibodies to IgM [89]. Human IL-4 cDNA was isolated from a T cell library by cross-hybridization with murine cDNA in 1986 [90]. Human IL-4 is a glycoprotein of 129 amino acids which is derived from a 153 amino acid precursor. IL-4 is a member of the helical cytokine family and its receptors have an extracellular, transmembrane, and intracellular domain structure common to other cytokine receptors [91].

IL-4 has a variety of activities and one review refers to it as a "problematic lymphokine" [92]. IL-4 has differential effects on T cells, B cells, macrophages and mast cells, and is dependent on a complex state of activation and the maturity of the target cell. In the early maturation of B-cells, IL-4 induces surface IgM expression and inhibits expression of CD5, a primitive B cell marker [93]. IL-4 stimulates B cell proliferation *in vitro* with upregulation of CD23, the low affinity IgE receptor, which, when secreted, acts as a mitogen for B cells [94]. Studies indicate that IL-4 upregulates MHC class II antigens on resting B cells which may be related to B cell antigen presentation pathways [95]. IL-4 may also stimulate or inhibit immunoglobulin production and isotype switching to favor IgE production [96]. IL-4 has a wide range of activities on other hematopoietic cells as well as endothelial cells, fibroblasts, myeloid, and epithelial cells. It may be stimulatory or inhibitory for myeloid progenitor cells when used with G-CSF, GM-CSF, or IL3.

IL-4 may stimulate or inhibit IL-2 induced LAK activity. Inhibition of LAK activity by IL-4 can be overcome by interferon-γ [97, 98]. IL-4 has important effects upon T-cells as well. It is expressed in thymocytes early in the development of the thymus [99] and can stimulate or inhibit expansion of T cells in the thymus [100, 101]. It acts as a proliferative stimulus on preactivated mature T cells [102]. IL-4 has direct effects against malignant cells as well. IL-4 can inhibit spontaneous proliferation of chronic lymphocytic leukemia cells [103].

Immunomodulatory anti-tumor effects of IL-4 have been demonstrated in animal models. When injected into the region of draining lymph node sites of transplanted murine fibrosarcoma or spontaneous mammary adenocarcinoma, IL-4 resulted in tumor regression and subsequent tumor immunity [104]. Inoculation of mice with tumors (B cell lymphoma, mammary adenocarcinoma and mastocytosis), transfection of tumor cells expressing of the IL-4 gene [105] or IL-4 and IL-2 genes (Pardoll, unpublished, cited by Spits [98]) all have resulted in tumor regression. These results coupled with similar findings following inoculation of tumor cells transfected and expressing IL-2 [106] or interferon-γ genes [107] suggest that peripheral tolerance of tumors may be overcome by elaboration of cytokines at tumor sites.

Human trials of IL-4 have been conducted. With the demonstration that IL-4 promoted the growth of tumor-infiltrating lymphocytes cytotoxic for human autologous melanoma cells [108], investigators at the NCI initiated a phase I trial of IL-4 in 48 patients with cancer. Mild toxicity was encountered for the most part and was most prominent at the higher doses (10–30 μg/kg administered 3 times a day). Significant toxicity included a vascular leak syndrome similar to that encountered with IL-2, nasal congestion, and gastritis with gastric ulceration, perhaps due to the indomethacin that these patients received. Rarely, liver toxicity characterized by transaminase elevations was observed.

Pharmacokinetic analysis suggested a distribution phase of about 8 minutes, and a clearance phase of about 48 minutes. No evidence of responses to IL-4 alone was seen in this trial. When combined with IL-2, severe renal dysfunction was dose limiting with serum creatinine levels reaching 8 mg/dl in some patients. At lower doses of the IL-4, IL-2 combination, some patients with renal cell carcinoma and melanoma achieved impressive tumor responses without major toxicity. The patient with a B cell lymphoma treated in this study did not have a response.

Gilleece et al. [109] reported on 9 patients receiving various doses of subcutaneous IL-4 up to 5 μg/kg/day. Flu-like symptoms and hepatic enzyme elevations were noted as well as confusion and other neurological symptoms in two patients. No evidence of an antitumor effect was seen. The one patient in this series with multiple myeloma had a fall in M-protein from 8.0 g/dl to 5.8 g/dl by day 15 following initiation of treatment. Treatment was discontinued because of toxicity and the patient's M-protein returned to pretreatment levels by day 30.

Interest in the possible effect of IL-4 in B cell derived malignancies such as multiple myeloma is from the observation that IL-4 suppresses the *in vitro* production of IL-6 which appears to be an important proliferative signal to B lymphocytes. Taylor, Grogan and Salmon [110] studied the effect of IL-4 on the growth of 35 fresh human lymphoid and plasma cell cultures. Growth inhibition occurred in 52% of myeloma and 60% of lymphoma cell suspensions. Importantly, growth was stimulated in 8.6% of the cultures. Herrmann et al. [111] studied IL-6 production in short-term cultures of bone marrow from patients with multiple myeloma. IL-4 inhibited the production of IL-6 in these cultures in a dose-dependent fashion. This was associated with a significant reduction in the plasma cell growth, and this growth reduction could be reversed by addition of exogenous IL-6. Plasma cells displayed negligible levels of IL-6 message. This study also presents evidence that the IL-6 produced in the cultures was derived from adherent bone marrow cells rather than plasma cells.

An effect of IL-4 on proliferation of cells derived from other B cell malignancies appears somewhat less clear than for myeloma cells. In a study of freshly isolated B cell lymphoma cells by Defrance et al. [112], IL-4 strongly suppressed anti-immunoglobulin and IL-2 induced proliferation. In addition, IL-5, IL-6 and TNF were not found to be proliferative signals in IL-2 responsive samples. In 1 of 10 specimens, proliferation occurred following culture with IL-4 and anti-Ig reagents, but not after IL-2. Other studies evaluating IL-6 as a growth factor have used Epstein-Barr virus (EBV) infected B cells. These cells show consistent proliferation to IL-6 stimulation [113]. The inconsistency of these findings may relate to the presence of the EBV.

The laboratory models suggest that IL-4 acts most commonly as an anti-proliferative signal but on occasion can act as a stimulatory signal for B-lymphocytic derived malignancies. Knowledge of the *in vitro* effect of IL-4 on short-term cultures will prove essential to the interpretation of the clinical results, and will provide insight into the mechanism of anti-tumor action of IL-4 if clinical responses occur.

5   Interleukin-6

Interleukin-6 (IL-6) was first recognized as a cytokine involved with B-lymphocyte differentiation and is now known to be involved with multiple immunologic pathways. The glycolylated molecule of 212 amino acids with a molecular weight of 21–30 kd may be produced by a variety of cells including T-lymphocytes, NK cells, monocytes/macrophages, neutrophils and epithelial cells [114, 115]. IL-6 binds to an 80 kDa transmembrane receptor which requires association with a second membrane glycoprotein (gp130) for signal transduction. Its activity can be divided into effects on: (1) growth regulation of hematopoietic progenitor cells; (2) immune regulation; (3) cellular proliferation; and (4) acute phase reactant [116, 117].

IL-6 alone or in conjunction with other cytokines will stimulate proliferation of early hematopoietic progenitor cells. The most pronounced effect has been observed on megakaryocytes and production of platelets [118, 119]. In addition, IL-6 will enhance the growth regulator aspects of granulocyte-monocyte colony stimulating factor (GM-CSF) demonstrated by an increase in the size of granulocyte-monocyte colonies [120]. Early phase I studies of IL-6 alone in humans have demonstrated a 2–8 fold increase in circulating $CD34^+$ cells, an early hematopoietic progenitor phenotype ($CD34^+$) [121].

IL-6 is involved with multiple immunologic pathways. IL-6 stimulates immunoglobulin secretion by B-cells and functions as a cofactor in T-lymphocyte proliferation and differentiation. Murine studies have demonstrated that IL-6 can induce tumor immunity and the development of tumor specific cytolytic T-cell capable of mediating regression of tumor metastases [122–124]. 3LL tumor cells transfected with IL-6 gene are capable of inducing protective immunity in mice demonstrated by rejection of subsequent challenges with the parent tumor. Although IL-6 can be shown to augment NK and LAK activity through IL-2 production, observation in human clinical trials suggests a suppressive role on NK and LAK activity [125, 126].

IL-6 has been implemented as an autocrine/paracrine growth regulatory molecule in a number of different malignancies. Human myeloma cell lines have been developed that require IL-6 as a proliferative signal, supporting a role for IL-6 as a stimulatory growth factor [127]. On the other hand, spontaneous high IL-6 production found in enriched bone marrow preparations from multiple myeloma patients is associated with low tumor burden, suggesting an inhibitory growth regulation in myeloma cells [128]. Renal cell carcinoma cell lines can be stimulated to grow using IL-6 and growth can be inhibited by IL-6 neutralizing antibodies or interferon gamma [129]. Other murine adenocarcinoma models have demonstrated tumor growth inhibition by IL-6 [130]. Thus, direct effects of IL-6 on tumor may be disease and model specific.

IL-6 has been employed in clinical trials as both an immunomodulator as well as a hematopoietic growth factor. The toxicity profile included fever, chills, fatigue, headache, thrombocytosis, proteinuria, decrease in renal function, elevation in liver function tests, cardiac arrhythmias and hyperglycemia. Dose-limiting toxicity occurs at dosage ranges from 1–30 mg/kg

and includes atrial fibrillation, centrolobular hepatic necrosis and elevation in acute phase reactants. Acute phase reactants such as CRP, fibrino-
gen and haptoglobin all increase in a dose-dependent manner. Antitumor
benefit has not yet been determined.

6   Interleukin-10

Interleukin-10 is a 35 kDa noncovalent homodimeric cytokine expressed
by a variety of cell types including T_H2 T-cells, B-cells, monocytes, macrophages and keratinocytes [131]. The 3-dimensional structure of IL-10
has been determined and is similar to INFγ [132, 133]. The IL-10 receptor has been characterized and it also shares structural similarity with the
interferon receptor [134]. IL-10 was originally described as "cytokine
synthesis inhibitory factor" for its apparent ability to inhibit the production of IL-1, IL-2, IL-3, IL-6, IL-8, TNF, INFγ and Granulocyte-Macro-
phage Stimulating Factor (GM-CSF) in a variety of cell types [135]. As a
result of the ability of IL-10 to inhibit the production of INFγ and IL-2
by activated T-cells, to suppress T-cell proliferation [136] and expression
of IL-1, IL-6, IL-8 and TNF by monocytes [137], IL-10 became the first
cytokine with true immunosuppressive activity *in vitro*. The biological
activities of IL-10 are complex, however, and some may actually be immunostimulatory [138]. Therefore, the potential value of IL-10 for immunosuppressive therapy in the treatment of inflammatory diseases such as
arthritis or for sepsis syndrome is difficult to predict. Trials of IL-10 have
begun and in healthy volunteers at least, single IV bolus doses of up to
25 µg/kg were well tolerated [139]. Evidence of immunosuppression was
detected, particularly in volunteers receiving the highest doses. T-cell
counts fell by 25% and mitogen-induced T-cell proliferation was suppressed along with *in vitro* production of TNF and IL-1 by endotoxin stimulated whole blood cells. Thus, the rationale for further clinical trials of
IL-10 has been established.

7   Interleukin-12

Interleukin-12 (IL-12) is a pleiotropic cytokine that consists of a disul-
fide-linked heterodimeric structure. It is composed of a 35 kDa light
chain (p35) that is homologous to other cytokines and a 40 kDa heavy
chain (p40) that is homologous to the extracellular portion of several
cytokine receptors [140]. IL-12 is produced primarily by stimulated mac-

rophages and dendritic cells [141] and seems to correlate with their function as antigen presenting cells (APC) [142]. IL-12 production is so variable that the same population of macrophages will produce high levels of IL-12 when stimulated with live Listeria or low levels when activated by avirulent or heat-killed pathogens. Macrophages produce high levels of endogenous IL-12 following exposure to non-virulent Listeria and small doses of IL-12 demonstrating an autostimulatory or self-priming effect [143].

IL-12 exerts a variety of biological effects on human T-cells and NK cells [144]. These include promoting cytolytic activity of NK cells toward cancer cells and pathogen-infected cells (Mycobacterium tuberculosis or HIV) [145], and priming γ-δ T-cell populations to produce IFN-γ which will induce tumor regression [146]. IL-12 appears to play a major role in regulating the immune response, by signaling naive T helper cells to differentiate toward the specific subset of Th1 lymphocytes. Thus, in the presence of tumor growth or in the early phase of infection, IL-12 appears to direct uncommitted T helper cells toward a Th1 response or cellular immunity. IL-4 appears to direct uncommitted T helper cells toward a Th2 or humoral response [147]. However, Delespesse et al. showed that even if IL-12 induces Th1 differentiation and priming for IFN-γ production in naive human cord blood T-cells, it also increases the IL-4 production from T-cells that have been committed previously by exposure to IL-4 [148]. In some instances, IL-2 also has been shown to stimulate the production of IL-4 and IFN-γ from spleen cells. Although neither IFN-γ nor IFN-α can induce Th1 development alone, IFN-γ will prime T-cells to respond to IL-12 with subsequent IFN-γ production.

Recently, it has become evident that the environment of cytokines during early T-cell activation and maturation can determine the dominant cytokine profile of the T-cell response. In fact, the Th1 cells are now defined by their production of interleukin-2 (IL-2), IFN-γ, and tumor necrosis factor-β (TNF-β) [149] and the Th2 cells are defined by their production of IL-4, IL-5, IL-6, IL-10, and IL-13. In this context, the role played by IL-12 becomes extremely important in shaping a Th1-type of immune response [142]. This especially enhances vaccine-induced immunity and limits or decreases Th2 cytokine production. In the anti-tumor or anti-parasite immune responses, cell-mediated pathways represent the keystone of the immune response. On the basis of these laboratory studies, several trials were recently initiated using IL-12 as adjuvant in schistosoma and leishmania vaccine in non-human primates in Africa by Scott et al. [150, 151]. More recently, interest has increased in experiments of mouse models against tuberculosis. In these models, IL-12 primes a greater Th1 response while at the same time it reinforces a preexisting Th2 response, boosting the immune system to maximum efficacy.

The molecular mechanisms of IL-12 are unknown; however, most recently Bacon et al. [152] showed that IL-12 and IL-2 are able to induce tyrosine phosphorylation of distinct members of the Janus family of protein tyrosine kinases in human T-lymphocytes. IL-12, but not IL-2, stimulates the tyrosine phosphorylation of TYK2 and JAK2, whereas JAK1 and JAK3, which are phosphorylated in response to IL-2, are not phosphorylated after IL-12 treatment. This indicates clearly that IL-2 and IL-12 have two different activation pathways in terms of signal transduction.

8   Interleukin-15

Interleukin-15 is a recently discovered cytokine [153] that has not yet reached the clinic but bears mentioning because of its unique properties. Although IL-15 shares no sequence homology with IL-2, it stimulates T-cell growth by interacting with both the β- and γ-subunits of the IL-2 receptor complex [154]. The spectrum of IL-15 bioactivity does not mirror that of IL-2, however, since IL-15 has a unique recognition receptor subunit that is structurally similar but not homologous to the IL-2 receptor alpha subunit [155]. In addition, IL-15 is not highly expressed by activated T-cells or monocytes [153]. Nevertheless, IL-15 is capable of mediating IL-2 like T-cell, B-cell and NK-cell activities [153, 156] and apparently can induce growth of some tumor-associated lymphocytes *in vitro* [157]. Combined with the preliminary preclinical finding that IL-15 may have a superior therapeutic index to IL-2 [158], these studies have provided sufficient evidence to warrant clinical trials in cancer therapy.

The outcome of these trials is difficult to predict since the role of IL-15 in the immune response has not been established. In fact, IL-15 may serve other physiologic functions such as mediating the growth of skeletal muscle fiber [159] and thus prove useful for clinical applications entirely separate from IL-2.

9   Interferons

Interferons (IFN) are a family of more than 20 related proteins. Initially described in 1957 by Isaacs and Lindenmann, IFN was found to be a protein produced in response to viral infection which was capable of inhibiting both viral replication and infectivity [160]. There are several broad classes of IFNs ($\alpha,\beta,\gamma,\delta,\varepsilon$) which have been cloned, sequenced and are commercially available. IFNs -α and -β are encoded on chromosome 9 and share 45% nucleotide homology while the gene for IFNγ, located on chromosome 12, manifests little sequence similarity but retains the functional capacity to induce resistance to viral replication [161, 162].

IFN-α is produced primarily by lymphocytes and macrophages in response to a number of antigenic or mitogenic stimuli and has seen the greatest use clinically. Fibroblast or IFN-β is principally produced by stimulated fibroblastic and mesenchymal cells [162]. Many normal and malignant cells have the capacity under appropriate conditions to produce IFNs implying local paracrine and autocrine function. IFN-α and -β transduce their signal via a common receptor [163]. By contrast, IFN-γ is produced by activated T-lymphocytes, binds a unique receptor and is involved with macrophage activation [164, 165].

The antitumor activities of the IFNs, though well described, are only partially understood. The IFNs have pleiotropic effects on gene expression, immune function, differentiation, angiogenesis and cellular proliferation. Consequently, the possibility for antitumor effects via enhanced tumor immunogenicity, decreased virulence and induction of immune responses either directly or through cytokine cascades needs to be considered [160–162, 166–168]. Broadly, it appears that IFN is capable of stimulating many components of the immune response which are involved in antitumor activity. Cytotoxic T-lymphocyte function of recognizing and lysing foreign cells in the context of appropriate MHC class I antigens is enhanced by all classes of IFN [162]. The expression of the requisite MHC antigens is upregulated as well [169]. Concomitantly, IFNs augment antibody-dependent cellular cytotoxicity mediated by a subpopulation of these cytolytic T-cells [170–172].

IFN-γ has been shown to be part of the regulatory pathway of phagocytic cells and is used therapeutically in the treatment of congenital and acquired deficiencies of granulocyte and macrophage activation [173]. IFNs also play a regulatory role on NK cells, a population of CD56+, CD16+ lymphocytes which have the unique ability to recognize and lyse foreign cells to which the host has not been previously immunized [174–176]. In general, the IFNs, particularly IFN-γ, appear capable of increasing the susceptibility of numerous targets to NK cell mediated lysis [177–180] and can reverse the depressed lytic activity associated with natural aging and malignancy. However, IFN induced inhibition of NK cell activity has been documented both *in vivo* and *in vitro* [181, 182]. These discrepancies likely arise from subtle variations in the subtypes of interferon employed as well as from paracrine cytokine effects elicited either directly or as a consequence of a more complex cytokine cascade.

Finally, it should be noted that the effects of the interferons on tumor growth are multiple and clearly not limited to immunomodulatory activities. The interferons, particularly IFN-α, have long been known to have direct antiproliferative actions on the growth of normal and neoplastic tissue including RCC [183, 184] and some reports suggest that IFN may actually function as a tumor suppressor [185–187]. The expression of tumor associated antigens including MHC molecules appears to be enhanced by the administration of IFN [167, 188–190]. Tumor neoangiogenesis may be inhibited by IFNs and is considered a new target for anti-cancer therapy [191–197].

Interferons have been used in clinical trials to treat a variety of malignant diseases, viral infections, and immune deficient states. Interferon-α was first found to play a major role in treating hairy-cell leukemia (HCL) and in severing the profound neutropenia associated with this illness [198]. Between 800 and 1,000 IFN-α receptors have been demonstrated on hairy cells [199] which are inhibited in their growth by exposure to the cytokine [200]. While not curative, IFN-α has made a significant contribution to the overall treatment and well being of patients with HCL. IFNs have also been used in the treatment of chronic myelogenous leukemias (CML). Initially used in chronic phase CML, IFN-α showed a high response rate and, in approximately 35% of patients, a reversion of expression of the Philadelphia chromosome, a marker for the disease [201]. Low doses of IFN-α (2–5 U/m^2) daily can produce partial or complete clinical remission in patients with chronic phase CML in 40–100%. About 25% of patients will have a duration of response of at least 1 year. Pilot studies of combination IFN-α and chemotherapy have not demonstrated significant improvement over either modality alone. IFN-γ monotherapy has also been piloted with initial studies suggesting non cross-resistance with IFN-α [202]. CML cells from patients sensitive and resistant to IFN-α treatment express interferon receptor, but only cells from sensitive patients have IFN inducible proteins produced following cytokine exposure [203, 204]. It is believed that IFN-a antitumor activity in CML is related to its antiproliferative effect and potentially from down regulation of c-myc [205].

The initial reports of the efficacy of IFN-α in RCC by Quesada, deKernion and Kirkwood were confirmed in short order by both these investigators and others [206, 207]. Several durable responses in excess of 200 days were observed in these early IFN-α studies [208]. Responses were observed most frequently among small lesions and pulmonary metastases and less commonly among bulky and extrapulmonary sites [209]. Neither the optimal dose nor schedule of IFN therapy have been clearly delineated. Preliminary studies by Kirkwood et al. [207] and Quesada et al. [207] suggested that high dose regimens (10×10^6 U daily, or 20×10^6 U/m^2 daily) were more effective than lower dose regimens.

The route by which the IFN is administered appears to have little impact on overall response or survival. A randomized trial of the subcutaneous versus intravenous routes of administration of IFN-α demonstrated essentially equal but low response rates [209]. Intramuscular administration at doses up to 36×10^6 U daily or brief IM courses of even higher doses, while effective, appears to confer little additional benefit [210, 211].

The addition of agents modulating interferon toxicity was undertaken to improve the tolerance to treatment. Aspirin at a dose of 600 mg qid was found ineffective in ameliorating the myalgias, nausea, fatigue and anorexia attendant upon treatment with IFN-α [212]. Similarly, while indomethacin is effective in the prevention of IFN-α induced febrile reactions (rarely dose-limiting) it like aspirin has little or no effect on the incidence of major constitutional complaints [213]. Prednisone, by contrast, may be effective in abrogating these flu-like symptoms [214] but its overall effect on immune response remains to be clarified. We undertook a small randomized study evaluating the effects of acetaminophen, indomethacin and dexamethasone on the IFN-γ. The use of acetaminophen to treat and prophylax against IFN-induced malaise appeared as good as the other agents and is commonplace [215].

Reports that recombinant human IFN-γ had anti-tumor activity against human RCC xenografts in nude mice led to subsequent human trials which have reported variable response rates (0–15%) [216–219]. The possibility that there exists an "optimum" dose for the administration IFN-γ above and below which biologic activity wanes has received considerable attention and was explored by Aulitzky et al. [220]. A biologically active dose of 100 µg SQ weekly was found to give a 30% response in 20 patients with primarily pulmonary metastases. As is often the case, a confirmatory study was less impressive [221]. Given the differing mechanisms of action of IFNs-α and -γ, the presence of distinct IFN receptors and in vitro data suggestive of synergistic activity [222], a theoretical rationale exists for trials of combination therapy. Various schedules of IFN-α and -γ have been assayed for potential synergism with generally disappointing results [223, 224]. By contrast, sequential administration is better tolerated and may in fact result in an additive clinical benefit though this remains to be convincingly demonstrated [225]. Immunologic studies of patients receiving sequential cytokine therapy are notable for a decrease in circulating CD8+

cells which may parallel treatment response and provocatively, these studies suggest that the order in which these cytokines are sequenced may in fact be crucial [226].

Interferons have also been administered in conjunction with cytotoxic chemotherapy, with disappointing results [227–240]. IFN-α with vinblastine, 5FU, mitomycin, Ifosfamide and vindesine have been used either alone or in combination.

In reference to renal cell cancer, the interferons clearly manifest clinical anti-tumor activity in metastatic renal cell carcinoma. However, results are generally modest and interpretation of the literature is complicated by the prevalence of studies which enroll statistically insignificant numbers of patients. It is not clear whether any one interferon preparation or dosage schedule is superior nor is there definitive evidence for the superior efficacy of interferon combinations or interferon in conjunction with chemotherapy. In a metanalysis of over 1,200 patients treated with IFN the 95% confidence interval for treatment response was 11–15%, with a 2% CR [241]. Higher response rates are generally seen among patients with better performance status and pulmonary lesions as the site of metastases. Consequently, selection bias may account for much of the variability in reported response rates. Recent reviews suggest that the use of interferon alone will have little long-term impact on the survival of the majority of patients with metastatic disease and that large multi-institutional studies more clearly reflect the response of this disease to treatment [241, 242]. As our understanding of the biology of RCC increases, we may in the future be able to better predict which patients' tumors are likely to respond to IFN-based therapies and thus spare unnecessary toxicity.

The effect of interferon on melanoma can be divided into direct antiproliferative effects as well as immunoregulatory control by effects on major histocompatibility molecules and tumor-associated antigens on the tumor cell as well as effects on the immune system [243–245]. As with the treatment of other solid tumors such as renal cell carcinoma, the optimal therapeutic dose has not yet been identified. Nevertheless, moderate doses of interferon given over a prolonged time appear to provide optimal therapeutic advantage except in the adjuvant setting [246]. More recently, the observation that high-dose interferon given over a period of 1 year in the setting of high risk melanoma (adjuvant therapy) provides both disease-free and overall survival advantage has led the FDA to approve high-dose interferon in this setting [247]. In this study, 287 patients were randomly assigned to receive either high-dose interferon (20 U/m^2 per day IV for 1 month followed by 10 U/m^2 at 3 times per week subcutaneously for 48 weeks) or observation. A significant prolongation of relapse-free survival and overall survival was observed with a median follow-up of 6.9 years. The benefit of treatment was greatest among node positive resected patients. Further confirmatory studies and combination treatments are currently being pursued. Interferon alpha-2b is the first agent to show significant benefit in relapse-free and overall survival of high risk melanoma patients.

10   Tumor necrosis factor

TNF-α (cachectin) and TNF-β (lymphotoxin) are two specific cytokines encoded by two separate genes. These genes reside on chromosome 6 in the region of the MHC genes. TNF-α and TNF-β share a 30% amino acid sequence homology and several biological activities.

TNF-α is a 157 amino acid cytokine that circulates as a non-glycosylated, non-covalently bound trimer composed of monomers that are rich in β-pleated sheets. Monocytes, macrophages, T-cells, B-cells, NK cells, Kupffer cells and glial cells of the central nervous system secrete TNF-α following exposure to endotoxins or other bacterial, viral, and parasitic products as well as inflammatory chemical agents [248].

Transcription of the gene-encoding TNF-α increases many fold after exposure of unstimulated cells to endotoxin. Serum levels of TNF-α increase in a few minutes after *in vivo* exposure to endotoxin and reach peak levels in about 1.5–2 hours, falling to baseline in 4–5 hours [249].

The highest levels of cytokine are observed during lethal endotoxemia following gram-negative bacteremia and are associated with induction of other cytokines such as IL-1 and IL-6. Increased levels of this cytokine lead to development of the shock syndrome pathway but, unlike IL-1, IL-6 does not enhance TNF lethality [250].

However, in this cascade of events, macrophage-derived TNF undoubtedly represents the most important host mediator in the pathogenesis of shock. Alone or in combination with endotoxin or IL-1, macrophage-derived TNF is capable of inducing lethal shock as well as venous occlusive disease, a less documented but no less devastating process that develops shortly after allogenic bone marrow transplantation.

In the last few years, attention has been focused on the debilitating effects of wasting, malnutrition, anemia and weight loss caused by chronically low levels of TNF in patients with cancer, chronic infections and HIV. Although the pathogenesis of cachexia in cancer and the wasting syndrome in AIDS is complex, several studies suggest that release of IL-1 from endothelial cells and TNF from macrophages are the major anorexigenic factors [251].

Finally, several studies have examined the antineoplastic activity of TNF-α on different tumors. The results suggest that TNF-α has potent necrotizing activity against solid tumors which seems to be derived from mechanisms related to the growth and differentiation of the tumor and not to direct cytotoxicity. TNF-α produced from either tumor or nontumor cells may function in paracrine fashion by inhibiting the growth of unmodified, tumor cells implanted at the same site [252]. These studies support the concept that TNF-α is involved with host immunity to defeat the cancer. In clinical studies, dose-limiting toxicity of TNF-α has been a particular problem. The maximal tolerated dose of TNF-α in humans (10 μg/kg) was 40-fold less (on a per kg basis) than the dose required to generate a significant antitumor response in mice (400 μg/kg) [253].

TNF-β is a glycosylated protein composed of 169 amino acids and has 30% homology to TNF-α. Like TNF-α, TNF-β is produced after antigen activation of cytotoxic CD8 T cells, a subset of CD4 T cells called TH1, and by several murine malignant cell lines that represent early stages of B cells, as well as human melanoma cells and human Epstein-Barr virus transformed B cells. The 3' end of the TNF-β gene is approximately 1 KBP from the transcription initiation site of the TNF-α gene. The direction of transcription through the TNF-complex is from TNF-β to TNF-α and occurs in the same coding strand. In contrast to TNF-α, which can be displayed as a membrane-bound molecule and then released, TNF-β is stored and transported through the cell in granules and then secreted. Several agents, including cyclosporin and prostaglandin E2, inhibit the TNF-β production from T cells by inhibition of mRNA accumulation [254].

The major biological role of TNF-β is to mediate the cellular killing activity of cytolytic T cells, "helper"-"killer" T cells, NK cells and LAK cells. After stimulation with antigen presented by MHC or by IL-2, the level of TNF-β production increases severalfold [255].

The cytolytic activity of TNF-β is mediated by the capacity to induce DNA fragmentation or apoptosis in the target cells as tumor cells. This mechanism probably contributes in large part to graft rejection and to manifestations of graft-versus-host reactions in bone marrow transplanted patients.

Like TNF-α, it is possible that TNF-β plays a major role in the clinical presentation of AIDS, particularly in the mechanism of T cell death and B cell activation in late-stage disease [256]. However, more studies must be carried out before we can fully understand all the intrinsic mechanisms of these two cytokines and their roles in all human pathologies. Without this knowledge to help circumvent the inherent toxicity of these proteins, effective therapeutic applications are unlikely.

11   Concluding remarks

The number of characterized cytokines continues to grow and as it does, the complexity of molecular communication within the immune system is beginning to be revealed. Each new cytokine presents an additional target for clinical investigation. Thus far, however, experience has demonstrated that the path to effective therapeutic application is often a difficult one. Toxicity and unpredictable efficacies are commonly encountered. Nevertheless, successes, although few when compared to the number of trials attempted, have had a major impact in the treatment of a variety of diseases. It is certain that strategies that combine multiple cytokines with other drugs and those that exploit genetic approaches will add to the clinical successes for immunostimulatory therapy.

12   Acknowledgments

The authors would like to acknowledge the editorial assistance of Suzanne E. Markloff. Support for this work was provided by the Norris Cotton Cancer (National Institutes of Health grant CA23108), the Veterans Administration and the National Institutes of Health.

References

1   B. Lee and T. L. Ciardelli: Clinical applications of cytokines for immunostimulation and immunosuppression. Prog. in Drug Res. *39*, 167 (1992).

2   T. Vail and J. Descotes: Immune-mediated side-effects of cytokines in humans. Toxicology *105*, 31 (1995).

3   M.A.S. Moore: Hematopoietic reconstruction: New approaches. Clin. Cancer Res. *1*, 3 (1995).

4   M.J. George: The present and future of hematopoietic cytokines in clinical practice. Stem Cells (Dayt) *12* S1., 249 (1994).

5   P.J. Quesenberry: Biotherapy in hematology: The next decade. Rev. Invest. Clin. *Apr. S.*, 8 (1994).

6   F. Takaku: Clinical application of cytokines for cancer treatment. Oncology *51*, 123 (1994).

7   R. Mertelsmann: Hematopoietic cytokines: from biology and pathophysiology to clinical application. Leukemia *7* S2, 168 (1993).

8   G.M. Clore, P.T. Wingfield and A.M. Gronenborn: High-resolution three-dimensional structure of interleukin 1 beta in solution by three- and four-dimensional nuclear magnetic resonance spectroscopy. Biochemistry *30*, 2315 (1991).

9   K. Ye, K.C. Koch, B.D. Clark and C.A. Dinarello: Interleukin-1 down-regulates gene and surface expression of interleukin-1 receptor type I by destabilizing its mRNA whereas interleukin-2 increases its expression. Immunology *75*, 427 (1992).

10   J. Smith, W. Urba, R. Steis, J. Janik et al.: Interleukin-1 alpha: Results of a phase one toxicity and immunomodulatory trial. Am. Soc. Clin. Oncol. *9*, 717 (1990).

11   C.A. Haworth, N.M. Ravindir and M. Feldman, Prospects for cytokines in human immunotherapy. The cytokine handbook (Academic Press, 1994).

12   C.A. Dinarello and S.M. Wolff: The role of interleukin-1 in disease. N. Engl. J. Med. *328*, 106 (1993).

13   C.A. Dinarello: The interleukin-1 family:10 years of discovery. FASEB J. *8*, 1314 (1994).

14   C.A. Dinarello: Interleukin-1. Adv. in Pharm. *25*, 21 (1994).

15   B.G. Redman, Y. Abubakr, T. Chou et al: Phase II trial of recombinant interleukin-1 beta in patients with metastatic renal cell carcinoma. J. Immunother. Emphasis Tumor Immunol. *16*, 211 (1994).

16   P.L. Triozzi, J.A. Kim, E.W. Martin et al: Phase I trial of escalating doses of interleukin-1β in combination with a fixed dose of interleukin-2. J. Clin. Oncol. *13*, 482 (1995).

17   J. Crown, A. Jakubowski and J. Gabrilove: Interleukin-1: biological effects in human hematopoiesis. Leuk. Lymphoma *9*, 433 (1993).

18   J.W. Smith 2nd, W.J. Urba, B.D. Curti et al.: The toxic and hematologic effects of interleukin-1 alpha administered in a phase I trial to patients with advanced malignancies. J. Clin. Oncol. *10*, 1141 (1992).

19   D. Weisdorf, E. Katsanis, C. Verfaillie et al.: Interleukin-1 alpha administered after autologous transplantation. Blood 84, 2044 (1994).

20   C.A. Dinarello: Blocking interleukin-1 receptors. Int. J. Clin. Lab. Res. *24*, 61 (1994).

21   W.P. Arend: Interleukin-1 antagonism in inflammatory disease. Lancet *16*, 155 (1993).

22   P. Ghiara, D. Armellini, G. Scapigliati et al.: Biological role of the IL-1 receptor type II as defined by monoclonal antibody. Cytokine *3*, 1423 (1991).

23   C.A. Jacobs, M.P. Beckman, K. Mohler et al.: Pharmacokinetic parameters and biodistribution of soluble cytokine receptors. Internat. Rev. Exp. Path. *34*, 123 (1993).

24   S.P. Eisenberg, R.J. Evans, W.P. Arend et al.: Primary structure and functional expression from complementary DNA of a human interleukin-1 antagonist. Nature *25*, 341 (1990).

25   C.H. Hannum, C.J. Wilcox, W.P. Arend et al.: Interleukin-1 receptor antagonist activity of a human interleukin-1 inhibitor. Nature *343*, 336 (1990).

26   E.V. Granowitz, R. Porat, J.W. Mier et al.: Pharmacokinetics, safety, and immuno-modulatory effects of human recombinant interleukin-1 receptor antagonist in healthy humans. Cytokine *4*, 353 (1992).

27   M.D. Mitchell, S.S. Edwin, R.M. Silver and R.J. Romero: Potential agonist action of the interleukin-1 receptor antagonist protein: implications for the treatment of women. J. Clin. Endocrin. Metab. *76*, 1386 (1993).

28   J.H. Antin, H.J. Weinstein, E.C. Guinan et al.: Recombinant human interleukin-1 receptor antagonist in the treatment of steroid resistant graft-versus-host disease. Blood *84*, 1342 (1994).

29   E. Abraham and T.A. Raffin: Sepsis Therapy Trial. JAMA *271*, 1876 (1994).

30   C.J. Fisher, J.A. Dhainaut, S.M. Opal et al.: Recombinant human interleukin-1 recep-

tor antagonist in the treatment of patients with sepsis syndrome. JAMA *271*, 1836 (1994).

31 S.A. Greenfeld, P. Nunes, L. Kwee et al.: Molecular cloning and characterization of a second subunit of the interleukin-1 receptor. J. Biol. Chem. *270*, 13757 (1995).

32 K.A. Smith: Interleukin-2: Inception, impact and implications. Science *240*, 1169 (1988).

33 Y. Minami, T. Kono, T. Miyazaki and T. Taniguchi: The IL-2 receptor complex. Annu. Rev. Immunol. *11*, 245 (1993).

34 T. Taniguchi and Y. Minami: The IL-2/IL-2 receptor system: a current overview. Cell *73*, 5 (1993).

35 J.N. Ihle: Cytokine receptor signalling. Nature *377*, 591 (1995).

36 S.M. Russell, J.A. Johnston, M. Noguchi et al.: Interaction of IL-2Rβ and γ_c Chains with Jak1 and Jak3: Implications for XSCID and XCID. Science *266*, 1042 (1994).

37 B.A. Witthuhn, O. Silvennoinen, O. Miura et al.: Involvement of the Jak-3 Janus kinase in signalling by interleukins 2 and 4 in lymphoid and myeloid cells. Nature *370*, 153 (1994).

38 T. Miyazaki, A. Kawahara, H. Fujii et al.: Functional Activation of Jak1 and Jak3 by Selective Association with IL-2 Receptor Subunits. Science *266*, 1045 (1994).

39 N. Stahl and G.D. Yancopoulos: The Alphas, Betas, and Kinases of Cytokine Receptor Complexes. Cell *74*, 587 (1993).

40 S.M. Gorsch and M.S. Ernstoff: Management of Metastatic Renal Cell Carcinoma: Chemotherapy, Hormonal Therapy and Interferons. In: Comprehensive Textbook of Genitourinary Oncology. N.J. Vogelzang, P.T. Scardino, W.U. Shipley and D.S. Coffey (eds). Williams & Wilkins, Baltimore (1996).

41 J.K. Bruton and J.M. Koeller: Recombinant interleukin-2. Pharmacotherapy *14*, 635 (1994).

42 M.H. Oppenheim and M.T. Lotze: Interleukin-2: Solid tumor therapy. Oncology *51*, 154 (1994).

43 D.R. Parkinson and M. Sznol: High-dose interleukin-2 in the therapy of metastatic renal-cell carcinoma. Seminars in Oncology *22*, 61 (1995).

44 S.S. Taneja, W. Pierce, R. Figlin and A. Belldegrun: Immunotherapy for renal cell carcinoma: the era of interleukin-2-based treatment. Urology *45*, 911 (1995).

45 L.T. Vlasveld and E.M. Rankin: Recombinant interleukin-2 in cancer: basic and clinical aspects. Cancer Treatment Reviews *20*, 275 (1994).

46 J. Wagstaff, J.W. Baars, G.-J. Wolbink et al.: Renal cell carcinoma and interleukin-2: A review. Eur. J. Cancer *31A*, 401 (1995).

47 C. Garbe: Perspectives of cytokine treatment in malignant skin tumors. Recent Results Cancer Res. *139*, 349 (1995).

48 R. Whittington and D. Faulds: Interleukin-2. a review of its pharmacological properties and therapeutic use in patients with cancer. Drugs *46*, 446 (1993).

49 S.A. Rosenberg, M.T. Lotze, L.M. Muul et al.: Observations on the systemic administration of autologous lymphokine-activated killer cells and recombinant interleukin-2 in patients with metastatic cancer. N. Eng. J. Med. *313*, 1485 (1985).

50 J.R. Ortaldo, A. Mason and R. Overton: Lymphokine activated killer (LAK) cells: analysis of progenitors and effectors. J. Exp. Med. *164*, 1193 (1986).

51 T. Nakarai, M.J. Robertson, M. Streuli et al.: Interleukin 2 Receptor γ Chain Expression on Resting and Activated Lymphoid Cells. J. Exp. Med. *180*, 241 (1994).

52 M. Caligiuri, A. Zmuidzinas, T.J. Manley et al.: Functional Consequences of Interleukin-2 Receptor Expression on Resting Human Lymphocytes. J. Exp. Med. *171*, 1509 (1990).

53 S.A. Rosenberg, M.T. Lotze, J.C. Yang et al.: Prospective randomized trial of high-dose interleukin-2 alone or in conjunction with lymphokine-activated killer cells for the treatment of patients with advanced cancer. J. Natl. Cancer Inst. 85, 622 (1993).

54 M.J. Koretz, D.H. Lawson, M. York et al.: Randomized study of interleukin-2 (IL-2) vs IL-2 plus lymphokine-activated killer cells for the treatment of melanoma and renal cell cancer. Arch. Surg. 126, 898 (1991).

55 P.A. Palmer, J. Vinke, P. Evers et al.: Continuous infusion of recombinant interleukin-2 with or without autologous lymphokine activated killer cells for the treatment of advanced renal cell carcinoma. Eur. J. Cancer 28A, 1038 (1992).

56 S. Legha , M.A. Gianan, C. Plager et al.: Evaluation of interleukin-2 administered by continuous infusion in patients with metastatic melanoma. Cancer 77, 89 (1996).

57 T.M. Law, R.J. Motzer, M. Madhu et al.: Phase III randomized trial of interleukin-2 with or without lymphokine activated killer cells in the treatment of patients with advanced renal cell carcinoma. Cancer 76, 824 (1995).

58 B. Fisher, B.S. Packard, E.J. Read et al.: Tumor localization of adoptively transferred Indium-111 labeled tumor infiltrating lymphocytes in patients with metastatic melanoma. J. Clin. Oncol. 7, 250 (1989).

59 C.D. Platsoucas: Human autologous tumor-specific T-cells in malignant melanoma. Metastasis Rev. 10, 151 (1991).

60 W.C. Pierce, A. Belldegrun and R.A. Figlin: Cellular therapy: scientific rationale and clinical results in the treatment of metastatic renal cell carcinoma. Semin. Oncol. 22, 74 (1995).

61 J.A. Thompson, M.C. Benyunes, J.A. Bianco and A. Fefer: Treatment with pentoxifylline and ciprofloxacin reduces the toxicity of high-dose interleukin-2 and lymphokine-activated killer cells. Semin. Oncol. 20, 46 (1993).

62 J.A. Anderson, T.M. Woodcock, J.I. Harty et al.: The effects of pentoxifylline on interleukin-2 toxicity in patients with metastatic renal cell carcinoma. Eur. J. Cancer 31A, 714 (1995).

63 M.R. Albertini, J.A. Sosman, J.A. Hank et al.: The influence of autologous lymphokine activated killer cell infusions on the toxicity and antitumor effect of repetitive cycles of interleukin-2. Cancer 66, 2457 (1990).

64 J.C. Yang, S.L. Topalian, D. Parkinson et al.: Randomized comparison of high-dose and low-dose intravenous interleukin-2 for therapy of metastatic renal cell carcinoma, an interim report. J. Clin. Oncol. 12, 1572 (1994).

65 P. Lissoni, S. Barni, A. Ardizzoia et al.: Prognostic factors of the clinical response to subcutaneous immunotherapy with interleukin-2 alone in patients with metastatic renal cell carcinoma. Oncology 51, 59 (1994).

66 L.T. Vlasveld, S. Horenblas, A. Hekman et al.: Phase II study of intermittent continuous infusion of low-dose recombinant interleukin-2 in advanced melanoma and renal cell cancer. Ann. Oncol. 5, 179 (1994).

67 R.P. Whitehead, D. Ward, L. Hemingway et al.: Subcutaneous recombinant interleukin-2 in a dose escalating regimen in patients with metastatic renal cell adenocarcinoma. Cancer Res. 50, 6708 (1990).

68 D.T. Sleifer, R.A. Janssen, J. Buter et al.: Phase II study of subcutaneous interleukin-2 in unselected patients with advanced renal cell cancer on an outpatient basis. J. Clin. Oncol. 10, 1119 (1992).

69 S. Sone and T. Ogura: Local interleukin-2 therapy for cancer, and its effector induction mechanisms. Oncology 51, 170 (1994).

70   P.M. Anderson and M.A. Sorenson: Effects of route and formulation on clinical phar-
      macokinetics of interleukin-2. Clin. Pharmacokinet. *27*, 19 (1994).
71   P.M. Anderson, E. Katsanis, S.F. Sencer et al.: Depot characteristics and biodistri-
      bution of interleukin-2 liposomes: importance of route of administration. J. Immu-
      nother. *12*, 19 (1992).
72   F.J. Meyers, C. Paradise, S.A. Scudder et al.: A phase I study including pharmacoki-
      netics of polyethylene glycol conjugated interleukin-2. Clinical Pharmacol. and
      Therap. *49*, 307 (1991).
73   L.P. Courtney, J.L. Phelps and L.M. Karavodin: An anti-IL-2 antibody increases serum
      halflife and improves anti-tumor efficacy of human recombinant interleukin-2. Immu-
      nopharmacology. *28*, 223 (1994).
74   R.P. Whitehead, K.D. Friedman and D.A. Clark: A phase I trial of subcutaneous inter-
      leukin-2 and interleukin-4. Proc. Ann. Meet. Am. Assoc. Cancer Res. *33*, A1381 (1992).
75   Y.C. Yang, L. Owen-Schaub, A. Mendiguren-Rodriquez et al.: Combination immu-
      notherapy for non-small cell lung cancer-results with interleukin-2 and TNFa. J.
      Thorac. Cardiovasc. Surg. *79*, 8 (1990).
76   U. Keilholz, C. Scheibenbogen, P. Brossart et al.: Interleukin-2-based immunotherapy
      and chemoimmunotherapy in metastatic melanoma. Recent Results Canc. Res. *139*,
      383 (1995).
77   M.S. Mitchell: Combining chemotherapy with biological response modifiers in the
      treatment of cancer. J. Natl. Cancer Inst. *80*, 1445 (1988).
78   A.C. Buzaid and S.S. Legha: Combination of chemotherapy with interleukin-2 and
      interferon-alpha for the treatment of advanced melanoma. Seminars in Oncol. *21*,
      23 (1994).
79   D.M. Pardoll: Paracrine cytokine adjuvants in cancer immunotherapy. Annu. Rev.
      Immunol. *13*, 399 (1995).
80   J. Triesman, P. Hwu, S. Minamoto, G.E. Shafer et al.: Interleukin-2-transduced lym-
      phocytes grow in an autocrine fashion and remain responsive to antigen. Blood *85*,
      139 (1995).
81   P.A. Cassileth, E. Podack, K. Sridhar et al.: Clinical protocol: Phase I study of trans-
      fected cancer cells expressing the interleukin-2 gene product in limited stage small
      cell lung cancer. Human Gene Ther. *6*, 369 (1995).
82   B. Gansbacher: A pilot study of immunization with IL-2 secreting allogeneic HLA-
      A2 matched renal cell carcinoma cells in patients with advanced renal cell carci-
      noma. Human Gene Therapy *3*, 691 (1992).
83   Clinical Protocols. Cancer Gene Ther. *1*, 289 (1994).
84   W. Schmidt, T. Schweighoffer, E. Herbst et al.: Cancer vaccines: The IL-2 dosage effect.
      Proc. Natl. Acad. Sci. USA *92*, 4711 (1995).
85   J.A. Kovacs, M. Basler, R.J. Dewar et al.: Increases in CD4 T lymphocytes with inter-
      mittent courses of interleukin-2 in patients with human immunodeficiency virus infec-
      tion. N. Engl. J. Med. *332*, 567 (1995).
86   Z.P. Bernstein, M.M. Porter, M. Gould et al.: Prolonged administration of low-dose
      interleukin-2 in human immunodeficiency virus-associated malignancy results in sel-
      ective expansion of innate immune effectors without significant clinical toxicity.
      Blood *86*, 3287 (1995).
87   R.G. Hewitt: Interleukin-2; Full circle in a decade. Infect. in Med. *July* 490 (1994).
88   J.R. Minor: Interleukin-2 in HIV. Am. J. Health-Syst. Pharm. *52*, 1345 (1995).
89   M. Howard, J. Farrar, M. Hilfiker et al.: Identification of a T cell derived B-cell gro-
      wth factor distinct from IL-2. J. Exp. Med. *155*, 914 (1982).

90   T. Yokota, T. Otsuka, T. Mosmann et al. Proc. Natl. Acad. Sci. USA *83*, 5894 (1986).
91   J. Banchereau, T. Defrance, J.P. Galizzi et al.: Human interleukin 4: Its agonistic and antagonistic effects on B lymphocytes and its receptor. In Cytokines: Basic Principles and Clinical Applications. S. Romagnani, A.K. Abbas (eds). Raven Press: New York 1990. 177–187.
92   M.T. Lotze: Role of IL-4 in the antitumor response. In IL-4 Structure and Function. H. Spits (ed). CRC Press: Boca Raton, 19XX.
93   F.M. Hofman, M. Brock, C.R. Taylor et al.: IL-4 regulates differentiation and proliferation of human precursor B cells. J. Immunol. *141*, 1185 (1988).
94   J. Gordon, M.J. Millsum, G.R. Guy et al.: Resting B lymphocytes can be triggered directly through the CDW40(Gp50) antigen. J. Immunol. *140*, 1425 (1988).
95   R. Noelle, P.H. Karmmer, J. Ohara et al.: Increased expression of Ia antigen on resting B cells: a new role for B cell growth factor. Proc. Natl. Acad. Sci. USA *81*, 6149 (1984).
96   C.M. Snapper, F.D. Finkelman, W.E. Paul: Differential regulation of IgG1 and IgE synthesis by interleukin 4. J. Exp. Med. *167*, 183 (1988).
97   X. Han, K. Hoh, C.M. Balch et al.: Recombinant interleukin 4 [RIL-4] inhibits interleukin-2 induced activation of peripheral blood lymphocytes. Lympho. Res. *7*, 227 (1988).
98   H. Spits, H. Yssel, X. Paliard et al.: Interleukin 4 inhibits interleukin 2 mediated induction of human lymphokine activated killer cells, but not the generation of antigen specific cytotoxic T lymphocytes in mixed leukocyte cultures. J. Immunol. *141*, 29 (1988).
99   S.R. Carding, E.J. Jenkinson, R. Kingston et al.: Developmental control of lymphokine gene expression in fetal thymocytes during T cell ontogeny. Proc. Natl. Acad. Sci. USA *86*, 2242 (1989).
100   J. Ransom, M. Fischer, T. Mosmann et al.: Interferon gamma is produced by activated immature mouse thymocytes and reverses the interleukin 4-induced proliferation of immature thymocytes. J. Immunol. *139*, 4102 (1987).
101   M.D. Mossalayi, J.C. Lecron, A.H. Dalloul, et al Soluble CD23 (FcE) and interleukin 1 synergistically induce early human thymocyte maturation. J. Exp. Med. *171*, 959 (1990).
102   J. Hu-Li, E.M. Sherach, J. Mizuguchi et al.: B cell stimulatory factor I (interleukin 4) is a potent costimulant for normal resting T lymphocytes. J. Exp. Med. *165*, 157 (1987).
103   H. Luo, M. Rubio, G. Biron et al.: Anti-proliferative effect of IL-4 in B chronic lymphocytic leukemia. J. Immunol. in press (ref from Spits).
104   M. Bosco, M. Giovarelli , M. Forni et al.: Low doses of IL-4 injected perilymphatically in tumor-bearing mice inhibit the growth of poorly and apparently non-immunogenic tumors and induce a tumor-specific immune memory. J. Immunol. *145*, 3136 (1990).
105   R.I. Tepper, P.K. Pattengale and P. Leder: Murine interleukin 4 displays potent antitumor activity *in vivo*. Cell *57*, 503 (1989).
106   E.R. Fearon, D.M. Pardoll, T. Itanya et al.: Interleukin 2 production by tumor cells bypasses T helper function in the generation of an anti-tumor response. Cell *60*, 397 (1990).
107   B. Gansbacher, R. Bannerji, B. Daniels et al.: Retroviral vector-mediated gamma interferon gene transfer into tumor cells generates potent and long lasting anti-tumor immunity. Cancer Res. *50*, 7820 (1990).

108 Y. Kawakami, S.A. Rosenberg and M.T. Lotze: Interleukin 4 promotes the growth of tumor-infiltrating lymphocytes for human autologous melanoma. J. Exp. Med. *168*, 2183 (1988).

109 M.H. Gilleece, J.H. Scarffe, A. Ghosh et al.: Recombinant human interleukin 4 (IL-4) given as daily subcutaneous injections – a phase I dose toxicity trial. Brit. J. Cancer *66*, 204 (1992).

110 C.W. Taylor, T.M. Grogan and S.E. Salmon: Effects of interleukin 4 on the *in vitro* growth of human lymphoid and plasma cell neoplasms. Blood *75*, 1114 (1990).

111 F. Herrman, M. Andreeff, H.J. Gruss et al.: Interleukin-4 inhibits growth of multiple myelomas by suppressing interleukin 6 expression. Blood *78*, 2070 (1991).

112 T. Defrance, A.C. Fluckiger, J.-F. Rossi et al.: Antiproliferative effects of interleukin 4 on freshly isolated non-Hodgkin malignant B-lymphoma cells. Blood *79*, 990 (1992).

113 T.E. Tanner and G. Tosato: Regulation of B-cell growth and immunoglobulin gene transcription by interleukin-6. Blood *79*, 452 (1992).

114 J. Van Snick: Interleukin-6: An overview. Annu. Rev. Immunol. *8*, 253 (1990).

115 T. Hirano, S. Akira, T. Tetsuya and T. Kishimoto: Biological and clinical aspects of interleukin 6. Immunol. Today *11*, 443 (1990).

116 K. Yamasaki, T. Taga, Y. Hirata et al.: Cloning and expression of the human interleukin-6 [BSF-2/IFNb2] receptor. Science *241*, 825 (1988).

117 T. Taga, M. Hibi, Y. Hirata et al.: Interleukin-6 triggers the association of its receptor with a possible signal transducer gp130. Cell *58*, 573 (1989).

118 T. Ishibashi, H. Kimura, Y. Shikama et al.: Interleukin-6 is a potent thrombopoietic factor *in vivo* in mice. Blood *74*, 1241 (1989).

119 J. Weber, J.C. Yang, S.L. Topalian et al.: Phase I trial of subcutaneous interleukin-6 in patients with advanced malignancies. J. Clin. Oncol. *11*, 499 (1993).

120 D. Caracciolo, S.C. Clark and G. Rovera: Human interleukin-6 supports granulocytic differentiation of hematopoietic progenitor cells and acts synergistically with GM-CSG. Blood *73*, 666 (1989).

121 T. Olencki, G.T. Budd, S. Murthy et al.: Phase IA/IB trial of rhIL-6 in patients with refractory malignancy: hematologic and immunologic effects. Blood *Suppl 1*, 89a (1992).

122 J.J. Mulé, J.K. McIntosh, D.M. Jablons et al.: *In vivo* administration of recombinant interleukin-6 mediates tumor regression in mice. J. Exp. Med. *171*, 629 (1990).

123 J.J. Mulé, S.G. Marcus, J.C. Yang et al.: Clinical applications of IL-6 in cancer therapy. Res. Immunol. *143*, 777 (1992).

124 A. Porgator, E. Tzehoval, A. Katz et al.: IL-6 gene transfection into 3LL tumor cells suppresses the malignant phenotype and confers immunotherapeutic competence against parental metastatic cells. Cancer Res. *52*, 3679 (1992).

125 C. Scheid, R. Young, R. McDermott et al.: Immune function of patients receiving recombinant human interleukin-6 (IL-6) in a phase I clinical study: induction of C-reactive protein and IgE and inhibition of natural killer and lymphokine-activated killer cell activity. Cancer Immunol. Immunother. *38*, 119 (1994).

126 J. Malejczyk, M. Malejczyk, A. Urbanski and T.A. Luger: Production of natural killer cell activity-augmenting factor (interleukin-6) by human epiphyseal chondrocytes. Arthritis Rheum. *35*, 706 (1992).

127 H. Goto, C. Shimazaki, T. Tatsumi et al.: Establishment of a novel myeloma cell line KPMM2 carrying t(3;14)(q21;q32), which proliferates specifically in response to interleukin-6 through an autocrine mechanism. Leukemia *9*, 711 (1995).

128 O.F. Ballester, L.C. Moscinski, G.H. Lyman et al.: High levels of interleukin-6 are

associated with low tumor burden and low growth fraction in multiple myeloma. Blood *83*, 1903 (1994).

129 H.J. Gruss, M.A. Brach, R.H. Mertelsmann and F. Herrmann: Interferon-gamma interrupts autocrine growth mediated by endogenous interleukin-6 in renal-cell carcinoma. International J. Cancer *11*, 770 (1991).

130 M. Rabau, H. Kashtan, S. Baron et al.: Inhibition of CT-26 murine adenocarcinoma growth in the rectum of mice treated with recombinant human interleukin-6. J. Immunother. Emphasis Tumor. Immunol. *15*, 257 (1994).

131 K.W. Moore, P. Vieira, D.F. Fiorentino et al.: Homology of cytokine synthesis inhibitory factor (IL-10) to Epstein-Barr virus gene BCRF1. Science *248*, 1230 (1990).

132 M.R. Walter and T.L. Nagabhushan: Crystal structure of interleukin-10 reveals an interferon gamma-like fold. Biochemistry *34*, 12118 (1995).

133 A. Zdanov, C. Schalk-Hihi, A. Gustchina et al.: Crystal structure of interleukin-10 reveals the functional dimer with an unexpected topological similarity to interferon gamma. Structure *3*, 591 (1995).

134 Y. Lui, S.H. Wei, A.S. Ho et al.: Expression cloning of the human IL-10 receptor. J. Immunol. *15*, 1821 (1994).

135 K.W. Moore, A.O'Garra, M. de Waal et al.: Interleukin-10. Ann. Rev. Immunol. *11*, 165 (1993).

136 K.Taga and G.Tosato: IL-10 inhibits T-cell proliferation and IL-2 production. J. Immunol. *148*, 1143 (1992).

137 M. de Waal, R.J. Abrams, B. Bennet et al.: Interleukin-10 (IL-10) inhibits cytokine synthesis by human monocytes: an autoregulatory role of IL-10 produced by monocytes. J. Exp. Med. *174*, 1209 (1991).

138 W.E. Carson, M.J. Lindemann, R. Baiocchi et al.: The functional characterization of interleukin-10 receptor expression on human natural killer cells. Blood *85*, 3577 (1995).

139 A.E. Chernoff, E.V. Granowitz, L. Shapiro et al.: A randomized, controlled trial of IL-10 in humans. J. Immunol. *154*, 5492 (1995).

140 H. Tahara and M.T. Lotze: Antitumor effects of interleukin-12 (IL-12): applications for the immunotherapy and gene therapy of cancer. Gene Therapy *2*, 96 (1995).

141 G.Trinchieri and P. Scott: The role of interleukin 12 in the immune response, disease and therapy. Immunol. Today *15* , 460 (1994).

142 F.D. Finkelman: Relationships among antigen presentation, cytokines, immune deviation, and autoimmune disease. J. Exp. Med. *182*, 279 (1995).

143 M.J. Skeen and H.K. Ziegler: Activation of γδ T cells for production of IFN-γ is mediated by bacteria via macrophage-derived cytokines IL-1 and IL-12. J. Immunol. *154*, 5832 (1995).

144 R.T. Gazzinelli, S. Hayashi, M. Wysocka et al.: Role of IL-12 in the initiation of cell mediated immunity by *Toxoplasma gondii* and its regulation by IL-10 and nitric oxide. J. Eukaryotic Microbiol. *41*, 9S (1994).

145 M. Denis: Interleukin-12 (IL-12) augments cytolytic activity of natural killer cells toward *Mycobacterium tuberculosis*-infected human monocytes. Cellular Immunol. *156*, 529 (1994).

146 C.L. Nastala, H.D. Edington, T.G. McKinney et al.: Recombinant IL-12 administration induces tumor regression in association with IFN-α production. J. Immunol. *153*, 1697 (1994).

147 A. Kelso: Th1 and Th2 subsets: paradigms lost. Immunol. Today *16*, 374 (1995).

148 T.A. Wynn, D. Jankovic, S. Hieny et al.: IL-12 exacerbates rather than suppresses T

helper 2-dependent pathology in the absence of endogenous IFN-γ. J. Immunol. *154*, 3999 (1995).

149 A. D'Andrea, X. Ma, M. Aste-Amezaga et al.: Stimulatory and inhibitory effects of interleukin (IL)-4 and IL-13 on the production of cytokines by human peripheral blood mononuclear cells: Priming for IL-12 and tumor necrosis factor a production. J. Exp. Med. *181*, 537 (1995).

150 T.A. Wynn, D. Kankovic, S. Hieny et al.: IL-12 enhances vaccine-induced immunity to *Schisotoma mansoni* in mice and decreases T helper 2 cytokine expression, IgE production, and tissue eosinophilia. J. Immunol. *154*, 4701 (1995).

151 S.S. Hall: IL-12 at the crossroads. Science 268, 1432 (1995).

152 C.M. Bacon, D.W. McVicar, J.R. Ortaldo et al.: Interleukin-12 (IL-12) induces tyrosine phosphorylation of JAK2 and TYK2: differntial use of Janus family tyrosine kinases by Il-2 and IL-12. J. Exp. Med. *181*, 399 (1995).

153 K.H. Grabstein, J. Eisenman, K. Shanebeck et al.: Cloning of a T cell growth factor that interacts with the beta chain of the interleukin-2 receptor. Science *264*, 965 (1994).

154 J.G. Giri, M. Ahdieh, J. Eisenmann et al.: Utilization of the beta and gamma chains of the IL-2 receptor by the novel cytokine IL-15. EMBO J. *13*, 2822 (1994).

155 J. Giri, S. Kumaki, M. Ahdieh et al.: Identification and cloning of a novel IL-15 binding protein that is structurally related to the alpha chain of the IL-2 receptor. EMBO J. *14*, 3654 (1995).

156 R.J. Armitage, B.M. Macduff, J. Eisenman et al.: IL-15 has stimulatory activity for the induction of B cell proliferation and differentiation. J. Immunol. *15*, 483 (1995).

157 W.M. Lewko, T.L. Smith, D.J. Bowman et al.: Interleukin-15 and the growth of tumor derived activated T-cells. Cancer Biother. *10*, 13 (1995).

158 W. Munger, S.Q. DeJoy, R. Jeyaseelan Sr. et al.: Studies evaluating the antitumor activity and toxicity of interleukin-15, a new T cell growth factor: Comparison with interleukin-2. Cellular Immunol. *165*, 289 (1995).

159 L.S. Quinn, K.L. Haugk and K.H. Grabstein: Interleukin-15: A novel anabolic cytokine for skeletal muscle. Endocrinology *126*, 3669 (1995).

160 E.C. Borden: Interferons. In: Cancer Medicine. J.F. Holland et al. (eds). 1993. Lea & Feabiger: Philadelphia.

161 S.E. Grossberg: Interferons: an overview of their biological and biochemical properties. In Mechanism of Interferon Actions. L.M. Pfeffer (ed). 1987. CRC Press, Inc: Boca Raton. p. 137.

162 A.A. Branca and C. Baglioni: Evidence that types I and II interferons have different receptors. Nature *294*, 768 (1981).

163 M. Aguet, Z. Dembic and G. Merlin: Molecular cloning and expression of the human interferon-g receptor. Cell *55*, 273 (1988).

164 R.D. Schreiber and M.A. Farrar: The biology and biochemistry of interferon-gamma and its receptor. Gastroenterol. Jpn. *4*, 88 (1993).

165 J.L. Pace and S.W. Russell: Activation of mouse macrophages for tumor cell killing. Quantitave analysis of interactions between lymphokine and lipopolysaccharide. J. Immunol. *126*, 1863 (1981).

166 L. Reid, N. Minato, I. Gresser et al.: Influence of antimouse interferon serum on the growth and metastasis of tumor cells persistently infected by virus and of human prostatic tumors in athymic mice. Proc. Natl. Acad. Sci. *78*, 1171 (1981).

167 I. Gresser, F. Belardelli, C. Maury et al.: Injection of mice with antibody to interferon enhances the growth of murine transplantable tumors. J. Exp. Med. *158*, 2095 (1983).

168 A.E. Maluish: Effects of recombinant interferon-alpha on immune function in cancer patients. J. Biol. Response Mod. *2*, 470 (1983).

169 M. Fellous, U. Nir, D. Wallach et al.: Interferon-dependent induction of mRNA for the major histocompatability antigens in human fibroblasts and lymphoblastoid cell lines. Proc. Natl. Acad. Sci. *79*, 3082, 1982.

170 R.C. van Schie, H.G. Verstraten, W.J. Tax et al.: Effect of rIFN-gamma on antibody-mediated cytotoxicity via human monocyte IgG Fc receptor II (CD32). Scand. J. Immunol. *36*, 385 (1992).

171 A.A. te Velde, R. de Waal Malefijt, R.J. Huijbens et al.: IL-10 stimulates monocyte Fc gamma R surface expression and cytotoxic activity. Distinct regulation of antibody-dependent cellular cytotoxicity by IFN-gamma, IL-4, and IL-10. J. Immunol. *149*, 4048 (1992).

172 W.M. Vuist, M.J. Visseren, M. Otsen et al.: Enhancement of the antibody-dependent cellular cytotoxicity of human peripheral blood lymphocytes with interleukin-2 and interferon alpha. Cancer Immunol. Immunother. *36*, 163 (1993).

173 V. Jendrossek, A.M. Peters, S. Buth et al.: Improvement of superoxide production in monocytes from patients with chronic granulomatous disease by recombinant cytokines. Blood *81*, 2131 (1993).

174 M.J. Robertson, T.J. Manley, C. Donahue et al.: Costimulatory signals are required for optimal proliferation of human natural killer cells. J. Immunol. *150*, 1705 (1993).

175 M.J. Robertson and J. Ritz: Biology and clinical relevance of human natural killer cells. Blood *76*, 2421 (1990).

176 J.R. Wunderlich and R.J. Hodes: Principles of Tumor Immunity: Biology of Cellular Immune Responses, in: Biologic Therapy of Cancer, V.T. Devita, S. Hellman, S.A. Rosenberg (eds). 1991. J. B. Lippincott: New York. p. 14.

177 N. Minato, L. Reid, H. Cantor et al.: Mode regulation of natural killer cell activity by intereferon. J. Exp. Med. *152*, 124 (1980).

178 C. Losinno, B.D. Wines, T.G. Johns et al.: Natural killer cell activity against cultured melanoma cells: a dye-reduction technique with studies on augmented activity by interferon subtypes. Nat. Immun. *11*, 215 (1992).

179 M.A. Giedlund, H. Orn and H. Wigzell: Enhanced NK cell activity in mice injected with interferon and interferon inducers. Nature *273*, 759 (1987).

180 E. Saksela, T. Timonen and K. Cantell: Cellular Interactions in the augmentation of human NK activity by interferon. Ann. N.Y. Acad. Sci. *350*, 102 (1980).

181 R.M. Welsh, K. Karre, M. Hansson et al: Interferon-mediated protection of normal and tumor target cells against lysis by mouse natural killer cells. J. Immunol. *1*, 219 (1981).

182 C. Garbe and K. Krasagakis: Effects of interferons and cytokines on melanoma cells. J. Invest. Derm. *100*, 239S (1993).

183 H. Matsuyama, S. Yoshihiro, Y. Ohmoto et al.: Direct and indirect effects of human interferon alpha on renal cell carcinoma: a new in vitro assay system for evaluating cytokine-mediated antitumor effects. Cancer Immunol. Immunother. *37*, 84 (1993).

184 Z. Reiter, S. Tomson, O.N. Ozes et al.: Combination treatment of 2-chlorodeoxyadenosine and type I interferon on hairy cell leukemia-like cells: cytotoxic effect and MHC-unrestricted killer cell regulation. Blood *81*, 1699 (1993).

185 E.F. Meurs, J. Galabru, G.N. Barber et al.: Tumor suppressor function of the interferon-induced double-stranded RNA-activated protein kinase. Proc. Natl. Acad. Sci. *90*, 232 (1993).

186   R. Godbout, J. Miyakoshi, K.D. Dobler et al.: Lack of expression of tumor-suppressor genes in human malignant glioma cell lines. Oncogene 7, 1879 (1992).

187   O.I. Olopade, D.L. Buchhagen, K. Malik et al.: Homozygous loss of the interferon genes defines the critical region on 9p that is deleted in lung cancers. Cancer Res. 53 (Suppl. 10), 2410 (1993).

188   C. Natoli, C. Garufi, N. Tinari et al.: Dynamic test with recombinant interferon-alpha-2b: effect on 90K and other tumour-associated antigens in cancer patients without evidence of disease. Br. J. Cancer 67, 564 (1993).

189   R.L. Scher, W.M. Koch and W.J. Richtsmeier: Induction of the intercellular adhesion molecule (ICAM-1) on squamous cell carcinoma by interferon gamma. Arch. Otolaryngol. Head Neck Surg. 119, 432 (1993).

190   H. Takahashi, Y. Okai, R.J. Paxton et al.: Differential regulation of carcinoembryonic antigen and biliary glycoprotein by gamma-interferon. Cancer Res. 53, 1612 (1993).

191   N. Weidner, J.P. Semple, W.R. Welch et al.: Tumor angiogenesis and metastasis – correlation in invasive breast carcinoma. N. Engl. J. Med. 324, 1 (1991).

192   N. Weidner, J. Folkman, F. Dozza et al.: Tumor angiogenesis: a new significant and independent prognostic indicator in early-stage breast carcinoma [see comments]. J. Natl. Cancer Inst. 84, 1875 (1992).

193   I. Saiki, K. Sato, Y.C. Yoo et al.: Inhibition of tumor-induced angiogenesis by the administration of recombinant interferon-gamma followed by a synthetic lipid-A subunit analogue (GLA-60). Intl. J. Cancer 51, 641 (1992).

194   J. Folkman and D. Ingber: Inhibition of angiogenesis. Semin. Cancer Biol. 3, 89 (1992).

195   C.W. White: Treatment of hemangiomatosis with recombinant interferon alfa. Semin. Hematol. 27, 15 (1990).

196   R.K. Maheshwari, V. Srikantan, D. Bhartiya et al.: Differential effects of interferon gamma and alpha on in vitro model of angiogenesis. J. Cell. Physiol. 146, 164 (1991).

197   D.C. Billington: Angiogenesis and its inhibition: potential new therapies in oncology and non-neoplastic diseases. Drug Des. Discov. 8, 3 (1991).

198   J.R. Quesada, J. Reuben, J.T. Manning et al.: Alpha interferon for the induction of remission in hairy-cell leukemia. N. Engl. J. Med. 310, 15 (1984).

199   R. Dadmarz, T. Evans, D. Secher et al.: Hairy cells possess more interferon receptors than other lymphoid cell types. Leukemia 1, 357 (1987).

200   J.D. Scharzmeier, M. Schwabe, L. Wagner et al.: Effect of alpha-2-interferon on hairy cells and cell lines. A role for type I interferon receptors and RNA synthesis. Leukemia 1, 361 (1987).

201   M. Talpaz, H.M. Kantarjain, K.B. McCerdie et al.: Clinical investigation of human alpha interferon in chronic myelogenous leukemia. Blood 69, 1280, (1987).

202   R. Kurzrock, M. Talpaz, H.M. Kantarjain et al.: Therapy of chronic myelogenous leukemia with recombinant interferon-gamma. Blood 70, 943 (1987).

203   B. Maxwell, M. Talpaz and J.U. Gutterman: Down regulation of peripheral blood cell interferon receptors in chronic myelogenous leukemia patients undergoing human interferon (HuIFN) therapy. Intl. J. Cancer. 36, 23 (1985).

204   M. Rosenblum, B. Maxwell, M. Talpaz et al.: In vitro sensitivity and resistance of chronic myelogenous leukemia cells to alpha interferon: Correlation with receptor binding and induction of 2'5' oligoadenylate synthetase. Cancer Res. 46, 4848 (1986).

205   E. Knight, Jr., E.D. Anton, D. Fahey et al.: Interferon regulates c myc gene expression in Daudi cells at the post-transcriptional level. Proc. Natl. Acad. Sci. USA 82, 1151 (1985).

206 J.R. Quesada, D.A. Swanson, A. Trindade et al.: Renal Cell Carcinoma: Antitumor effects of leukocyte interferon. Cancer Res. *43*, 940 (1983).

207 J.M. Kirkwood, J.E. Harris, R. Vera et al.: A randomized study of low and high doses of leukocyte alpha-interferon in metastatic renal cell carcinoma: The American Cancer Society Collaborative Trial. Cancer Res. *45*, 863 (1985).

208 T. Umeda and T. Niijima: Phase II study of alpha interferon on renal cell carcinoma. Cancer *58*, 1231 (1986).

209 H.B. Muss, J.J. Costanzi, R. Leavitt et al.: Recombinant alfa interferon in renal cell carcinoma: A randomised trial of two routes of administration. J. Clin. Oncol. *5*, 286 (1987).

210 Figlin, R.A., J.B. deKernion, E. Mukamel et al.: Recombinant interferon alfa-2a in metastatic renal cell carcinoma. J. Clin. Oncol. *6*, 1604 (1988).

211 D. Vugrin, L. Hood, W. Taylor and J. Laslo: Phase II study of human lymphoblastoid Interferon in patients with advanced renal carcinoma. Cancer Treat. Reports *69*, 817 (1985).

212 E.T. Creagan, J.C. Buckner, R.G. Hahn et al.: An evaluation of recombinant leucocyte interferon with aspirin in patients with metastatic renal cell cancer. Cancer *61*, 1787 (1988).

213 R.L. Miller, R.G. Stess, J.W. Clark et al.: Randomized trial of recombinant alpha 2b-interferon with or without indomethacin in patients with metastatic malignant melanoma. Cancer Res. *49*, 1871 (1989).

214 S.D. Fosså, G. Lehne, R. Gunderson et al.: Recombinant interferon alpha-2A combined with prednisone in metastatic renal-cell carcinoma: treatment results, serum interferon levels and the development of antibodies. Intl. J. Cancer *50*, 868 (1992).

215 T.F. Logan, M.S. Ernstoff, J.M. Kirkwood, B. Gerich, D. Friberg, T. Whiteside, B. Eddy, P. Witman, J. Schindler, R.B. Herberman and S. Reich: Changes in natural killer cell (NK) phenotype in peripheral blood (PB) of patients (PT) with renal cell carcinoma and melanoma treated with recombinant interferon gamma (IFN-gamma). Proc. Am. Assoc. Cancer Res. *78*, 2520A (1987).

216 M.B. Garnick, S.D. Reich and B.E.A. Maxwell: Phase I/II study of recombinant interferon gamma in advanced renal cell carcinoma. J. Urol. *139*, 251 (1988).

217 J.R. Quesada, R. Kurzrock, S.A. Sherwin et al.: Phase II studies of recombinant human interferon gamma in metastatic renal cell carcinoma. J. Biol. Response Mod. *6*, 20 (1987).

218 J.J. Rinehart, L. Malspeis, D. Young et al.: Phase I/II Trial of human recombinant interferon gamma in renal cell carcinoma. J. Biol. Response Mod. *5*, 300 (1986).

219 U. Otto, S. Conrad, A.W. Schneider et al.: Recombinant interferon gamma in the treatment of metastatic renal cell carcinoma. Drug Res. *38*, 1658 (1988).

220 W. Aulitzky, G. Gastl, W.E. Aulitzky et al.: Successful treatment of metastatic renal cell carcinoma with a biologically active dose of recombinant interferon-gamma. J. Clin. Oncol. *7*, 1875 (1989).

221 U. Bruntsch, P.H. de Mulder, W.W. ten Bokkel Huinink et al.: Phase II study of recombinant human interferon-gamma in metastatic renal cell carcinoma. J. Biol. Response Mod. *9*, 335 (1990).

222 C.W. Czarniecki, C.W. Fennie, D.B. Powers et al.: Synergistic antiviral and antiproliferative activities of E coli derived human alpha, beta and gamma interferons. J. Virol. *49*, 490 (1984).

223 K. Foon, J. Doroshow, E. Bonnem et al.: A prospective randomized trial of alpha2b interferon/gamma interferon or the combination in advanced metastatic renal cell carcinoma. J. Biol. Response Mod. *7*, 540 (1988).

224 J.R. Quesada, L. Evans, S.R. Saks et al.: Recombinant interferon alpha and gamma in combination as treatment for metastatic renal cell carcinoma. J. Biol. Response Mod. 7, 234 (1988).

225 M.S. Ernstoff, S. Nair, R.R. Bahnson et al.: A phase IA trial of sequential administration recombinant DNA-produced interferons: combination recombinant interferon gamma and recombinant interferon alfa in patients with metastatic renal cell carcinoma. J. Clin. Oncol. 8, 1637 (1990).

226 M.S. Ernstoff, W. Gooding, S. Nair et al.: Immunological effects of treatment with sequential administration of recombinant interferon gamma and alpha in patients with metastatic renal cell carcinoma during a phase I trial. Cancer Res. 52, 851 (1992).

227 J.P. Kuebler, G.A. Godette, D.J. Bock et al.: Synergistic effects of vinblastine and recombinant interferon-beta on renal tumor cell lines. J. Interferon Res. 10, 281 (1990).

228 R.A. Figlin, J.B. deKernion, J. Maldazys et al.: Treatment of renal cell carcinoma with alpha(human leukocyte) interferon and vinblastine in combination: A phase I-II trial. Cancer Treat. Reports 69, 263 (1985).

229 S.D. Fosså and S.T. de Garis: Further experience with recombinant interferon alfa-2a with vinblastine in metastatic renal cell carcinoma: a progress report. Intl. J. Cancer Suppl 1, 36 (1987).

230 M.R. Sertoli, I. Brunetti, A. Ardizzoni et al.: Recombinant alpha-2a interferon plus vinblastine in the treatment of metastatic renal cell carcinoma. Am. J. Clin. Oncol. 12, 43 (1989).

231 S.D. Fosså, N. Raabe and B. Moe: Recombinant interferon-alpha with or without vinblastine in metastatic renal carcinoma. Results of a randomised phase II study. Br. J. Urol. 64, 468 (1989).

232 S. Palmeri, V. Gebbia, A. Russo et al.: Vinblastine and interferon-alpha-2a regimen in the treatment of metastatic renal cell carcinoma. Tumori 76, 64 (1990).

233 D.L. Trump, P.M. Ravdin, E.C. Borden et al.: Interferon-alpha-n1 and continuous infusion vinblastine for treatment of advanced renal cell carcinoma. J. Biol. Response Mod. 9, 108 (1990).

234 L.P. Kellokumpu and E. Nordman: Recombinant interferon-alpha 2a and vinblastine in advanced renal cell cancer: a clinical phase I-II study. J. Biol. Response Mod. 9, 439 (1990).

235 M. Rizzo, R. Bartoletti, C. Selli et al.: Interferon alpha-2a and vinblastine in the treatment of metastatic renal carcinoma. Eur. Urol. 16, 271 (1989).

236 O. Merimsky and S. Chaitchik: Interferon plus vinblastine in renal carcinoma patients who had failed on interferon alone [letter]. Eur. J. Cancer 26, 8 (1990).

237 O. Merimsky, B.I. Shnider and S. Chaitchik: Does vinblastine add to the potency of alpha interferon in the treatment of renal cell carcinoma? Mol. Biother. 3, 34 (1991).

238 A. Sella, C.J. Logothers, K. Fitz et al.: Phase II study of interferon-alpha and chemotherapy (5-fluorouracil and mitomycin C) in metastatic renal cell cancer. J. Urol. 147, 573 (1992).

239 H.J. Konig, W. Gutmann and J. Weissmuller: Ifosfamide, vindesine and recombinant alpha-interferon combination chemotherapy for metastatic renal cell carcinoma. J. Cancer Res. Clin. Oncol. 117, S221 (1991).

240 A. Falcone, C. Cianci, S. Ricci et al.: Alpha-2B-interferon plus floxuridine in metastatic renal cell carcinoma. A phase I-II study. Cancer Diag. Treat. Res. 72, 564 (1993).

241   H.B. Muss: Renal Cell Carcinoma. In: Biologic Therapy of Cancer, V.T. Devita, S. Hellman, S.A. Rosenberg (eds). 1991. J.B. Lippincott: New York. p. 298–309.

242   L.M. Minasian, R.J. Motzer, L. Gluck et al.: Interferon alfa-2a in advanced renal cell carcinoma: treatment results and survival in 159 patients with long-term follow-up. J. Clin. Oncol. *11*, 1368 (1993).

243   S.E. Salmon, B.G. Durie, L. Young et al.: Effects of cloned human leukocyte interferons in the human tumor stem cell assay. J. Clin. Oncol. *1*, 217 (1983).

244   P.P. Trotta and S.D. Harrison, Jr.: Evaluation of the anti-tumor activity recombinant human gamma interferon employing human melanoma xenografts in athymic nude mice. Cancer Res. *47*, 5347 (1987).

245   M.S. Ernstoff, D. Chee, G. Witman et al.: The expression of p97, kd250, DR and beta-2 microglobulin cell surface antigen in cycling melanoma cells in culture (Abstract). Clin. Res. *32*, 345A (1984).

246   J.M. Kirkwood and M.S. Ernstoff: Melanoma: therapeutic options with recombinant interferons Semin. Oncol. *12*, 7 (1985).

247   J.M. Kirkwood, M.H. Stawderman, M.S. Ernstoff et al.: Interferon alpha-2b adjuvant therapy of high risk resected cutaneous melanoma: The Eastern Cooperative Oncology Group Trial EST1684. J. Clin. Oncol. *14*, 7 (1996).

248   B. Beutler, D. Greenwald, J.D. Hulmes et al: Identity of tumour necrosis factor and the macrophage-secreted factor 'cachectin'. Nature *316*, 552 (1985).

249   K.J. Tracey and A. Cerami: Tumor necrosis factor: an updated review of its biology. Crit .Care Med. *21* (10 Suppl), S415 (1993).

250   A.S. Dofferhoff, E. Vellenga, P.C. Limburg et al.: Tumour necrosis factor (cachectin) and other cytokines in septic shock: a review of the literature. Nether. J. Med. *39*, 45 (1991).

251   K.J. Tracey and A. Cerami: Metabolic responses to cachectin/TNF. A brief review. Ann. NY. Acad. Sci. *587*, 325 (1990).

252   P. Vassalli: The pathophysiology of tumor necrosis factor. Ann. Rev. Immunol. *10*, 411 (1992).

253   B.B. Aggarwal and J. Vilcek (eds.): Tumor Necrosis Factor: Structure, Function and Mechanisms of Action. 1992. New York: Marcel Dekker.

254   E. Ottaviani, E. Caselgrandi and C. Franceschi : Cytokines and evolution: *in vitro* effects of IL-1 alpha, IL-1 beta, TNF-alpha and TNF-beta on an ancestral type of stress response. Biochem. Biophys. Res. Commun. *207*, 288 (1995).

255   D. Adamthwaite and M.A. Cooley : CD8+ T-cell subsets defined by expression of CD45 isoforms differ in their capacity to produce IL-2, IFN-gamma and TNF-beta. Immunol. *81*, 253 (1994).

256   C. Jassoy, T. Harrer, T. Rosenthal et al.: Human immunodeficiency virus type 1-specific cytotoxic T lymphocytes release gamma interferon, tumor necrosis factor alpha (TNF-alpha), and TNF-beta when they encounter their target antigens. J. Virol. *67*, 2844 (1993).

Progress in Drug Research, Vol. 47 (E. Jucker, Ed.)
© 1996 Birkhäuser Verlag, Basel (Switzerland)

Alternative therapeutic modalities.
Alternative medicine

By Pushkar N. Kaul

Clark Atlanta University, Brawley Drive at Fair Str. S.W., Atlanta, Georgia 30314, USA

1   Introduction

Commonly known as Alternative Medicine (AM) in the current literature, treatment of diseases by approaches other than those of allopathic or conventional medicine has feverishly caught on in the United States of America (USA) during the current decade. Public and political pressures on the government to address the escalating costs of health care under the conventional system, which incidentally cannot be afforded by over forty million Americans, finally resulted in the establishment of the Office of Alternative Medicine (OAM) early 1992 within the well-known National Institutes of Health (NIH). With an initial token budget of $ 2 million, the OAM was charged with examining and promoting the alternative therapeutic modalities from acupressure to acupuncture to yoga, a formidable task indeed, if the medical and scientific communities are to assess these modalities the same way as new treatments or procedures are viewed under the rigid guidelines of the U.S. Federal Food and Drug Administration (FDA).

The media in the USA appears to describe AM as something new. However, those in the field of pharmaceutical and medical sciences are well aware of the fact that use of naturally occurring medicinal plants (herbs) to treat ailments has been practiced ever since the cave man era. In fact the origin of most of the allopathic drugs and surgical practices can be traced back to Ayurveda, the system of medicine practiced in India eight thousand years B.C. [1]. Perhaps it is more appropriate to call this current AM movement as a revisitation to nature or "back to nature", rather than new approaches to treating diseases. Some authors have termed it as "complimentary medicine" [2], but the term is misleading since an allopathic physician would not allow simultaneous use of an ayurvedic or homeopathic treatment he is neither knowledgable about nor has any faith in.

There is no denying that aggressive application of basic scientific knowledge, methods and tools to the ancient systems of medical practices helped evolve the modern science-based allopathic medical practice. It was the Flexner Report of 1910 which led to a total reorganization of medical education in the USA, and which in turn helped develop an upgraded version of medicine in the current health care system [3]. Emphasizing the basic physiological and biochemical processes in health and disease, the allopathic medicine made exponential strides during the twentieth century in both the American and the European continents. Finally, the medical professional organizations, e.g., American Medical Association, adopted, endorsed and secured this allopathic system of medical practice [4].

Critical analyses of the overall effectiveness of modern medicine reveals that it is very effective for treating trauma, infections of various types, and surgeries, but is not good for treating chronic illnesses which constitute 85% of the total health care costs in the USA [5]. Historically, until the fourth decade of this century, health was always believed to be a balance or harmony and disease an imbalance/disharmony of body and mind. Even the father of modern medicine, Hippocrates, believed more in hygiene, calm and balanced mental state, proper diet, exercise, and sound environment at home as well as at work, the key elements commonly found in Ayurvedic medicine of India and Chinese herbal medicine [6]. It is only after the antibacterials such as sulpha drugs and antibiotics appeared on the medical scene that feverish search for new drugs began for treating diseases and/or symptoms. If one takes a critical look at all of the allopathic treatments available, it would be very difficult to find a drug, other than antibiotics and vaccines, which can truly cure a disease. Most drugs treat symptoms rather than the cause, especially when we deal with chronic diseases involving metabolic machinery of the body.

The USA is probably the only country in the world that resisted the spread of any alternative approaches to treating diseases during the latter half of this century. This is partially due to very rigid FDA regulations and partly because the American Medical Association is quite powerful in protecting the interests of its members who are almost entirely allopathic physicians. However, some startling developments have occurred in recent years. The prevalence and patterns of use of unconventional medicine (AM) studied and reported upon by Eisenberg et al. [7] reveal that over 30% of Americans choose to use AM. One of the reasons given by patients for their decision was the uncontrolled escalating costs of health care under modern medicine which has been indulging in extensive and at times unnecessary clinical diagnostic testings and expensive drugs, driven largely by the physician's fear of malpractice suits that prevailed during the seventies and eighties.

The current wave of spreading acceptance of AM in the USA is too strong to be stopped. It is therefore mandatory for the biomedical research and the health care communities to begin taking a pragmatic, unbiased and in-depth look at some of the more established and practiced alternative modalities of medicine. This review is an attempt to collate the basic concepts and the available evidence in support or otherwise of such modalities.

2   Alternative therapeutic modalities

Alternative medicine includes over 150 different approaches from "acupressure" to "yoga" to "zero balancing" [8]. In this review, however, only those approaches will be discussed which have either a very long history of successful practice or are amenable to scientific reasoning acceptable within the knowledge base today.

2.1   Acupuncture

According to ancient Chinese medical practice, insertion and twisting of fine needles at specific points in the body to relieve pain and other disease symptoms is called acupuncture. A Korean team of researchers in the sixties demonstrated evidence that in addition to the vascular and lymphatic systems there exists a specialized system of ducts termed "meridians"[9]. A French scientist, de Vernejoul [10], is believed to have further confirmed the existence of meridians by injecting radioactive isotopes at specific points along the meridians called acupoints and subsequently finding that the isotopes traveled 30 cm along the acupunctured meridians. Isotopes injected into the blood vessels at random did not show the type of specific distribution found in the meridians. Since then, it has been shown that a relationship exists between the acupuncture points, the meridians, and the electrical activity of the body. Studies have shown that acupoints have a higher level of conductance than the non-acupuncture sites [11]. Becker and colleagues [12] have since demonstrated that electrical currents do flow along the meridians and that at least 25% of all acupoints exist on these ducts. They suggest that the inserted needles interfere in the flow of this electric current and thereby block the afferent component of the pain circuit [13].

Although used as a part of the Chinese system of medicine since the 27th century B.C., acupuncture came to North America around the end of 19th century A.D. when a Canadian physician, Sir William Osler (1849–1919) used it to treat lower back pain [8]. It was only in 1972 that acupuncture began to be known in the USA when a journalist, James Reston, accompanying U.S. President Nixon on his visit to China, underwent an appendectomy in Beijing under acupuncture-induced anesthesia. Subsequent formalized medical exchange between the USA and China the same year resulted in 30 Chinese acupuncturists visiting the University of California at Los Angeles (UCLA) School of Medicine. For the past 25 years, the UCLA pain center has been using acupuncture as one of its primary treatments for pain [8].

The World Health Organization (WHO) has listed over 100 different physical conditions treatable by acupuncture, including narcotic addiction, myopia, duodenal ulcer, trigeminal neuralgia, bursitis, osteoarthritis, and pains of all other sorts [14]. In the USA today, there are 30 schools of acupuncture providing a curriculum of 2,400 hours of instruction over a period of 3–4 years. The prerequisites for admission to these schools include anatomy, physiology and biochemistry. Currently, there are over 5,000 acupuncture practitioners. All of these developments have occurred only since 1972.

2.1.1   Clinical evaluation of acupuncture

The most common use of acupuncture is in treating pain. In a study on 20,000 patients at UCLA clinics, acupuncture reduced the severity as well as frequency of headaches, migraines and muscle tensions [15]. In another study involving 204 patients with chronic pain, 74% showed a significant pain relief for over 3 months following acupuncture [16]. Sodipo [17] has reported that younger patients with various types of pain respond better to acupuncture.

Although the exact mechanism of analgesic action of acupuncture is not known, it has been demonstrated that release of cortisol, endorphins and enkephalins is stimulated during acupuncture [18]. There is also evidence that acupuncture influences the synthesis and distribution of neurotransmitters and neuromodulators, and that this reduces the impact of afferent impulse arising from the abnoxious pain stimulus [19, 20].

Holder received the prestigious Albert Schweitzer Prize in medicine for his work demonstrating over 80% success rate in treating withdrawal symptoms of addicts consuming nicotine, alcohol, cocaine and heroin [21]. In 1993, there were 300 acupuncture-based substance abuse programs in the USA and similar detoxication programs in Canada, Mexico, United Kingdom, Sweden, Germany, Hungary, Romania, Spain and Saudi Arabia [6]. Resch and Ernst [22] have analyzed 39 clinical studies on acupuncture published between 1987 and March 1994. They believe that most of the reported studies lacked good designs and controls, and that perhaps that is why acupuncture has not been universally accepted. However, their interpretation is contrary to the experiences at the UCLA pain center in Los Angeles, California.

Studies currently in progress under the funding from OAM of NIH may further substantiate the clinical effectiveness of acupuncture and possibly also the mechanism of its action, which can only further validate this alternative therapeutic modality and pave a way for its universal adoption by the allopathic, or better stated, by the health care systems of the twenty-first century.

2.2   Ayurveda

Derived from the Sanskrit words 'Ayur' meaning life and 'Veda' meaning knowledge, ayurveda is the art and science of the holistic system of
medicine practiced in India since the Aryan time, eight thousand years
B.C.[1]. The oldest system of medicine known to man, ayurveda is recognized by WHO and is still practiced around the world [23]. In India, there
are over 300,000 practicing ayurvedic physicians and over 100 ayurvedic
colleges providing a five-year degree program. Recently, a revised version, Maharishi Ayurved, was introduced globally under the direction of
Maharishi Mahesh Yogi [24, 25], with his headquarters in Holland.
Ayurveda emphasizes a balanced harmony between the mind, the body
and the spirit. The diagnosis of ill-health is based on the concept that all
people belong to three metabolic types known in Sanskrit as 'Vata', 'Pitta'
and 'Kapha'. Most people actually fall into categories of combinations of
these three traits in varying proportions. By approximation, the three types
can be compared to the body types thin, muscular and fat, respectively.
Each trait is known as 'dosha', and together they constitute the ayurvedic
concept of 'tridosha'. The quality of pulse and its rate, the texture of tongue,
the appearance of nails and skin, and urinalysis are used to support the
diagnosis of the tridosha body type.
Once the mind-body-spirit imbalance (disease) is diagnosed, the treatment may call for 'shodan' (cleansing and detoxication), or 'shaman' (pal-
liation), or 'rasayana' (rejuvenation), and/or 'satvajaya' (mental and spir-
itual hygiene), or all of these procedures in sequence or in some combination. The cleansing and detoxication involves a process of rinsing and
purging the stomach by emesis, the bowels by purgatives and oil lavage,
the rectum by enema, the blood by herbal tonics, and the nasal passage
by douching. These five procedures together are known as 'panchakarma'.
An herbal oil massage of the skin is also a part of the total package. The
palliative treatment, 'shaman', is usually a combination of the use of herbs,
fasting, chanting of certain words or phrases repeatedly, deep breathing,
physical exercises, and meditation. This treatment may be prescribed to
a patient that is either too weak or too ill to withstand the more aggressive 'panchakarma'.
Rejuvenation, usually done after the 'panchakarma', is a process of physiological tune up. By using ayurvedic herbal products in the form of pills,
powders, jellies, jams, etc., overall vitality and the immune system of the
body are strengthened. Ayurvedic medicinal plants and their products,
described in books called the 'Samhitas' compiled by ayurvedic physicians
Charaka and Sushruta around 1500 B.C., number in the thousands, includ-

ing *Rauwolfia serpentina* and *Digitalis purpurea* well known to the Western world [26]. Rasayanas are made from those described herbs by specific procedures under well-controlled conditions of collection, drying, pharmaceutical processing and preservation.

Interestingly, an all out effort and commitment on the part of one Swiss drug company during the late forties on just one ayurvedic herb, *B. serpentina*, led to the isolation of two sets of alkaloids represented by reserpine and rescinamine, the former a very potent antihypertensive agent and the latter a potent antipsychotic drug. Rauwolfia roots have been used in ayurvedic medicine for thousands of years to treat both hypertension and insanity.

2.2.1 *Pharmacology and clinical evaluation*

Sharma et al. [27] have described two 'rasayanas', Maharishi Amrit Kalash 4 and 5 (MAK-4, MAK-5) studied at various universities in the USA. Both of these products were found to reduce chemically-induced mammary carcinoma up to 88% in animals. The MAK-5 was found to enhance lymphoproliferative response in antigen-stimulated animals and to also reduce thrombocyte aggregation induced by adenosine diphosphate, collagen and epinephrine [28]. Other studies reported that MAK-4 and MAK-5 showed protection against adriamycin-induced lipid peroxidase activity in the rat liver microsomal preparations and against lethality in mice [29–31]. They also exhibited free radical scavenging [32], antineoplastic [33–37], and antioxidant [38–40] properties. Clinical studies on these 'rasayanas' have shown that they cause an increase in the substance-P concentration in plasma, suggesting a reduction in psychiatric depression and/or distress [41], and an increase in visual discrimination [42]. Detailed reviews on Maharishi Ayurveda, a revitalized version of ancient ayurveda, by Sharma [43, 44] provide a fairly good account of the essentials of ayurvedic medicine. A good review on some of the ayurvedic herbal preparations has also been published [45].

Mental hygiene, 'satvajaya', is an essential part of ayurvedic approaches to treating disease. A healthy body is recognized as being in total harmony with mind and vice versa. The mind is regarded as consciousness based on physiology rather than some abstraction. Stimulating consciousness of the patient through mental techniques to release and reduce stress is one of the more common approaches used by ayurvedic physician. One of the well-publicized techniques of this type is the transcendental meditation (TM) developed by Maharishi Mahesh Yogi and being taught globally. Several hundred scientific studies have been carried out on TM during the past two decades [25]. Evidence has been put forth suggesting metabolic changes characteristic of a "restful alertness" [46]. Increased longevity, reduced anxiety, reduction of blood pressure and of cholesterol levels in hypertensives are some of the other benefits of TM [47].

International conferences on ayurvedic medicine have taken place in recent years in India, Brazil, Poland, Hungary and Czechoslovakia. In Moscow, Russia, the Ministry of Public Health Research Center for Preventive Medicine looks after the Institute of Ayurveda where more than one thousand Russian physicians have received training in ayurvedic medicine [48].

It thus appears that ayurvedic medicine, though overshadowed by the allopathic system during the past two centuries, is experiencing a global revival. Perhaps the extensive and wider clinical investigations currently under way or in the planning stage in various countries will yield enough clinical data to convince the skeptics of the real value of this alternative therapeutic modality.

2.3   Biofeedback training

Prior to 1962, most of the allopathic physicians and scientists believed that autonomically regulated functions, e.g., cardiac and vascular tones, gastrointestinal activity, brain waves, etc., could not be affected by voluntary attempts. In fact the biomedical scientists in the USA would laugh at any claims made by practitioners of yoga, called 'yogis' in India, that through meditational methods they could voluntarily control their heartbeat, breathing and other vital activities. It was only in 1962 that Barbara Brown published the first book on Biofeedback Training based on her own experiments in California and those of Greens at the Menninger Foundation in Kansas, in which the EEG patterns of subjects were monitored and visually fed back to them in order to have the subjects recreate the patterns by voluntarily reprocessing their thoughts [6]. Since the sixties, considerable research in this field has led to a wide acceptance of biofeedback training as a mode of treating hypertension, asthma, muscular dysfunction and various gastrointestinal disorders. In the USA, both the AMA and the health insurance companies for reimbursement purposes accept biofeedback as a treatment modality for all stress-related disorders.

In principle, the person using biofeedback technique makes use of a biomedical device which sends out visual and/or auditory signals relative to a particular thought or relaxation mode. By learning to recreate the thought pattern or any other body activity with the help of the signal-based feedback of the monitored physiological activity, one can subtly learn to control heart rate and other autonomic activities [49]. The skill once learnt is retained by the subject for daily use. The more one practices with it, the more perfection one achieves.

Although the Western world calls this idea of learning to control visceral organ functions new [6], its practice can be traced back thousands of years B.C. in the ayurvedic system of medicine. Moreover, our current knowledge of physiology and biochemistry of the brain clearly shows that various autonomic control centers in the medulla oblongata are controlled by the hypothalamus, which in turn is affected by cerebral cortex of the frontal lobe believed to be responsible for reasoning, biological intelligence, intuition and will. Thus, there clearly is a physiological basis for the biofeedback training as a valid, and perhaps the most natural, approach to treating disorders amenable to it.

2.4   Chelation therapy

Chelation therapy involves removal of divalent metals, e.g., lead, calcium etc., from the circulating blood by intravenous infusion of ethylenediamine tetraacetic acid (EDTA) that forms a metal-complex chelate which is then excreted via the urine. Although quite successful in treating lead and other heavy metal poisonings, its wider use to treat atherosclerosis and other diseases remains questionable.

Chelation therapy has been used relatively safely on over half a million chronically ill patients in the USA for the last five decades [50], but to date no formal approval for the use of EDTA for such diseases has come forth from the FDA. In spite of this, there are at least one thousand physicians who use chelation therapy for cardiovascular diseases.

2.4.1   Clinical evaluation of chelation
Based on a treatment protocol developed by the American College of Advancement of Medicine (ACAM) and the American Board of Chelation Therapy, the FDA approved clinical trials, in 1993, to assess the safety and tolerance of EDTA. The final status as to the general use of EDTA remains to be determined. The protocol, however, involves administration of 50 mg/kg of EDTA in 0.5 to 1.0 liter of saline, containing 20 g of ascorbic acid and a reasonable amount of B group of vitamins, as an intravenous drip over 3.5 to 4.0 hours, up to a total of 20 to 30 such slow infusions being a recommended regimen.

The largest earlier study involved 2,870 cardiac patients with peripheral- and cerebro-vascular diseases who received NaMgEDTA over three months [51]. The authors claimed that 93% of the patients with coronary blockage showed a significant improvement. No serious side effects were observed in any of the patients. A subsequent and the only well-controlled double-blind study on EDTA was carried out in New Zealand on 32 atherosclerotic patients with plaques in the leg arteries [52, 53]. The ACAM protocol for chelation therapy was used in the study conducted in 10 weeks. The changes in the plaques, if any, were measured by X ray. No conclusive evidence for the plaque reduction was observed, but after 3 months a better arterial pulsation was seen in the legs of the EDTA-treated patients. No side effects occurred in the patients receiving chelation therapy.

Olivieri et al. [54] have recently reported on the beneficial effects of chelation therapy with deferoxamine in 21 patients suffering from thalassemia major. An editorial in the New England Journal of Medicine [55] has endorsed the use of deferoxamine as a chelating agent for the removal of excess iron which occurs in the genetically inherited disease, beta thalassemia, characterized by unstable erythrocytes. However, a newer drug, deferiprone, an orally effective chelating agent has been recommended to increase patient compliance.

Similarly, Zucker [56] has indicated the usefulness of EDTA and vitamins in treating Alzheimer's disease. In other claims on chelation in atherosclerosis, the removal of calcium by the chelating agent has been proposed as the mechanism by which the plaques are reduced [57], although the New Zealand study revealed no reduction in the plaques [55]. A short-term efficacy without any side effects of oral dimercaptosuccinic acid has been shown in lead toxicity cases in children [58]. The American Academy of Pediatrics Committee on Drugs has recently published guidelines for treating lead poisoning in children [59]. Chelation in a hospital environment has been recommended for cases showing blood levels of lead between 45 and 70 mcg/dcl.

Cranton [61], an advocate of preventive medicine, has boldly criticized all coronary by-pass surgeries and has proposed chelation therapy as a viable and superior alternative [60]. In contrast to this and similar other advocates [51], a report in a medical communication [61] questions the beneficial effect of chelation therapy in atherosclerotic patients.

One of the most critical rebuttals to chelation therapy has been put forth by Green [62] who has discussed and analyzed both pro and con literature on it. He claims that the ACAM founded in 1973 and with a membership of 450 physicians has a primary goal of not advancing medicine but only chelation therapy. He rejects most of the clinical claims on the basis that no large-scale, randomized and well-controlled trials have been carried out. It may be pointed out here again that the New Zealand study on 32 patients, which is the only well-controlled study known since Green's analysis, did not show any significant benefit of chelation therapy in atherosclerosis [52, 53]. Green further claims that expert committees of various prestigious health and biomedical organizations of the USA, e.g., FDA, NIH, CDC, AMA etc., have also concluded in agreement with his analysis.

In spite of all these controversial accounts on chelation therapy, this alternative modality continues to be recommended by its supporters. In the USA, about 300,000 coronary by-passes and 250,000 angioplasties are carried out annually, with about 20,000 fatalities occurring during these procedures [6]. In 1991, $10 billion was spent on by-pass surgeries alone. Considering all this, argument in favor of a non-invasive (oral) or least invasive (intravenous infusion) chelation therapy becomes a compelling alternative. However, unless its benefit is proven by well-controlled studies, its use will continue to be questionable.

2.5   Chiropractic

Based upon manipulation of the spine and the spinal nerves, chiropractic was established in September of 1895 by Daniel David Palmer, an ardent reader of anatomy and physiology in Iowa, USA, when he examined a deaf custodian who had lost his hearing after hurting his back some years earlier [8]. Palmer found one of the vertebrae displaced and tried to put it back in place by manual manipulation. The custodian began to regain his hearing. Palmer opened the first chiropractic school in Devenport, Iowa in 1897. Since then, an enormous expansion and refinement of this alternative modality has occurred. Today it is applied to all types of musculoskeletal disorders, e.g., whiplash injuries, neck problems, lower back pain, sciatica, bursitis etc., and to organic disorders including hypertension, migraine, neuritis, and other nervous diseases in patients of all ages.

The chiropractic degree, Doctor of Chiropractic (D.C.), is a 4-year postgraduate program similar to the doctor of medicine. The practitioner, chiropractor, must also pass both the state and the national board examinations in order to practice. Like medicine, the admission to a chiropractic school requires an undergraduate background in the sciences. The professional training emphasizes anatomy and physiology, especially of the nervous and the musculoskeletal systems.

2.5.1   Clinical assessment of chiropractic
One of the most common ailments amenable to chiropractic is lower back pain. In a 2-year study by the British Medical Council, chiropractic was found to be better than the conventional hospital outpatient care, and during the subsequent years chiropractic-treated patients suffered less pain

than those treated otherwise [63]. An editorial in Lancet gave a clear and strong advantage to chiropractic over conventional care [64]. Likewise, another 2-year study sponsored by the Ontario Ministry of Health in Canada showed that lower back pain is treated better and less expensively by chiropractic than by conventional medicine [65].

A more recent randomized comparison of chiropractic and hospital outpatient care for lower back pain in UK revealed that chiropractic achieved superior results [66]. In this study, 741 patients were randomly assigned to the two types of care. Both groups had similar pain scores at entry into the study. The patients were evaluated at 6 weeks, 6 months, and at 1, 2 and 3 years. Chiropractic care consistently produced superior results at every evaluation.

Chiropractic once considered quackery by the AMA is clearly finding more acceptance. In fact, chiropractors in the USA rank third in numbers behind the physicians and the dentists, and they actually see twice the number of backache patients as do the allopathic physicians [67]. In 1989, 3 out of 4 patients treated by a chiropractor said that they were happy with the treatment [68]. In 1994, as also today indeed, chiropractors constitute the third largest group of primary care physicians in the USA where at least 15 million seek this alternative modality of health care [69]. Several reports appeared during 1995 declaring chiropractors as being more popular than the allopaths and the osteopaths among backache patients [70]. In fact, the U.S. federal guidelines on health care, published recently, strongly recommend chiropractic as a preferred therapeutic modality for treating lower back pain [71].

Although there have been plenty of critics [72, 73], especially the AMA, discrediting chiropractic, court rulings have permanently debarred AMA from interfering in the development of chiropractic medicine [73]. Despite criticism, it is noteworthy that U.S. hospitals are granting clinical privileges to chiropractors in record numbers [74]. This may be so because of the fever of escalating health care costs; hospitals desirous of cutting costs are bringing the chiropractors into their fold, believing that they not only provide cost-effective care but also constitute an additional source of revenue, since more and more patients are seeking chiropractic care. A survey by the American Chiropractic Association on 16,000 of its members revealed that at least 100 conventional hospitals have chiropractic departments now [74].

2.5.2   Cost analysis of chiropractic care
The only published economic comparison of chiropractic care with conventional care dates back to 1993 [75]. The annual cost of chiropractic care

in the USA was $ 1.19 billion in 1980 and $ 4.2 billion in 1988. In another study over a 2-year period, 395,164 patients with 15 different ailments were randomly divided into two groups. One group received only conventional therapy, whereas the other group received either chiropractic alone or both chiropractic and conventional together. The group on only the conventional therapy consumed $ 1,138 per patient more and also showed 60% more hospitalizations costing an additional 35% [76].

2.6   Homeopathy

Homeopathy, derived from the Greek word 'homoios', meaning similar, and 'pathos' meaning disease, is based on the law of similars, which states that a drug capable of causing symptoms similar to those of a disease can cure the disease [77, 78]. Although a German physician, Samuel Hahnemann, in the 19th century is being credited for the birth of homeopathy, it was Hippocrates in the 4th century B.C. who said "Through the like, disease is produced, and through the application of the like it is cured" [77, 79].
The principles of homeopathy were first described by Hahnemann in 1880 in Materia Medica Pura [77]. The first principle is the principle of "similars" which states that a drug will heal the symptoms similar to those it is known to cause. For example, a fever-producing drug can in small doses cure the fever. The second principle is that the diagnosis is made by studying a "pattern of symptoms" rather than just one or a few symptoms, and the patient is considered as a particular type exhibiting a specific body-mind pattern. The third principle believes in the safety of medication by using the smallest dose possible. A series of dilutions (potentizations) of the drug are made to arrive at a dose that may be only a few hundred molecules. It is interesting to point out that our current scientific knowledge supports the concept that drugs finally work at the molecular level by interacting with biological molecules such as enzymes and nucleic acids in our cells. The fourth and final principle deals with understanding the healing process at physical, emotional, and mental levels, a holistic approach. It is believed that the "healing first benefits the internal initial functions and then progresses to the external functions" [78].
An estimated 500 million people in the world receive homeopathic medicine [6]. The WHO has stated homeopathy as one of the traditional alternative medicines that if integrated with modern medicine may provide adequate health care globally by the end of this century [48]. A survey done during 1985 and 1992 showed that, in contrast to only 3% Americans, 56% Belgians, 20% Danish, 32% French, 15% Swedes, 16% British

and 31% Dutch were using homeopathic care [80]. Another survey in 1986 showed that 42% of British allopaths referred patients to homeopaths [81], an interesting trend indeed and one that must have increased in more recent years.

There are over 6000 homeopathic practitioners in Germany, 5000 in France, 25,000 in India, and over 3000 in the USA [6]. In the UK, homeopathic outpatient clinics and hospitals are a part of the national health care system. British royalty has patronized homeopathy at least for a century, and in the UK, homeopathy is regarded as a well-accepted postgraduate medical specialty. In Europe, pharmacies are required to carry homeopathic medications. The FDA recognizes the Homeopathic Pharmacopeia of the United States first published in 1897 and considers homeopathic medicines as official drugs, regulating their manufacture, labeling and dispensing. It is also interesting that the first professional association of practicing physicians in the USA was that of homeopathy, the American Institute of Homeopathy, not the American Medical Association formed three years later [82].

A recent analysis in the USA revealed that the use of homeopathy and other alternative modes of therapy appears to be increasing rapidly on the one hand, while strong movements to stop this development are under way on the other hand [83]. The sale of homeopathic medicines in 1988 was $ 100 million, but it grew at an annual rate of 25% to $ 200 million in 1992 as per the data from the National Center for Homeopathy in Alexandria, Virginia. More independent pharmacists are increasing their homeopathic inventories. However, a group of allopathic physician protesters have filed a petition asking the FDA to enforce proper regulation of ineffective homeopathic medicines [84]. Also, the National Council Against Health Fraud (NCAHF) in its newsletter has made a strong position statement against homeopathy, declaring it to be quackery and an ineffective health care system [85]. The council has urged the public to abandon homeopathy and has asked the FDA to apply to the homeopathic drug formulations the same rigid standards that are applied to the allopathic drugs. According to the Council's expert opinion, the homeopathic principles have been refuted by the basic concepts of chemistry and pharmacology.

Curiously, in the USA, claims have been made in favor of homeopathic superiority over conventional medicine in dealing with epidemics of cholera in 1849 and yellow fever in 1879 [86]. Of course, one could argue that the knowledge base in allopathic medicine was very primitive and limited during the 19th century. Perhaps therefore, by the end of that century, there were 22 homeopathic schools, over 100 homeopathic hospitals, and nearly 15% of all physicians as homeopaths [87]. By the beginning of the 20th century, however, AMA and pharmaceutical companies had made a formidable alliance which did not help the continued development of homeopathy. Nonetheless, the last decade or two have witnessed a resurgence of homeopathy as a viable alternative therapeutic modality.

2.6.1   Clinical assessment of homeopathy

Several placebo-controlled randomized clinical studies have been reported in the last two years. In a study on 28 allergic asthmatic patients assigned randomly to a placebo or a treatment group, the patients were asked to keep their own diaries of their symptoms while the physicians evaluated their respiratory function and bronchial reactivity after 4 weeks of treatment. Nine out of 11 patients on homeopathic treatment improved significantly as compared to only 5 out of 13 on placebo. These data together with data from two other earlier studies, making a total of 202 patients, showed a clear effectiveness of homeopathic treatment [88].

A randomized trial in Nicaragua on 81 children suffering from diarrhea and kept on oral hydration showed that the group receiving homeopathic care recovered in only 2 days as against 4 days needed by the placebo group [89]. The homeopathic medicines used in this study included arsenic, mercury, chamomile, sulphur and May-apple. In contrast to these two positive studies, a placebo-controlled randomized trial on 170 boys and girls with recurring upper respiratory tract infections, showed only a marginal difference between the treated and the placebo groups [90]. Similarly, no difference was observed between the treatment and the placebo groups of patients suffering from pain following wisdom teeth extraction [91]. In Europe of course several clinical studies on homeopathic medicines have been carried out and published in prestigious journals including The Lancet, British Medical Journal, British Journal of Clinical Pharmacology, Human Toxicology, the European Journal of Pharmacology, etc. [77]. It should be of historical noteworthiness for homeopathy in the USA that the first U.S. government funding was awarded for clinical evaluation of homeopathy to Linda Johnson in 1994 [92]. A conventional allopathic physician, Johnson, began practicing homeopathy in 1986, opened the Academy of Homeopathic School in 1990, and has trained and graduated 70 allopathic physicians with a 2-year postgraduate training in homeopathy. The *Materia medica* of a homeopath includes some of the most potent drugs and toxins, e.g., Aconite, Arsenic, Belladonna, Ignatia, Bushmaster snake venom, Mercury, Poison ivy, *Nux vomica*, etc. [77]. Although liquid extracts and solutions of several potencies are available, the preferred dosage forms are small pills made of powdered sucrose or lactose to which the liquid medication has been added.

The pills may be as small as cake sprinkle granules, but the largest size is as big as a pea. The formulated medications are not to be touched by hand, exposed to sunlight, or kept at temperatures above 38 degree Celsius. The diseases claimed to be treatable by homeopathy include most disorders known to man, but fevers, dermatological diseases, asthma and allergies are believed to respond better than infections.

Although homeopathy has been extensively used in Europe and India during the past century, it is only recently that it has become somewhat popular in the USA. It is extremely difficult for allopathic physicians to understand and accept homeopathy, since the principles of allopathy are diametrically opposite to those of homeopathy. Allopathy is derived from two Greek words; Alloe means "against" and Pathos means "disease"; in other words, contrary to the homeopathic principle of similars. The drug used in allopathy creates symptoms opposite (against) of the symptoms caused by the disease. Also, allopathy believes that a larger dose (nontoxic) treats disease better than a small dose, quite contrary to the potentization principle of homeopathy. Thus one can understand why homeopathy has not expanded in the USA, especially during the recent decades of this century.

A little digression into fundamentals of pharmacology would suggest that drugs do work finally at a molecular level by interacting with the biological molecules or their receptors. For this interaction, only a few molecules of the drug are needed at the biophase to elicit a response. Most allopathic drugs consumed in large doses do undergo metabolism and excretion (elimination) simultaneously while being distributed to create an effective concentration at the biophase. One wonders if the homeopathic medicines might not undergo any elimination, thus providing a reasonable explanation for why small doses of homeopathic medicines might work.

3   Global development

Herbal medicine in recent years appears to have grabbed a center stage worldwide [93]. Over the counter sales of herbal medicines in Northern America in 1990 were $ 861 million. In the European market, this figure for Germany alone was $ 1.5 billion. The West European countries showed an increase of 22% in the annual sales of herbal medicines. In Norway, National Research Foundation on Alternative Medicine was established in 1991 with the help of government funds. In Japan, the traditional medicine called "Kampoh" increased 15-fold between 1979 and 1989, as against only a 2.6-fold increase in modern medicine. Furthermore, 65% of Japanese physicians in 1989 administered both Kampoh and allopathic medicines, a trend that must have increased further by now. Over 140 Kampoh medicines are eligible for reimbursement under the national health insurance scheme of Japan.

In 1993, the herbal remedies in the USA sold at $ 1.13 billion, almost double the sales in 1985, and the sales are projected to increase at a rate of 10 to 15 percent annually through 1997 [94]. An estimated 400 herbs are in the market. The Herb Research Foundation in Boulder, Colorado receives 20,000 and the American Botanical Council in Austin, Texas 6,000 enquiries per year on herbal medicine. Apparently in 1989, an estimated 100,000 physicians worldwide wrote 10 million prescriptions on Gingko, a Chinese medicinal herb [94].

Xue [95] has recently drawn the attention of the American scientific community to the clinical effectiveness of chinese herbal medicine. He has suggested that the FDA ought to consider the long history of their clinical use as the proof of safety and efficacy of chinese herbal preparations. Xue and several others have suggested that the FDA should take advantage of and guidance from the European regulating agencies that have experience in allowing so many herbal preparations in the clinical market.

Dictamnus dasycarpus, a herb used in Chinese medicine for over one thousand years has been claimed by many investigators as hepatotoxic, but a double-blind clinical study showed it to be non-toxic [96]. More recently, Saw [97] has also defended the herb and countered the claim of those labeling it toxic.

Clinical Research Methodology [98], a collection of 30 articles published during the late eighties and early nineties is a valuable compendium in that it establishes standards for clinical studies on alternative therapies and gives valuable research designs and protocols addressing some of the difficult issues arising out of the on-going debate between allopathic and alternative practitioners [99]. Knipschild [100] created a series of controversial debates on expressing his viewpoint that data on clinical trials of alternative therapies is abundant and blaming the biased allopaths for not accepting the data generated by such trials. Grotzche [101] has raised an issue of bias in the interpretation of positive clinical trials pointed out by Knipschild. A more categorical challenge has come from Renckens [102] who is willing to bet with Knipschild on the non-existence of meridians the acupuncturists believe in. Ernst [103], however, has put forth a more balanced viewpoint that today allopathic physicians around the world are admitting potential benefits of alternative medicine, and has suggested that the alternatives be dealt with and evaluated in a fair and unbiased way.

Gaus and Hogel [104] have proposed an interesting approach to the evaluation of unconventional therapies. They suggest that new trial designs and study components must be found to meet the specific requirements of a particular alternative therapy. This approach implies that the FDA will have to modify its rigid protocols of clinical trials when dealing with the assessment of AM approaches.

Complementary Therapies in Medicine, a journal with an international advisory board, was established in 1993. Its uniqueness, among other holistic and alternative medicine journals, has been claimed to be that it provides a forum for allopaths to explore and discuss AM [105].

Although illegal during the communist rule, the practice of AM in Russia has skyrocketed in the short time since the dismantling of the Soviet Union. There are over 300,000 practitioners from faith healers to herbalists which are seen by over 80% of the Russian population [106]. A similar picture is imminent also in the Eastern European Countries.

3.1   Development in North America

Chronologically [107], homeopathy came to the USA from Germany in the 1800s, and the general rise of naturopathy, chiropractic and osteopathy occurred during the century. The back-to-nature movement of 1960s and the holistic health movement of the 1970s including the introduction of acupuncture, was followed by an emergence of new respectability for acupuncture and chiropractic in the current decade [107].

On November 21, 1991 the U.S. Congress passed a bill creating a National Office of Alternative Medicine (OAM) within the NIH, largely in response to public pressure in the midst of escalating health care costs of conventional medicine. The OAM become operative in 1992. During 1993 and 1994, various divisions of the NIH funded a total of 147 different research projects in the area of alternative medicine (AM) totalling $ 26.54 million. During the same period, the OAM also funded 43 projects totaling $ 1.25 million. In addition, two NIH Exploratory Study Coordinator Centers for AM Research were established at Bastyr University in Seattle, Washington and at Minneapolis Medical Research in Minneapolis, Minnesota. The primary function of these centers is to gather and analyze clinical data on AM and to organize workshops and postgraduate training programs in AM [108]. Also, the OAM has established 10 AM Research Centers at various universities in the USA with an initial annual funding at $ 860,000 to $ 1,103,486 each, beginning September 1994. These centers are investigating the effectiveness of AM in treating pain, neurological conditions, cancer, general medical condition, addiction, asthma, allergy, aging, etc. [108].

A Harris poll on AM in 1986 conducted for the U.S. Department of Health and Human Services revealed that 90% of respondents who had used AM were satisfied with it. In a poll in 1991, 84% said they would go back to an AM practitioner [107, 109]. In a telephone interview with 1539 adults, a group of allopathic physicians and researchers found that 34% of the respondents had used unconventional therapy. Back pain, anxiety and depression were the prominent conditions seeking AM, with a total national projected out-of-pocket expenditure on AM of $ 13.7 billion in 1990, nearly half of out-of-pocket expenditure for all physicians services which was $ 23.5 billion for that year [7]. The foundation for the Advancement of Innovative Medicine in New York and a few politicians succeeded in having the State Assembly pass an act called the Alternative Medical Practicing Act in 1994, which provides legal protection for physicians using AM. Similar legislation is apparently underway in California, Wisconsin, and several other states in the USA [110].

Beliefs and attitudes of 400 general practitioners in Ontario and Alberta (Canada) were obtained through a questionnaire in which 200 responded [111]. The results showed that 56% believed that conventional physicians would benefit from the ideas and approaches of the AM, 54% referred patients to AM practitioners, and 15% practiced some form of AM. This picture is very much like what one observes in the UK.

In Quebec, the largest province of Canada, 4 out of 5 physicians believe in a distinct benefit from complimentary health care services, and it has been suggested that AM should be integrated with the conventional system for the good of the public [112]. Another similar study in Quebec indicated 60% of allopathic practitioners knew of at least one AM practitioner, and 59% referred patients to other allopathics who practice AM and 68% referred patients to non-allopathic AM practitioners [113]. Also, 48% expressed a desire to receive training in AM.

The first International Congress on AM and complimentary medicine, organized by Mary Ann Liebert, the publisher of the Journal of Alternative and Complementary Medicine, was held in Arlington, Virginia early 1995 [114]. One of the stimulating events that occurred was a detailed discussion on a congressional bill being drafted at that time and to be called the Access to Medical Treatment Act. This legislation would give the patient freedom to choose any method of treatment involving a procedure or drug, even if it is not approved by the FDA. However, the new

Director of OAM, Dr. Wayne Jonas emphasized that controlled clinical trials are essential for accepting any evidence in favor of an alternative therapy. This Congress is likely to become an annual event.

3.2   Development in the United Kingdom

The British Library data base held in the Library of Royal Society of Medicine, and other establishments are believed to have 55,000 publications on AM research and some 200–300 are being added each month. Over 60 journals dedicated to AM and largely unknown to the conventional physicians are the resource for such publications [115]. Apparently, there are 300 methods of diagnosis and treatments in AM being used in the UK. In order to bring some order to all that is available out there, it has been suggested that a fair evaluation of these AM methods must be carried out to bring them into the national health care programs [115].

As a model of integration perhaps worthy of emulation, an urban practice with 6000 patients has been working closely with nine AM practitioners since 1991 [116]. The cooperative inquiry and cross referral of patients between allopathic and AM practitioners enhanced the mutual understanding of the two groups. The model has been suggested as a good one for adoption by any enthusiastic general practice. There are an estimated 50,000 AM practitioners in the UK. A large number of allopathic general or family practice physicians either have further training in one or two modalities of AM or interact with and refer their patients to AM practitioners [117]. Based on the evidence available in the literature and the history of the nature of democratic governance in the UK, it is quite conceivable that a real integration of AM with the ongoing conventional health care system may first occur in that country. This trend is perhaps best portrayed in the book on complementary medicine recently published by the British Medical Association [118].

Both in England and Ireland, non-medically qualified practitioners are free to practice health care, except treating venereal diseases, dental disorders and animals. The UK Faculty of Homeopathy was established by an act of the British parliament in 1950 to set standards for training and testing homeopathy. The UK is the only EEC country where complimentary medicine hospitals exist in London, Glasgow, Liverpool and Bristol [2].

3.3   Alternative Medicine in Europe

Europe has the largest tradition of AM. Two years ago, Fisher and Ward [2] compiled a valuable pool of information on the practice of AM in

Europe. Of interest is the comparison made between how the European countries used to look at each other as foreigners and how they now have learnt to look as partners in the emergence of a common European market. About 60% of the public in the Netherlands and Belgium are willing to pay extra health insurance premium to have access to AM. The data available shows 20–50% of general population uses complimentary therapies and the popularity seems to be growing rapidly. In France, homeopathy is the most common AM used, its use increasing from 16% of the population in 1982 to 36% in 1992. Reflexology, akin to acupuncture but without any needle insertion, is used by 39% of the AM users in Denmark [2].

In the whole of Europe, over-the-counter sales of homeopathic medicines were L 590 million in 1991 as against L 1.45 billion for herbal medicines. The world's largest homeopathic market is France, where 80% of all homeopathic medications are sold on prescription. The over-the-counter market for homeopathic medicines is increasing by 30% per year in Greece and Portugal [119].

Introduced in 1939, the German Heilpraktiker system licenses health practitioners who have passed a test for basic medical knowledge and are registered. Since the system is regulated at provincial levels, actual practice of AM may vary considerably from place to place. The health practitioners, however, are not allowed to indulge in obstetrics and dentistry [2].

The statistics of European physicians indulging in AM is interesting [2]. In Belgium, 84% of homeopathy and 74% of acupuncture are practiced by allopathic physicians, while in France over 30% of half a million allopathic general practitioners use AM. In the Netherlands, homeopathy is practiced by 47% of physicians, whereas other modalities of AM are practiced by practitioners not qualified medically. In Germany, 77% of pain clinics use acupuncture. Nearly 50% of Dutch physicians believe acupuncture to be effective for chronic pain, and homeopathy for upper respiratory tract problems.

The governments of UK, Germany, Denmark, Italy, Norway and Spain have joined Switzerland which proposed an European initiative COST Project B4, a research program on unconventional medicine designed to establish credibility of AM modalities and to contain health care costs [2]. A more recent analysis shows that European medical practitioners prefer natural cures for ailments over the conventional drugs [120]. Not alternative therapies but health promotion and health consciousness seem to be the latest wave in Europe. In a recently published [121] survey of 522 polyarthritic patients conducted in Germany between 1987 and 1992 to see the trends, the use of AM appeared to decrease over the years somewhat but the consumption of a vegetarian diet remains constant.

4   Conclusion and future scope

Human experience has shown that every generation looks upon the knowledge of the previous generations with skepticism and cynicism. Only thirty years ago we used to laugh at "Fakirs" and "Sadhus" who would claim that they could reduce their heart rate to near zero, their metabolism to near hibernation, and perform unbelievable physical acts through Yoga. It took some modern experimentation and coining of the term "bio-feedback training" by the current biomedical and scientific community of the world to convince the skeptics that man does have the ability to do what the "Fakirs" and "Sadhus" were claiming. A more recent episode in a similar vein was that The American Medical Association (AMA) in 1966 issued a policy statement labeling chiropractic "an unscientific cult whose practitioners lack the necessary training and background to diagnose and treat human disease" [121]. Fourteen years later in 1980, the AMA as well as the Health Insurance Industry for reimbursement purposes accepted the fast growing chiropractic health services. Thus it is expected that the current wave of AM will meet with resistance for sometime, at least until some success stories emerge. It should be emphasized that a critical and thorough evaluation of the AM modalities is necessary before they are integrated within the modern health care system. The length of time required for this integration depends on the magnitude of research effort and funding dedicated to this cause by the biomedical research community in the governments, academia and the health industry of the affluent world.

In the meantime, however, controversies and debates [122–128] will continue on all modalities of AM. Clearly, the initial challenge for those interested in improving health care of man lies in developing an innovative clinical methodology to evaluate some of the widely used alternative therapeutic approaches described in this review. What would facilitate an objective outlook on the part of emerging allopathic physicians would be a curricular revision of the medical education globally, for then more physicians may get involved in both assessing and thereafter accepting those alternative modalities whose data would warrant it.

This curricular revision is expressly needed for the medical schools in the USA, for in French, Dutch and German medical schools the undergraduate courses include a curriculum in complementary medicine. Perhaps the best established AM curriculum in Europe is the "Münchner Modell" developed at the Faculty of the Ludwig Maximilian University in Munich. The British Medical Association has also recently recommended that complementary medicine be taught in the undergraduate medical curriculum. In the USA, the Montefiore Medical Center in New York established the first AM teaching program in the seventies [129]. Also, at the Tufts University School of Medicine, Boston, a course on complementary healing systems has become a popular elective. However, there has to be a much wider spread of this trend. Hopefully, the European initiatives will prompt the American Council on Medical Education and more medical schools in the USA to also follow suit.

One very exciting development within the past month in the USA is that the FDA has approved an accelerated review process to facilitate quicker introduction of new drugs or therapies into market for life-threatening diseases such as cancer and AIDS. This may be the beginning of some hope for alternative therapeutic modalities seeking approval of the FDA.

References

1   J. Walton, J.A. Barondess and S. Lock, Eds.: The Oxford Medical Companion, Oxford Univ. Press, Oxford, p. 586, 1994.
2   P. Fisher and A. Ward: B.M.J. *309* (6947), 107 (1994).
3   H.S. Berliner: Int. J. Hlth. Services *5*, 573 (1975).
4   J.W. Salmon: Alternative Medicine, popular and policy perspectives, Travistock/Methuen, New York 1984.
5   P. Bergner and K. Kail: Presented at the Amer. Asscn. Naturopathic Physicians convention, Sept. 1992.
6   B. Goldberg: The Definitive Guide, Future Medicine Publishing, Puyallup 1993.
7   D.M. Eisenberg, R.C. Kessler, C. Foster and F.E. Norlock: N. Engl. J. Med. *328*, 246 (1993).
8   M. Kastner and H. Boroughs: Alternative Healing, Halcyon Publishing, La Mesa, California 1993.
9   R. Gerber: Vibrational Medicine, Bear & Co. Santa Fe, New Mexico 1988.
10   P. de Vernejoul, P. Abarade and J.L. Darras: Bull. Acad. Natl. Med. *189*, 1071 (1985).
11   Z. Zhu: Am. J. Acupuncture *9*, 203 (1981).
12   R.O. Becker: The Promise of Electromedicine, Jeremy P. Tarcher, Los Angeles 1990.
13   R.O. Baker and G. Sheldon: The Body Electric: electro-magnetism and the foundation of life, William Morrow & Co. New York, p. 235, 1985.
14   A. Jayasuraiya: Text Book on Acupuncture, Open University Press, Sri Lanka 1987.
15   B. Millman: Ann. Rev. Med. *28*, 223 (1977).
16   J. Cheung: Am. J. Chinese Med. *13*, 33 (1985).
17   J. Sodipo: Pain *7*, 359 (1979).
18   K.B. Chatfield: "Scientific Basis of Acupuncture", in: J.E. Pizzorno and M.T Murray (Eds.), Textbook for Natural Medicine, Bastyr Publications, Seattle 1988.

19   D. Eisenberg: Encounters with Qi; exploring Chinese medicine, Penguin, New York, p. 77, 1987.
20   G.T. Lewith and D. Machin: Pain *16*, 111 (1983).
21   J. Holder: New Auricular Therapy Formula to Increase Retention of the Chemically Dependent in Residential Treatment, a Resaerch Study Funded by Florida Department of Health and Rehabilitative Services 1991.
22   K.L. Resch and E. Ernst: Fortschr. Med. *113*, 45 (1995).
23   H. Zaman: The South-East Asia Region, in: R.H.Bannerman (Ed.), Traditional Medicine, W.H.O., Geneva 1974.
24   D. Chopra: Perfect Health, Harmony Books, New York 1990.
25   D. Chopra: Quantum Healing, Exploring the mind-body medicine, Bantam Books, New York 1989.
26   R.N. Chopra, I.C. Chopra, K.L. Honda and L.D. Kapur: Indigenous Drugs of India, Academic Publishers, Calcutta 1982.
27   H.M. Sharma, B.D. Triguna and D. Chopra: J.A.M.A. *265* (20), 2633 (1991).
28   H.M. Sharma, Y. Feng and R.V. Panganamala: Clinica & Terapia Cardiovscolare *8*, 227 (1989).
29   F.N. Engineer, H.M. Sharma and C. Dwivedi: Biochem. Arch. *8*, 267 (1992).
30   C. Dwivedi, H.M. Sharma, S. Dobrowski and F.N. Engineer: Pharmacol. Biochem. Behav. *39*, 649 (1991).
31   H.M. Sharma, A.N. Hanna, E.M. Kaufman and H.A.I. Newman: Pharmacol. Biochem. Behav. *43*, 1175 (1992).
32   Y. Niwa: Ind. J. Clin. Pract. *1*, 23 (1991).
33   H.M. Sharma, C. Dwivedi, B.C. Satter and H. Abou-issa: J. Res. Edu. Ind. Med. *10*, 1 (1991).
34   H.M. Sharma, C. Dwivedi, B.C. Satter, K.P. Gudehithlu, H. Abou-issa, W. Malarkey and C.A. Tejwani: Pharmacol. Biochem. Behav. *35*, 767 (1990).
35   K.N. Prasad, J. Edward-prasad, S. Kentroti, C. Brodie and A. Vernadakis: Neuropharmacol. *31*, 599 (1992).
36   V.K. Patel, J. Wang, R.N. Shen, H.M. Sharma and Z. Brahmi: Nutr. Res. *12*, 51 (1992).
37   K.N. Dileepan, S.T. Verghese, J.C. Page and D.J. Stechschulte: Biochem. Arch. *9*, 365 (1993).
38   S.C. Bondy, T.M. Himandez and C. Mattia: Biochem. Arch *10*, 25 (1994).
39   A.F. Hanna, H.M. Sharma, E.M. Kaufman and H.E.I. Newman: Pharmacol. Biochem. Behav. *48*, 505 (1994).
40   H.M. Sharma, A.N. Hanna, E.M. Kaufman and H.A.I. Newman: Free Rad. Biol. Med. *18*, 687 (1995).
41   H.M. Sharma, S. Hanissian, A.K. Rattan, S.L. Stern and G.A. Tejwani: J. Res. Edu. Ind. Med *10*, 1 (1991).
42   P. Gelderloos, H.H.B. Ahlstrom, D.W. Orme-Johnson, D.K. Robinson, R.K. Wallace and J.L. Glaser: International J. Psychosomatics *37*, 25 (1990).
43   H.M. Sharma: Alt. Complem. Therap. *1*, 364 (1995).
44   H.M. Sharma, in: M. S. Micozzi (Ed.), Fundamentals of Coplementary and Alternative Medicine, Churchill, New York, p. 243, 1996.
45   R.K. Wallace: The Physiology of Consciousness, MIU Press, Fairfield, Iowa, USA, p. 110, 1993.
46   R.K. Wallace: Science *167*, 1751 (1970).
47   C.N. Alexander, E.J. Langer, J.L. Davies, H.M. Chandler and R.I Newman: J. Pers. Soc. Psychol. *57*, 950 (1989).

48   R.H. Bannerman, J. Burton and W. Chieh (Eds.): Traditional Medicine and Health Care Coverage, W.H.O., Geneva 1983.
49   D.G. Danskin and M. Crow: Biofeed, an Introduction and Guide, Mayfield Publishing, Palo Alto 1981.
50   E. Olczewer and J.P. Carter: Med. Hypotheses 27, 41 (1988).
51   E. Olczewer and J.P. Carter, in: E.M. Cranton (Ed.), EDTA Chelation Therapy, Human Services Press, New York, p. 197, 1989.
52   Harvard News Letter 5, 3 (1995).
53   A.M. van Rij, C. Solomon, S.G. Packer and W.G. Hogkins: Circulation 90, 1194 (1994)
54   N.F. Olivieri, G.N. Briltenham, D. Matsui, M. Berkowitch, L.M. Blendis, R.G. Cameron, R.A. McClelland, P.P. Liu, D.M Templeton and G. Koren: N. Engl. J. Med. 232, 918 (1995).
55   G.J. Dover and D. Vallo: N. Engl. J. Med. 331, 609 (1994).
56   M. Zueker: Let's Live 63 (8), 24 (1995).
57   M. Abramowicz: Med. Lett. Drugs and Therep. 36, 48 (1994).
58   J.B. Besunder, R.L. Anderson and D.M. Super: Pediatrics 96, 683 (1995).
59   American Academy of Pediatrics Committee on Drugs: Pediatrics 96, 155 (1995).
60   E. Cranton: Bypassing By-Pass: The new technique of chelation therapy, 2nd edition, Hampton Roads Publishing, Norfolk 1992.
61   Medical Letter on Drugs and Therapeutics 36, 48 (1994).
62   S. Green: Nutrition Forum 10, 33 (1993).
63   T.W. Meede: B.M.J. 300 (6737), 1431 (1990).
64   Editorial: The Lancet 336, 220 (1990).
65   S.A. Arria and C.I. Staley: Muscle & Fitness 55, 222 (1994).
66   T.W. Meede, D. Dyer, W. Browne and A.V. Frank: B.M.J. 311 (7001), 349 (1995).
67   B. Kallen: Shape 14, 100 (1994).
68   G. Maleskay: Prevention 41, 60 (1994).
69   Feature article in Good Housekeeping 21, 100 (1994).
70   The Back Letter 10, 109 and 111 (1995).
71   D.J. Cichoke: Total Health 17, 14 (1995).
72   G. Dunea: B.M.J. 307, 71 (1993).
73   National Council Against Health Fraud (NCAHF) Newsletter 16, 1 (1993).
74   The Back Letter 10, 51 (1995).
75   The Back Letter 8, (1993).
76   M. Stand: J. Manipulation and Physical Therapy 16, (1993).
77   S. Cummings and D. Ullman: Everybody's Guide to Homeopathic Medicine, Tarcher/ Putnam, New York 1992.
78   D. Ullman: Homeopathic Medicine for Children and Infants, Tarcher/Putnam, New York 1992.
79   T. Dixon: Special Delivery 18, 13 (1995).
80   Better Nutrition for Today's Living 56, 26 (1994).
81   R. Wharton and G. Lewith: B.M.J. Clinical Research Edition 292 (6534), 1498 (1986).
82   H.L. Coulter: Divided Legacy: A History of Schism in Medical Thought, 4 volumes, Wehawken Book Co., Washington 1973–1994.
83   Drug Topics 138, 102 (1994).
84   A.A. Sklonick: J.A.M.A. 272 (15), 1154 (1994).
85   NCAHF Newsletter 17, 1 (1994).
86   D. Ullman: Discovering Homeopathy, Medicine for 21 st Century, North Atlantic Books, Berkeley 1991.

87   T. Cook: Samuel Hahnemann, The Founder of Homeopathic Medicine, Thorsons, Wellingborough (UK) 1981.

88   D.Reilly, M.A. Taylor, N.G.M. Beattie, J.H. Campbell, C. McSharry, T.C. Aitchison, R. Carter and R.D. Stevenson: The Lancet *344*, 1601 (1994).

89   J. Jacobs, L.M. Jimenez, S.S. Gloyd, J.L. Gale and D.Crothers: Pediatrics *93*, 719(1994).

90   E.S.M. de Lange de Klerk, J. Bloomers, D.J. Kuik, P.D. Bezemer and L. Feenstra: B.M.J. *309* (6965), 1329 (1994).

91   P. Lokken, P.A. Stransheim, D. Tveiten, P. Skjelbred and C.F. Borchgrevink: B.M.J. *310* (6992), 1439 (1995).

92   R. Smith: Total Health *16*, 36 (1994).

93   Eastern Pharmacist *37* (6), 110 (1994).

94   B.C. Coleman: Alternatives *7* (11), 1 (1996).

95   T. Xue: The Scientist *10* (4), 9 (1996).

96   M.P. Sheehan, M.H.A. Rustin, D.J. Atherton, C. Buckley, D.J. Harris and J. Brostoff: The Lancet *340*, 3 (1992).

97   R.H.M. Saw: B.M.J. *312* (7023), 122 (1996).

98   G.T. Lewith and D. Aldridge (Eds.): Clinical Research Methodology for Complementary Medicine, Hodder & Stoughton, London 1993.

99   H. McGourty: The Lancet *342*, 668 (1993).

100 P. Knipschild: The Lancet *341*, 1135 (1993).

101 P.C. Gotzsche: The Lancet *341*, 1533 (1993).

102 C.N.M. Renckens: The Lancet *341*, 1533 (1993).

103 E. Ernst: The Lancet *341*, 1626 (1993).

104 W. Gaus and J. Hogel: Arzneimittelforschung *45*, 88 (1995).

105 D.D. McKee and J.S. Zenan: J.A.M.A. *272* (7), 570 (1994).

106 The Economist *337* (7932), 55 (1995).

107 Congressional Quarterly Researcher (USA) *2* (4), 75 (1992).

108 S.E. Clay, Office of Alternative Medicine, NIH (USA), personal communication dated Jan. 22, 1996.

109 The TIME *138* (18), 75 (1991).

110 F. Murray: Nutr. Today's Living *57*, 8 (1995).

111 M.J. Verhoef and L.R. Southerland: Can. Fam. Physician *41*, 1005 (1995).

112 J.W. LaValley and M.J. Verhoef: Can. Med. Assoc. J. *153*, 45(1995).

113 M. Goldszmidt, C. Levitt, E. Duarte-Franco and K. Kaczorowski: Can. Med. Assoc. J. *153*, 29 (1995).

114 C. Marwick: J.A.M.A *274* (2), 106 (1995).

115 C.R.B. Joyce: The Lancet *344*, 1279 (1994).

116 C. Paterson and W. Peacock: Br. J. Gen. Pract. *45*, 255 (1995).

117 P.C. Pietroni: B.M.J. *305* (6853), 564 (1992).

118 British Medical Association: Complementary Medicine; new approaches to good practice, Oxford Press, Oxford 1993.

119 EEC Market for Homeopathic Remedies, McAlpine, Thorpe and London, London 1992.

120 J. Harris: Conde Nest Traveler *30*, 98 (1995).

121 B.J. Culliton and W.K. Waterfall: B.M.J. *1* (6161), 467 (1979).

122 J.O. Neher and J.M. Borken: Arch. Fam. Med. *3*, 859 (1994)

123 C. Marwick: J.A.M.A, *273* (8), 607 (1995).

124 Office of Alternative Medicine: Health Facts *20*, 1 (1995).

125 J.W. LaValley and M.J. Veerhoef: Can. Med. Assoc. J. *153*, 45 (1995).

126 M.C. Sutter: Can. Med. Assoc. J. *154*, 14 (1996).
127 J.S. McGoey: Can. Med. Assoc. J. *154*, 14 (1996).
128 J. Lynn: Prof Nurse *11*, 266 (1996).
129 M. Abrams: Good Housekeeping *218* (3), 99 (1994).

Progress in Drug Research, Vol. 47 (E. Jucker, Ed.)
© 1996 Birkhäuser Verlag, Basel (Switzerland)

Calcium channel blockers in psychiatry

By Leo E. Hollister[1] and Enrique S. Garza-Trevino[2]

[1]University of Texas, Houston Medical School and Harris County Psychiatric Center, 2800 South MacGregor Way, Houston, TX 77021, USA; and [2]San Antonio (Tex) Mood Disorders Clinic

1   Introduction

The influence of calcium in mental disorders has been considered over time. For example, intravenous calcium gluconate was used for treatment of periodic psychosis as late as the 1970s. Also, mental symptoms may be prominent in patients with hypercalcemia of various causes. The role of serum calcium in the switch process of manic-depressive disorder was studied in the late 1970s. Increases in serum calcium and phosphorus induced by treatment of bipolar-1 depressed patients with dihydrotachysterol-increased symptoms of hypomania. On the other hand, treatment with salmon calcitonin, which has the opposite effect, mitigated mania. Abrupt changes in serum calcium were implicated in the rapid changes in periodic psychosis [1]. A rationale for the employment of calcium channel blocking drugs was proposed after the observation that antipsychotic drugs of the diphenylbutylpiperidine type (pimozide, penfluridol, fluspiriline) were also potent inhibitors of calcium channels of the nitrendipine type. This pharmacological action, beyond the classical one of blocking D2 dopamine receptors, was implicated in the beneficial effects of these drugs on negative symptoms of schizophrenia [2].

The role of calcium as an almost universal intracellular messenger, however, provided the strongest rationale for use of calcium channel blocking drugs. Since membrane-bound "pumps" drive calcium out of the cell, the concentration of calcium ions is generally 10,000 times greater in the fluid surrounding the cell than in the cytosol. Calcium serves as an "on-off" switch in several transient cellular responses, influencing neurotransmitters and hormone secretion as well as the contraction of skeletal and cardiac muscle cells [3]. The rise in calcium ion concentration initiates the response, and its fall terminates it. By blocking calcium influx, the release of various neurotransmitters involved in mental disorders might be modulated presynaptically rather than by blocking post-synaptic receptors. Since 1982, scattered reports in the literature have explored the use of calcium channel blocking drugs in various psychiatric and neurological syndromes. It is our purpose to review, as completely as possible, this literature and to try to evaluate the evidence for the use of this class of drugs in these disorders.

2   Bipolar disorders

Because more studies of calcium channel blockers have been accomplished in patients with mania, we shall consider this work first. Lithium is still the drug of choice for acute manic episodes, but 20%–40% of patients do not respond well, and side effects impair many patients [4]. Lithium may affect calcium metabolism, and patients with bipolar disorder may have abnormalities in calcium metabolism as a characteristic of this disorder [5]. Thus, some initial rationale for using calcium channel blocking drugs in mania existed prior to the first trials. Studies will be cited in chronological order in all subsequent discussions. By doing this, one may gain some sense of the activity of research in the various areas at any given period.

A brief 1982 report related the treatment of 5 purely manic patients with diltiazem. Significant improvement was noted in 3 following doses up to 360 mg/day. In another, such improvement might have been spontaneous and in the fifth patient no improvement was noted [6]. Treatment with verapamil of a single manic patient who could not tolerate lithium due to tremor was reported the same year. A dose of 160 mg/day provided good control, which was lost when she was switched to placebo [7].

No additional reports were made during 1983, but by the next year further studies were reported. A brief letter told of good to excellent results of treatment of patients with bipolar disorder using nifedipine [8]. A controlled trial in 12 patients compared 320 mg/day of verapamil with lithium (doses titrated to adequate serum levels) using a 10-day placebo washout period between treatments with a cross-over design in which verapamil was always given during the first 30-day trial. Results indicated that both drugs were better than placebo in mild to moderate mania but that no differences between them could be found [9].

A single case reported suggested the use of verapamil as maintenance treatment of mood swings. A 32-year-old woman obtained some relief of mania from lithium but became depressed. Adding the anti-depressant amoxapine caused a reoccurrence of mania. She was similarly intolerant of most antidepressants other than trazodone, which in a dose of 450 mg/day combined with lithium 1500 mg/day produced partial relief. After verapamil 160 mg/day was added, she exhibited marked improvement which was maintained for one year during which she was on both verapamil 240 mg/day and the previous dose of trazodone [10].

In 1985, a second report of treatment of mania with diltiazem described significant improvement in 4 of 7 manic patients treated with diltiazem in doses of 210 to 360 mg/day. One patient had what was thought to be spontaneous improvement. Two others with mania presumed to be secondary to chronic brain syndromes failed to respond [11]. It is uncertain whether 5 of these patients were previously described in an earlier publication by the same author [6]. Verapamil 320 mg/day was compared with clonidine 17 μg/kg in a cross-over study of 20 manic patients who had previously shown a poor response to lithium. Each treatment period was for 20 days with a 5-day placebo wash-out between treatments. Verapamil was superior to clonidine on a number of measures [12]. However, in view of the uncertain efficacy of clonidine for mania, the results did not provide strong evidence of efficacy for verapamil.

1986 was a peak period with 5 reports. A double-blind cross-over study compared verapamil with placebo in 7 acutely manic patients. Patients were treated for 24 days; doses of verapamil were gradually increased to a maximum of 480 mg/day; those who received verapamil were switched to placebo and vice versa for another 24 days. Five of the 7 patients improved significantly while taking verapamil as compared with placebo [13]. Six acutely manic patients were treated by the addition of doses of 240 to 320 mg/day of verapamil. All patients showed a prompt reduction in their manic symptoms [14]. However, because of the open nature of the trial and the use of concomitant treatment with antipsychotics or lithium the value of verapamil was indeterminate.

Eight manic patients were treated in a double-blind cross-over study in which they received first placebo, then a period of verapamil treatment followed by placebo. Doses of verapamil were 320–480 mg/day for 7 days. Five patients were improved while on the drug and showed slight relapse when placebo was substituted. Two patients improved while on verapamil but did not relapse when switched to placebo. One patient was unimproved. A 5 to 7 day delay in response to drug was noted [15].

Two patients with depressive episodes complicating treatment with verapamil were treated successfully by the addition of trazodone. It was concluded that such a combination was safe and effective in such patients [16].

The most unfavorable report was contained in a letter which described two cases of mania previously unresponsive to lithium or carbamazepine. Both were treated with 320 mg/day of verapamil with response. These two cases were said to be "typical of a number" of patients treated with poor results [17].

Three reports were added in 1987. A long-term cross-over study compared lithium with verapamil in 20 patients. Ten patients each were assigned either to lithium treatment with plasma concentrations of 0.8 to 1.0 mEq/l or verapamil 320 mg/day. During the first 180-day period, patients on verapamil improved after 60 days of treatment while those on lithium required 180 days. After cross-over, lithium patients did not improve further but those assigned to verapamil once again showed improvement after 60 days of treatment [18].

A report which damned verapamil with faint praise used the drug in 14 outpatients unresponsive to lithium, adding the drug to existing treatment. None of 8 patients treated for acute mania responded. Two of four patients treated prophylactically showed a mildly favorable response. Verapamil was of some help in 2 patients with drug-induced mania [19]. A single case of a 20-year-old man who had numerous complications of other antimanic drug therapy responded well to verapamil 320 mg/day and stayed in remission for 6 months [20].

Two small studies were reported in 1988, neither highly supportive. Two of 4 patients with bipolar illness responded to 320 mg/day of verapamil and 2 of 3 schizoaffectives improved. However, 3 patients developed acute depression after 12 to 15 days of treatment [21]. Five of 6 manic episodes showed decreased psychopathology following treatment with 320 to 400 mg/day of verapamil. However, a tendency to relapse was noted during the third week of treatment [22].

No studies were reported in 1989, but 1990 produced two small reports. Another dihydropyridine calcium channel blocker, nimodipine, was tried as a treatment for mania. Improvement was found in all 6 patients treated with 360 mg/day for 7 days. Few side effects were noted [23]. Another report suggested usefulness of verapamil in cases of drug-induced mania. A 44-year-old man with chronic bipolar illness, mainly consisting of episodes of depression, had manic attacks precipitated by treatment with antidepressants. On verapamil 320 mg/day he went into remission. A partial relapse occurred when he was taken off verapamil but remission followed its resumption [24].

A case report appeared to document an aggravating effect of nifedipine on a patient with bipolar depression. This 59-year-old woman had been treated unsuccessfully with amitriptyline 150 mg/day, tryptophan 1 g/day and 14 ECT sessions. Nifedipine, 200 mg/day had been started 6 weeks prior to the present episode for treatment of associated hypertension and continued throughout the course of antidepressant treatment. Because of its close proximity to the current depressive episode and the fact that it was the only drug not previously used with success in this patient, it was stopped. Improvement was obtained almost immediately upon cessation, which suggested that it had aggravated the depression [25].

A 1992 study was the only test of verapamil using a clinical parallel group double-blind control in 20 severely manic patients. Verapamil, in doses gradually increased to 320 mg/day, was compared with lithium in doses required to maintain serum levels of 0.75 to 1.5 mEq/l. No significant differences in clinical response were found between the two treatments. Although the p values were nonsignificant between the two treatments, there was a trend favoring lithium at week 4. The small sample size of this study and the absence of a placebo control does not eliminate the possibility of a type II error. The improvement in these patients, while statistically significant, was not impressive [26].

1993 was another peak year, with 5 reports. Flunarizine, a calcium channel blocking drug unrelated chemically either to verapamil or the dihydropyridines, was used in 20 episodes of mania/depression either unresponsive to lithium or intolerant of side effects. A dose of 10 mg/day was said to cause remission in all [27].

Eighteen mentally retarded blind persons who suffered episodes resembling acute mania were unresponsive to usual treatments. With valproate 2750 mg/day, partial control was achieved but the addition of verapamil 320 mg/day afforded remission for over a year. Lowering the dose of valproate was followed by partial relapse which was aborted by resuming the full dose [28]. Whether such patients can truly be classified as having bipolar disorder may be questioned. A letter reported results in 7 patients with neuroleptic-resistant mania or schizoaffective disorder treated with nifedipine 120 mg/day added to their ongoing dose of neuroleptic. Two of 7 patients responded rapidly, 3 improved more slowly and 2 remained unchanged. Nifedipine was suggested as an adjunct to treatment with neuroleptic [29]. Three cases of pregnant bipolar women were taken off lithium or carbamazepine because of fear of teratogenesis. Verapamil was able to control manic symptoms during pregnancy and able to prevent relapse during post-partum as well [30].

Nimodipine was used in 12 patients with "treatment-refractory affective dysregulation". Doses ranged between 90 and 360 mg/day. An initial period of placebo was followed by active drug and then another period of placebo. Five of 9 patients who completed the entire sequence responded with leveling of the mood swings [31].

No reports appeared during 1994, but in 1995 an additional study evaluated nimodipine. Two cases were reported in which nimodipine was successful in stabilizing the mood in rapid cycling bipolar disorder. A 53-year-old woman presented with severe depression in a pattern of increasing manic-depressive cycles. Lithium carbonate 1200 mg/day, valproate 750 mg/day, verapamil 360 mg/day, thyroid and other antidepressants all failed. All medication was stopped after hospitalization, and nimodipine 90 mg/day was started. The dose was increased to 180 mg/day with stabilization of mood. This improvement lasted for 12 months on the same dose. Another patient, a 59-year-old man had a similar history. Lithium, carbamazepine, and antidepressants provided temporary help. All medications were stopped, and nimodipine alone quickly stabilized his mood. However, when nimodipine was stopped and the other medications restarted, he became worse. After two months, he was re-hospitalized and the other medications were tapered while the nimodipine dose was increased incrementally to 180 mg/day. He remained mood-stable for 5 months on nimodipine alone [32].

3   Unipolar depression

Ordinarily, one would expect a drug useful for treating mania to be more effective in treating bipolar depression. However, some suggestions have been made that calcium channel blockers might be useful in unipolar depression as well.

A case report in 1983 raised a question about the use of verapamil in depression. A 53-year-old woman who had many depressive episodes was resistant to all antidepressants. She was treated with verapamil 240 mg/day in a series of three placebo-drug sequences. Improvement was noted on the Hamilton Depressive Rating Scale during active drug treatment as compared with placebo [33].

A report in 1985 used flunarizine in a mixed, ill-defined group of "cerebral circulatory disturbances". Whether or not any of these patients were truly unipolar depressions was undetermined [34]. Another case of successful use of verapamil in unipolar depression was reported in 1987 for a 35-year-old woman with many episodes of depression who had been unresponsive to lithium and imipramine.

Verapamil in doses starting at 80 and increasing to 320 mg/day was followed by a remission for one year. For the last six months of this trial she was on verapamil alone [35].

In 1988, two reports cast considerable doubt on the use of nifedipine for depression. Six depressed men who had previously responded to antidepressants failed to show any improvement after treatment with nifedipine 60 mg/day for 4 weeks [36]. Four cases were reported in which depressive episodes followed use of nifedipine for angina pectoris. Two had previous episodes of depression but two did not. Remission followed quickly after nifedipine was discontinued [37]. These reports seemed to indicate that not only was nifedipine without benefit for depressed patients but also that it was depressogenic.

In 1989, a parallel-group controlled comparison was made in 86 depressed patients of verapamil, amitriptyline, placebo and elective treatment. The four groups were treated over a period of five weeks. Amitriptyline and elective treatment (physicians' choice) was more effective than verapamil or placebo [38]. The following year another case report suggested that nifedipine might worsen depression. A 67-year-old man with a 40-year history of unipolar depression was unresponsive to antidepressants and 2 ECT treatments; the latter had to be stopped prematurely because of cardiac complications. Just prior to the present episode he had been started on nifedipine for hypertension. Gradual reduction of the dose from 45 to 15 mg/day resulted in prompt remission [39].

The efficacy of verapamil was cited in a report of an 82-year-old man suffering his first episode of depression. He was treated with fluvoxamine 300 mg/day for 16 weeks without improvement. ECT was complicated by supraventricular tachycardia and heart failure. He became euthymic two weeks after starting verapamil 320 mg/day [40].

A 1995 open-label study of nimodipine reported that 9 of 10 patients with unipolar depression responded to doses gradually increased to 180–270 mg/day. Improvement was maintained during the 36-day observation period of the trial. These remarkable results were obtained despite the fact that oral nimodipine has a large first-pass metabolism which decreases bioavailability, and short (1 hr) plasma half-life [41].

4   Schizophrenia

The first test of verapamil in 1986 in schizophrenia was disappointing. Eight chronic schizophrenics (treated-resistant) were given verapamil 400 mg/day (one received only 160 mg/day) for 6 to 8 weeks in a double-blind cross-over design (placebo-drug-placebo). No benefit was observed but these were difficult patients in which to show the efficacy of any drug [42]. In 1987, an antipsychotic effect of verapamil was reported in 18 patients with schizophrenia. Three treatment groups of 6 each were studied; one group received verapamil 320 mg/day, another haloperidol in doses ranging from 10 to 40 mg/day, and the third a placebo control. Verapamil was found to be as effective as haloperidol after some statistical manipulations [43]. Use of the Bunney-Hamburg Global Rating Scale made this report unreliable, since only 5 out of 24 of the items of this instrument refer to psychotic symptoms. Thus, the alleged improvement could have reflected other symptoms unrelated to the core manifestations of schizophrenia. Seven chronic schizophrenics were first treated with placebo and then with verapamil 240 mg/day increasing to 480 mg/day at the end of the first week. No beneficial effects were noted [44]. Another study also used chronic schizophrenics. Twelve patients with high ratings on negative symptoms were assigned either to verapamil 320 mg/day or placebo for 4 to 6 weeks.

No beneficial effects were noted either on negative symptoms or on global measurement [45].

The most favorable report was a study which used 22 chronic schizophrenics who had been partially responsive to antipsychotic drugs. Verapamil 240 mg/day was added for 28 days to their existing treatment. Three of 22 were globally improved; no effect was noted on patients with tardive dyskinesia [46].

5   Panic disorder

Only two studies, both in 1988, evaluated the effect of verapamil in patients with panic disorder. Seven patients were treated with verapamil 240 mg/day for 180 days. Four experienced total remission although other drugs were not specified. The other three showed no benefit [47]. Another report was a double-blind cross-over study involving 11 patients treated with verapamil 480 mg/day. Six patients became panic-free while on the drug although 5 of these patients had only 5 panic attacks or less during the 4 weeks preceding their treatment. Three patients improved somewhat and 2 became slightly worse [48].

6   Tourette syndrome, tardive dyskinesia and Huntington disease

The first report in 1984 regarding the use of calcium channel blockers to control the tics of Tourette syndrome was favorable. A 12-year-old boy became tic-free 30 minutes after a test dose of 10 mg of nifedipine. After two weeks on a dose of 30 mg/day he became 90% improved [49]. A 22-year-old man given a test dose of 10 mg of nifedipine showed a decrease in obsessions within 30 minutes with the effects lasting 6 hours. He was placed on a dosage regime of 10–5 mg for six weeks with continued benefit [50]. Two cases of response to calcium channel blockers were reported in 1986. An 11-year-old with Tourette showed a marked reduction in symptoms following 60 mg/day of verapamil. The drug was discontinued after 6 months with relapse; re-starting the drug once again afforded remission. A 19-year-old man had been treated with little benefit and many side effects with haloperidol. Ten days after starting nifedipine 30 mg/day, he improved. When nifedipine was stopped after 4 months he relapsed but on its resumption again remitted [51].

A single case reported in 1986 told of the efficacy of verapamil 320 mg/day in the treatment of tardive dyskinesia. Relief of symptoms followed soon after starting the drug; the patient became worse when the dose was lowered but remission resumed following restoration to the original level [52]. The effects of single doses of 60 mg were studied in 6 schizophrenics with tardive dyskinesia. Doses were given of drug or placebo spaced at intervals of three days. Involuntary movements were significantly decreased 30, 60 and 90 minutes following the acute dose but not at 120 minutes, indicating a short span of action [53].

Verapamil 320 mg/day was given to 9 schizophrenics with tardive dyskinesia for 2 to 5 days. A mean decrease in AIMS scores of 19% was observed over this short period of time [54].

Diltiazem had only minimal benefits for 11 patients with Huntington disease. A dose of 240 mg/day was compared with placebo over a 7 to 12-month period. The differences between drug and placebo were not statistically significant. The 2 youngest patients in the series did the best [55].

7   Dementia

Two studies have considered nimodipine as a potential treatment for Alzheimer disease. A dose of 90 mg/day or placebo was given for 12 weeks to 178 elderly patients with cognitive decline. Results were superior to placebo on all outcome measures with nimodipine being equally effective in Alzheimer patients as in those with multi-infarct dementia [56]. In another study, 90 mg/day was given for 12 weeks to 227 patients with Alzheimer disease and compared with placebo. Disease progression in the placebo-treated patients was significantly greater [57].

8   Discussion

After 14 years of reports on the use of calcium channel blocking drugs for various psychiatric disorders, what can be said? First, considering that the majority of reports have been positive, remarkably little activity has followed up these claims. The frequency of yearly reports involving three major psychiatric disorders, manic-depressive disorder, unipolar depression and schizophrenia indicates that, rather than increasing as might be expected with a promising new treatment, reports seem to be decreasing.

Several possible reasons for this trend can be considered. One might be that reporting has shown selection bias, with only those reports claiming benefit reaching the literature while unreported clinical experience has been largely negative or at least unenthusiastic. Another reason is that none of the drug companies which sell the various drugs under discussion have shown much desire to pursue studies of efficacy with the goal of obtaining a New Drug Application. One of us (LEH) remembers proposing such a study in 1984 to the director of clinical investigation of the company then selling verapamil. The proposal was met with polite inattention. Is such reticence based on private information counseling conservatism, or the possibility that patent protection might have been lost before the new indications could be established, or simply marketing considerations?

In any case, without a sponsoring drug company actively pursuing a new indication, reports on the drug might be expected to be relatively few. The diffidence of drug companies has been commented upon elsewhere, with the suggestion that a joint private-governmental approach be attempted to settle the issue [58].

Another reason for lack of enthusiasm has been the fact that most of the reports involved only a few cases and were published as letters or brief case reports. The two largest studies involved 20 patients. Both were blind studies but only one was a classified double-blind comparison of parallel groups treated with verapamil or lithium. Even this study, which was probably the best to date, had severe deficiencies. Thus, the scientific basis for asserting the value of verapamil is tenuous.

Verapamil has been the calcium channel blocking drug most often tested. Although other drugs of this same class have been used, the number of instances of use of diltiazem, nifedipine, nimodipine or flunarizine have been too small to provide evidence suggesting that other drugs in this class might be equally effective. Not all calcium channel blockers are useful for the same indications, which could suggest that verapamil might be especially well-suited for use in psychiatric indications.

Thus, at this moment, not enough evidence is available to lead to the acceptance of verapamil as an effective therapeutic agent for psychiatric disorders. Nor is there any reason to believe that this situation might soon change. No new drug applications are on file for pursuing these possible indications. Yet, enough interest in these drugs has been promoted so that a chapter in one of the recent texts on psychopharmacology was devoted to these drugs [59].

The issue needs to be settled, as it is customarily done, by a large double-blind parallel-group design-study in which verapamil is compared with a standard treatment, most likely lithium. Recent policy of the NIMH granting programs has generally looked askance at funding of such drug studies. However, the possibility of overlooking an effective treatment for mental illnesses might mitigate this policy. Until that happens, we shall all have to live with uncertainty, or our own experience in trying these drugs in a non-experimental way.

References

1   Carman, J.S. and Wyatt, R.J.: Calcium: pacesetting the periodic psychoses. Am. J. Psychiatry 136, 1035–9 (1979).
2   Gould, R.J., Murphy, K.M., Reynolds, I.J. and Syder, S.H.: Antischizophrenic drugs of the diphenylbutylpiperidine type act as calcium channel antagonists. Proc. Natl. Acad. Sci. USA. 80, 5122–5125 (1983).
3   Rasmussen, H..: The cycling of calcium as an intracellular messenger. Scientific American (Oct), 66–73 (1989).
4   Swann, A.: Practical management of depressive and manic episodes. In: Garza-Trevino (Ed.): Medical Psychiatry: Theory and Practice 1, 8. River Edge, N.J., World Scientific, 1989.
5   Tan, C.H., Javors, M.A., Seleshi, E., Lowrimore, P.A. and Bowden, C.L.: Effects of lithium on platelet ionic intracellular calcium concentration in patients with bipolar disorder and healthy controls. Life Sci. 46, 1175–1180 (1990).
6   Caillard, V. and Masse, G.: Traitement de la manie par un inhibiteur calcique. Etude preliminaire, L'encephale VVI, 587–594 (1982).
7   Dubovsky, S.L., Franks, R.D., Lifschitz, M. and Coe, P.: Effectiveness of verapamil in the treatment of mania. Am. J. Psychiat. 139, 502–504 (1982).
8   Goldstein, J.A.: Calcium and neurotransmission. Biol. Psychiatry 19, 406 (1984).
9   Giannini, A.J., Houser, W.L. Jr., Loiselle, R.H., Giannini, M.C. and Price, W.A.: Antimanic effects of verapamil. Am. J. Psychiatry 141, 1602–1603 (1984).
10   Gitlin, M.J. and Weisse, J.: Verapamil as maintenance treatment in bipolar illness: A case report. J. Clin. Psychopharmacol. 4, 341–343 (1984).
11   Caillard, V.: Treatment of mania using a calcium antagonist-preliminary trial. Neuropsychobiology 14, 23–26 (1985).
12   Giannini, A.J., Loiselle, R.H., Price, W.A. and Giannini, M.C.: Comparison of antimanic efficacy of clonidine and verapamil. J. Clin. Pharmacol. 25, 307–308 (1985).
13   Dubovsky, S., Franks, R.D., Allen, S. and Murphy, J.: Calcium antagonists in mania: A double-blind study of verapamil. Psychiatry Res. 18, 309–320 (1986).
14   Brotman, A.W., Farhadi, A.M. and Gelenberg, A.J.: Verapamil treatment of acute mania. J. Clin. Psychiatry 47, 136–138 (1986).
15   Dose, M., Emrich, H.M., Cording-Tommel, C. and von Zerssen, D.: Use of calcium antagonists in mania. Psychoneuroendocrinology 11, 241–243 (1986).
16   Solomon, L. and Williamson, P.: Verapamil in bipolar illness. Can. J. Psychiatry 31, 442–444 (1986).
17   Kennedy, S., Ozersky, S. and Robillard, M.: Refractory bipolar illness may not respond to verapamil. J. Clin. Psychopharmacol. 6, 316–317 (1986).
18   Giannini, A.J., Taraszewski, R. and Loiselle, R.H.: Verapamil and lithium as maintenance therapy of manic patients. J. Clin. Pharmacol. 27, 980–982 (1987).
19   Barton, B.M. and Gitlin, M.J.: Verapamil in treatment-resistant mania: An open trial. J. Clin. Psychopharmacol. 7, 101–103 (1987).

20   Patterson, J.F.: Treatment of acute mania with verapamil. J. Clin. Psychopharmacol. 7, 206 (1987).

21   Mathis, P., Schmitt, L. and Moron, P.: Efficacité du verapamil dans les accès maniaques. Encephale XIV, 127–132 (1988).

22   Dinan, T.G., Silverstone, T. and Cookson, J.C.: Cortisol, prolactin, and growth hormone levels with clinical ratings in manic patients treated with verapamil. Int. Clin. Psychopharmacol. 3, 151–156 (1988).

23   Brunet, G., Cerlich, B., Robert, P., Dumas, S., Souetre, F. and Darcourt, G.: Open trial of a calcium antagonist, nimodipine, in acute mania. Clin. Neuropharmacol 13, 224–228 (1990).

24   Deichen, R.F.: Verapamil treatment of bipolar depression. J. Clin. Psychopharmacol. 10, 148–149 (1990).

25   Johnson, B.A. and Cowen, P.J.: Calcium channel blockade and resistant bipolar depression. Irish J. Psychological. Med. 8, 50–51 (1991).

26   Garza-Trevino, E.S., Overall, J.E. and Hollister. L.E.: Verapamil versus lithium in acute mania. Am. J. Psychiatry 149, 121–122 (1992).

27   Lindelius, R. and Nilsson, C.G.: Fluanrizine as maintenance treatment of a patient with bipolar disorder. Am. J. Psychiatry 149, 139 (1992).

28   Kastner, T. and Freidman, D.L.: Verapamil and valproic acid treatment of prolonged mania. J. Am. Acad. Child Adolesc. Psychiatry 31, 271–275 (1992).

29   de Beaurepaire, R.: Treatment of neuroleptic resistant mania and schizoaffective disorders. Am. J. Psychiatry 149, 1614 (1993).

30   Goodnick, P.J.: Verapamil prophylaxis in pregnant women with bipolar disorder. Am. J. Psychiatry 150–156 (1993).

31   Pazzaglia, P.J., Post, R.M., Ketter, T.A., George, M.S. and Marangell, L.B.: Preliminary controlled trial of nimodipine in ultra-rapid cycling affective dysregulation. Psychiatry Res. 49, 257–272 (1993).

32   Goodnick, P.: Nimodipine treatment of rapid cycling bipolar disorder. J. Clin. Psychiatry 56, 330 (1995).

33   Hoschl, C.: Verapamil for depression? Am. J. Psychiatry 140, 1100 (1983).

34   Eckmann, F.: Clinical double-blind study with the calcium antagonist flunarizine in cerebral circulatory disturbances. Arzneimittelforschung 35, 1276–1279 (1985).

35   Pollack, M.H. and Rosenbaum, J.F.: Verapamil in the treatment of recurrent unipolar depression. Biol. Psychiatry 22, 779–782 (1978).

36   Kramer, M.S., Caputo, K., Di Johnson, C, et al.: Negative trial of nifedipine in depression. Biol. Psychiatry 24, 958–959 (1988).

37   Hullett, F.T., Potkin, S.G., Levy, A.B. and Ciasc,a R.: Depression associated with nifedipine-induced calcium channel blockers. Am. J. Psychiatry 145, 1277–1279 (1988).

38   Hoschl, C. and Kozemy, J.: Verapamil in affective disorders: A controlled, double-blind study. Biol. Psychiatry 25, 128–140 (1989).

39   Eccleston, D. and Cole, A.J.: Calcium Channel blockade and depressive illness. Br. J. Psychiatry 156, 889–891 (1990).

40   Jacques, R.M. and Cox, S.J.: Verapamil in major (psychotic) depression. Br. J. Psychiatry 158, 124–125 (1991).

41   Walden, J., Fritze, J., VanCalker, D., Berger, M. and Grunse, H.: A calcium channel antagonist for the treatment of depressive episodes: Single case reports J. Psychiatric Research 29, 71–76 (1995).

42   Grebb, J.A., Shelton, R.C., Taylor, E.H. and Bigelow, L.: A negative double-blind

placebo-controlled clinical trial of verapamil in chronic schizophrenia. Biol. Psychiatry *21*, 691–694 (1986).

43   Price, W.A.: Antipsychotic effects of verapamil in schizophrenia. Hillside J. Clinical Psychiatry *9*, 225–230 (1987).

44   Pickar, D., Wolkwitz, O., Doran, A., Labarco, R., Roy, A., Breier, A. and Narong, P.C.: Clinical and biochemical effects of verapamil administration to schizophrenic patients. Arch. Gen. Psychiatry *44*, 113–119 (1987).

45   Urh, S.B., Jackson, K. and Berger, P.A.: Effects of verapamil administration on negative symptoms of chronic schizophrenia. Psychiatry Res. *23*, 551–352 (1988).

46   Bartko, G., Horvath, S., Zador, G. and Frecska, E.: Effects of adjunctive verapamil administration in chronic schizophrenic patients. Prog. Neuro-Psychopharmacol. Bio. Psychiatry *15*, 343–349 (1991).

47   Klein, E. and Uhde, T.W.: Controlled study of verapamil for treatment of panic disorder. A. J. Psychiatry, 431–434 (1988).

48   Goldstein, J.A.: Calcium channel blockers in the treatment of panic disorders. J.Clin. Psychiatry *46*, 546 (1985).

49   Goldstein, J.A.: Nifedipine treatment of Tourette's syndrome. J. Clin. Psychiatry *45*, 360 (1984).

50   Berg, R.: A case of Tourette's syndrome treatment with nifedipine. Acta Psychiatrica Scandinavica *72*, 400–401 (1985).

51   Walsh, T.L., Lavenstein, B., Licamele, W.I., Bronheim, S. and O'Leary, J.: Calcium antagonists in the treatment of Tourette's disorder. Am. J. Psychiatry *143*, 1467–1468 (1986).

52   Barrow, N. and Childs, A.: An anti-tardive dyskinesia effect of verapamil. Am. J. Psychiatry *143*, 1485 (1986).

53   Leys, D., Vermersch, P., Daniel, T., Comgras, S., Goudemand, M., Caron, J. and Petit, H.: Diltiazem for tardive dyskinesia. Lancet *1*, 250–251 (1988).

54   Reiter, S., Adler R. and Angrist, B.: Effect of verapamil on tardive dyskinesia and psychosis in schizophrenic patients. J. Clin. Psychiatry *50*, 26–27 (1989).

55   Walter, F.O., Young, A.B. and Rodnitsky, R.L.: Diltiazem in Huntington's disease. Neurology *25* (Suppl. 1), 177 (1985).

56   Ban, T.A., Morey, I., Aguglia, E., Azzserelli, O., Balsana, F., Masrigliano, V., Caglieris, N., Sterlicchio, M., Apurso, A., Tomsi, N.A., Crepaldi, G., Volpe, D., Palmieri, G. Ambrosi, G., Polli, E., Cortellaro, M., Zanussy, C. and Froldi, M.: Nimodipine in the treatment of old age dementia. Prog. Neuro-Psychopharmacol. & Biol. Psychiat. *14*, 525–551 (1990).

57   Tollefson, G.D.: Short-term effects of the calcium channel blocker nimodipine (Bay-e-9736) in the management of primary degenerative dementia. Biol. Psychiatry *27*, 1133–1142 (1991).

58   Dubovsky, S.L.: Why don't we hear more about the calcium antagonists? Biol. Psychiatry *35*, 149–150 (1994).

59   Dubovsky, S.L.: Calcium channel antagonists as novel agents for manic-depressive disorder, in: Schatzberg, A.F. and Nemeroff, C.B. (Eds.): Textbook of Psychopharmacology. American Psychiatric Press, Washington, DC. 1995. pp 377–390.

Index Vol. 47

The references of the Subject Index are given in the language of the respective contribution.
Die Stichworte des Sachregisters sind in der jeweiligen Sprache der einzelnen Beiträge aufgeführt.
Les termes repris dans la Table des Matières sont donnés selon la langue dans laquelle l'ouvrage est écrit.

Index of titles
Verzeichnis der Titel
Index des titres
Vol. 1–47 (1959–1996)

Author and paper index
Autoren- und Artikelindex
Index des auteurs et des articles
Vol. 1–47 (1959–1996)

Reactivity of bentonite flocculation, indirect haemagglutination and Casoni tests in hydatid disease *19*, 75 (1975)	R. C. Mahajan N. L. Chitkara
Characteristics of catechol O-methyltransferase (COMT) and properties of selective COMT inhibitors *39*, 291 (1992)	P.T. Männistö I. Ulmanen K. Lundström J. Taskinen J. Tenhunen C. Tilgmann S. Kaakkola
Interaction of cancer chemotherapy agents with the mononuclear phagocyte system *35*, 487 (1990)	Alberto Mantovani
Mechanisms of fibrinolysis and clinical use of thrombolytic agents *39*, 197 (1992)	Maurizio Margaglione Elvira Grandone Giovanni Di Minno
Drugs affecting plasma fibrinogen levels. Implications for new anti-thrombotic strategies *46*, 169 (1996)	M. Margaglione E. Grandone F. P. Mancini G. Di Minno
Epidemiology of diphtheria *19*, 336 (1975)	L. G. Marquis
Biological activity of the terpenoids and their derivatives *6*, 279 (1963)	M. Martin-Smith T. Khatoon
Biological activity of the terpenoids and their derivatives – recent advances *13*, 11 (1969)	M. Martin-Smith W. E. Sneader
Antihypertensive agents 1962–1968 *13*, 101 (1969) Fundamental structures in drug research – Part I *20*, 385 (1976) Fundamental structures in drug research – Part II *22*, 27 (1978) Antihypertensive agents 1969–1980 *25*, 9 (1981)	A. Marxer O. Schier
Relationships between the chemical structure and pharmacological activity in a series of synthetic quinuclidine derivatives *13*, 293 (1969)	M. D. Mashkovsky L. N. Yakhontov